A Complex Systems Approach to Epilepsy

A Complex Systems Approach to Epilepsy

Concept, Practice, and Therapy

Edited by

Rod C. Scott
Nemours Children's Hospital, Delaware
University of Delaware
Thomas Jefferson University

J. Matthew Mahoney
The Jackson Laboratory
University of Vermont

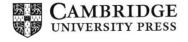

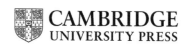

Shaftesbury Road, Cambridge CB2 8EA, United Kingdom

One Liberty Plaza, 20th Floor, New York, NY 10006, USA

477 Williamstown Road, Port Melbourne, VIC 3207, Australia

314–321, 3rd Floor, Plot 3, Splendor Forum, Jasola District Centre, New Delhi – 110025, India

103 Penang Road, #05–06/07, Visioncrest Commercial, Singapore 238467

Cambridge University Press is part of Cambridge University Press & Assessment, a department of the University of Cambridge.

We share the University's mission to contribute to society through the pursuit of education, learning and research at the highest international levels of excellence.

www.cambridge.org
Information on this title: www.cambridge.org/9781009258081

DOI: 10.1017/9781108582285

First published 2023

Printed in the United Kingdom by TJ Books Limited, Padstow Cornwall

A catalogue record for this publication is available from the British Library.

Library of Congress Cataloging-in-Publication Data
Names: Scott, Rod, editor. | Mahoney, J. Matthew, editor.
Title: A complex systems approach to epilepsy : concept, practice and therapy / edited by Rodney C. Scott, J. Matthew Mahoney.
Description: Cambridge ; New York, NY : Cambridge University Press, 2022. | Includes bibliographical references and index.
Identifiers: LCCN 2022024925 (print) | LCCN 2022024926 (ebook) | ISBN 9781009258081 (hardback) | ISBN 9781108582285 (epub)
Subjects: MESH: Epilepsy | Systems Analysis | Systems Biology
Classification: LCC RC372 (print) | LCC RC372 (ebook) | NLM WL 385 | DDC 616.85/3–dc23/eng/20220615
LC record available at https://lccn.loc.gov/2022024925
LC ebook record available at https://lccn.loc.gov/2022024926

ISBN 978-1-009-25808-1 Hardback

．．．

Contents

Contributors

Fraser Aitken
Department of Biomedical Engineering, Kings College London, London, UK

Eleonora Aronica
Amsterdam UMC, University of Amsterdam, Department of (Neuro)Pathology, Amsterdam Neuroscience, Amsterdam, the Netherlands; Stichting Epilepsie Instellingen Nederland (SEIN), Heemstede, the Netherlands

Andrea Bernasconi
Montreal Neurological Institute, Montreal, Quebec, Canada

Neda Bernasconi
Montreal Neurological Institute, Montreal, Quebec, Canada

Anika Bongaarts
Amsterdam UMC, University of Amsterdam, Department of (Neuro)Pathology, Amsterdam Neuroscience, Amsterdam, the Netherlands

Jeffrey L. Brabec
Department of Neurological Sciences, Robert Larner MD School of Medicine, University of Vermont, USA

David Carmichael
Department of Biomedical Engineering, King's College London, London, UK

Adrià Tauste Campo
Universitat Pompeu Fabra, Spain

Aswin Chari
Department of Developmental Neurosciences, Institute of Child Health, University College London, London, UK

Mircea I. Chelaru
Department of Neurobiology and Anatomy, University of Texas Health Science Center at Houston, Houston, USA

Fatemeh Fadaie
Montreal Neurological Institute, Montreal, Quebec, Canada

Niels Alexander Foit
Montreal Neurological Institute, Montreal, Quebec, Canada

Jagoda Glowacka
The Faculty of Electronics and Information Technology, Warsaw University of Technology, Warsaw, Poland

Viktor K. Jirsa
Institut de Neurosciences des Systèmes, UMR Inserm 1106, Aix-Marseille Université, 9 Faculté de Médecine, 27, Boulevard Jean Moulin, Marseille, France

Giridhar P. Kalamangalam
Department of Neurology, College of Medicine, University of Florida, USA

Montana Kay Lara
Department of Neurological Sciences, Robert Larner MD School of Medicine, University of Vermont, USA

J. Matthew Mahoney
The Jackson Laboratory, Bar Harbor, Maine, USA; Department of Neurological Sciences, Robert Larner MD School of Medicine, University of Vermont, USA

James D. Mills
Amsterdam UMC, University of Amsterdam, Department of (Neuro)Pathology, Amsterdam Neuroscience, Amsterdam, the Netherlands

Angelika Mühlebner
Amsterdam UMC, University of Amsterdam, Department of (Neuro)Pathology, Amsterdam Neuroscience, Amsterdam, the Netherlands

Rory J. Piper
Department of Developmental Neurosciences, Institute of Child Health, University College London, London, UK; Department of Biomedical Engineering, King's College London, London, UK

Maria Luisa Saggio
Institut de Neurosciences des Systèmes, UMR Inserm 1106, Aix-Marseille Université, 9 Faculté de Médecine, 27, Boulevard Jean Moulin, Marseille, France

Gabrielle Marie Schroeder
Interdisciplinary Computing and Complex BioSystems Group, School of Computing, Newcastle University, UK

Rod C. Scott
Nemours Children's Hospital, Delaware; University of Delaware; Thomas Jefferson University, USA

Nishant Sinha
Interdisciplinary Computing and Complex BioSystems Group, School of Computing, Newcastle University, UK; Institute of Neuroscience, Faculty of Medical Science, Newcastle University, UK

Peter Neal Taylor
Interdisciplinary Computing and Complex BioSystems Group, School of Computing, Newcastle University, UK; Institute of Neuroscience, Faculty of Medical Science, Newcastle University, UK; Institute of Neurology, University College London, UK

Anna L. Tyler
The Jackson Laboratory, Bar Harbor, Maine, USA

Manel Vila-Vidal
Universitat Pompeu Fabra, Barcelona, Spain

Yujiang Wang
Interdisciplinary Computing and Complex BioSystems Group, School of Computing, Newcastle University, UK; Institute of Neuroscience, Faculty of Medical Science, Newcastle University, UK; Institute of Neurology, University College London, UK

Konrad Wojdan
Warsaw University of Technology, Institute of Heat Engineering, Warsaw, Poland

Introduction

Rod C. Scott and J. Matthew Mahoney

This book takes a view of the brain as a *complex adaptive system* and seeks to identify mechanisms underlying the clinical outcomes as well as the therapeutic opportunities for epilepsy using this framework.

Complex systems theory is a nebulous field whose overarching goal is to understand the dynamical behavior of systems consisting of many interconnected component parts. It has attracted widespread interest from many domains that study examples of such systems, including ecologists, sociologists, engineers, artificial intelligence researchers, condensed matter physicists, neuroscientists, and many others. The results of these collected, multi-disciplinary efforts have not been so much a comprehensive theory of Complex Systems (capital-C, capital-S), but rather a set of techniques, analogies, and attitudes toward problem solving that emphasize interactions and dynamics over individual components and their functions. The chapters are written in a complex adaptive systems frame and therefore it is useful to provide a provisional theoretical description of such systems. Following Holland [1], a generalizable description of complex adaptive systems is that they are collections of relatively simple *agents* that have the property that they can *aggregate*, so that collections of agents can form meta-agents (and meta-meta-agents etc.) with higher-order structure. These aggregates interact *nonlinearly*, so that the aggregate behavior of a collection of agents is qualitatively different from the behavior of the individual agents. The interactions among agents mediate *flows* of materials or information. Finally, the agents are typically *diverse* with distinct specialties that are optimized through adaptation to selective pressures in their environments.

To manifest these properties, complex adaptive systems have mechanisms that underpin the formation and function of the whole system. In full generality, these mechanisms may seem unnecessarily abstract or obscure for application to a specific system, like the neural circuits of the brain. Nevertheless, the abstraction is precisely what accounts for the cross-disciplinarity of complex systems theory, and the applicability of its approaches across biological length scales from subcellular structures to whole brains. The first mechanism is *tagging*, which allows diverse agents in the system to signal their identities to other agents thus enabling complex self-organization into aggregates. The second mechanism is the ability to generate *internal models* that approximate and anticipate the world external to the system, which enables adaptive behavior by the aggregate system.

From the above description, brains are clearly complex adaptive systems par excellence. There are several hierarchical layers of agents. A diversity of genes aggregates into gene networks that form a diversity of proteins that aggregate from a diversity of cells (e.g., neurons and glia) that aggregate and form a diversity of brain regions that aggregate and form the brain with a diversity of emergent phenomena. Indeed, individual cells themselves are complex adaptive systems, where biomolecules as agents interact through electrostatic fields generated by patterns of charges (tags) that facilitate aggregation into complexes and structures. These structures implicitly compute models of the world outside the cell and generate an appropriate transcriptional response. For example, the presence of a phosphorylated signaling molecule inside a cell carries information about the concentration of particular ligands outside the cell. This organization is approximately repeated at the level of neural networks. Neurons as agents use a variety of biochemical and electrical cues (tags) to form into circuits that mediate the flow of sensory information into motor output, memory etc., through massively parallel nonlinear dynamics. These dynamics implicitly compute internal models of the external world to generate adaptive behavioral responses.

The brain is one of the guiding metaphors of complex systems science, so that other examples – economies, ecological systems, social networks, transportation networks – are often conceptualized as "brain-like" in one way or another within complex systems theory. However, these other systems repay the favor and invite tantalizing metaphors of their own. For example, the synchronous blinking of fireflies has long fascinated mathematical biologists [2]. In this system, nonlinear interactions among blinking fireflies causes a spontaneous synchronized blinking that spans a whole swarm. Intriguingly, a lone firefly does not even display periodic blinking, so the drive to synchronous blinking is fully mediated by the network of interactions. In the 1990s, as mathematical tools and computer simulations began to clarify these dynamics, the potential connection to synchronous brain activity, and specifically epilepsy, began to be seriously considered [3]. One of the major discoveries in complex systems theory over the last few decades was the "small-world" phenomenon in many real-world networks [4]. Small-world networks have the property that most nodes are not directly connected to each other, but nevertheless most pairs of nodes can be connected by short paths. In their seminal paper on small-world networks, Watts and Strogatz showed that the synchronizability of a network is highly sensitive to the structure of connections – the *topology* – of the network, where small-world networks synchronize more readily than other patterns of connections, and they speculated that this may underlie the synchronizability of physically distant pairs of neurons in the visual cortex. There has since been a wealth of research on small-world and other topological properties of many kinds of brain networks in health and disease (see, for example, Chapters 9 and 10). It is interesting from the "complex systems perspective" that the early luminaries in the mathematics of synchronization were inspired as much by brains as by firefly swarms.

The example of synchronizing fireflies highlights a dictum in complex systems coined by the physicist Philip Anderson in the title of a classic essay "More is Different" [5]. The essential point of that essay, beyond the particular physical examples given, is that aggregates of many things can have qualitatively distinct collective behavior from any of the parts (whole brains do not behave like big neurons). For the fireflies, a network of interacting, asynchronous fireflies becomes a wave of synchronous blinking over length scales many orders of magnitude larger than an individual firefly blinking. This *emergence* of new phenomena has achieved highly refined mathematical description in condensed matter physics, but has echoes across many disciplines, and forms an organizing metaphor in complex systems thinking [6–8].

But how can we put these ideas to work in understanding clinical phenomena and designing new treatments for epilepsy? Said more stridently, what is the added value of taking this abstract, complicated, and potentially sterile perspective? Or more sympathetically, how does complex systems theory help us understand clinical variability and design new interventions in the brain to produce desired outcomes?

An interesting observation among genetic epilepsies is that mutations in a single gene can result in vastly different phenotypes. Specific examples include variability in outcomes in tuberous sclerosis even within single families [9], and the wide clinical variability associated with sodium channel mutations [10]. Given that patients with identical mutations can have outcomes ranging from cognitively normal and medically tractable epilepsy to developmental delay, intellectual disability, and intractable epilepsy, within a complex systems framework it is clear that the individually variable adaptation of the whole brain system to the same genetic perturbation is a critical driver of outcomes. Understanding the nature of the adapted network that predicts good vs. poor outcomes will provide extremely important pathophysiological information that cannot be inferred from the mutation per se. The same ideas can be applied to acquired epilepsies. For example, the variability of outcomes following traumatic brain injury [11] is partly a function of the injury itself but also a function of network adaptation that is likely to be influenced by the nature of the individual pre-injury networks.

In terms of treatment, a few analogies help emphasize the perils of ignoring complexity and the promise of embracing it. The networks in which humans intervene most deliberately and totally are traffic networks. The purpose of any traffic network is to facilitate the efficient transfer of people and goods in space. All else being equal, we would expect that adding more roads to a network would necessarily add efficiency – there is more room for cars to drive, more possible paths from point A to point B. Alas, this is not so, as described in what is now known as Braess' "paradox." This classic argument shows that adding roads (under reasonable assumptions about driver behavior) can cause the overall traffic within the network to slow down. Conversely, there have been several real-world examples in which a temporary shutdown of major roads in cities has actually improved traffic flow [12]. The key point is that the overall traffic flow is a function of the whole network's topology. Thus, local heuristics, like "adding an expressway between two popular points will improve traffic flow," can have highly counterintuitive, negative consequences. A "toy" example of this effect can be seen in the ancient Hindu game Snakes and Ladders, where the addition of some ladders can lengthen the expected game length, while the strategic addition of snakes can actually shorten the expected length [13].

Now let us operationalize this analogy for epilepsy. Instead of cars on roads, the brain transports information along connectomes. Among the major therapeutic decisions in epilepsy is the strategic resection of some brain tissue or, more recently, the implantation of a neurostimulator device. However, if we take the traffic network analogies seriously, we must accept that local heuristics can lead us badly awry. If the emergent dynamics of the brain are determined by the whole connectome, then we must treat the whole connectome. Like adding or shutting down roads in a city center, adding or removing electrical pathways in the brain can have potent positive effects on whole brain function, but only if the rest of the brain is considered. Advances in imaging, machine learning, and dynamical modeling are facilitating such a holistic view, where virtual surgeries can be used to predict outcomes based on patient-specific network data (see Chapter 4).

Considering drug interventions, we can again consult far flung metaphors. The purpose of a drug in epilepsy is to suppress seizures. Medications do not directly influence the emergent phenomenon of seizures, but rather interact with a set of target molecules within cells and tissues in the body. In response, cells change their physiology, ideally toward a non-seizure-prone state. As is well known, however, the fraction of patients who are seizure free on any medication has remained stuck at around two-thirds for decades [14], and existing medications can have debilitating side effects, particularly when multiple treatments are prescribed simultaneously. The ability to predict what kinds of novel molecules will interact in just the right ways to normalize and stabilize the ceaseless molecular activity of the brain to prevent seizures is a goal of therapy development in a complex systems framework.

This problem is at least as hard as intervening in an ecosystem to normalize and stabilize population dynamics. Analogous to molecules within cells, organisms in ecosystems have diverse interactions forming a trophic network defining energy and material flows. There is an ignoble history of abject failures and a few instructive successes of human intervention into ecological systems. Canonical among the failures is the introduction of cane toads to Australia to control cane beetles; a strategy that had broad scientific consensus at the time. Not only did the toads fail to control cane beetles, they also destabilized the native ecosystem, endangering several species that did not coevolve with them [15]. In contrast, the reintroduction of wolves to Yellowstone National Park in the United States was successful beyond expectations [16]. Unlike the cane toads, the Yellowstone ecosystem evolved with wolves as an apex predator, who were extirpated by human activities. The reintroduced wolves had a number of salutary effects. Principally, as apex predators, they induced significant changes in behavior in their main prey species, elk, who no longer ventured out into the open to graze exclusively on the most desirable plants. This change in behavior had the downstream effect of allowing multiple plant populations to recover from overgrazing, which in turn allowed their roots to stabilize the soil, which arrested the erosion that was causing rivers to change course and further disrupt other niches. Furthermore, the availability of elk carcasses helped restore other scavenger species. Overall, biodiversity and population stability are both markedly improved.

The critical point to take away from the toads versus the wolves is that the wolves succeeded and the toads failed because of where they each sat within the trophic network. The wolves had an evolved function and a critical topological location within the trophic network as the apex predator. In contrast, the toads were speculatively introduced as a totally new node within a network. Importantly, both interventions had the proximal goal of controlling a target species (elk for the wolves, beetles for the toads), but it was network effects that determined success. In epilepsy terms,

3

these examples ask us to think deeply about how and why we choose molecular targets for anti-seizure drugs, and our strategies for targeting them. It is interesting to speculate at this level of generality whether we think any of our modern anti-seizure medications are wolves or toads. Like the traffic and ecological examples, the effects of introducing a molecule depends in highly nontrivial ways on the dynamics of the whole network of interactions. Systems biological approaches to genetic risk prediction and drug discovery, therefore, treat molecular networks and their emergent functions as fundamental, alongside individual molecule-trait associations (see Chapters 2 and 3).

The foregoing discussion has briefly highlighted the character of complex systems theory and sought preliminary connections to the main topic of this book. We hope this inspires interested readers to seek out comprehensive treatments of complex systems theory (as can be found in [1,8,17]), and keep these analogies and principles in mind as they go through the chapters. Overall, we have chosen to organize the book by physical scale within the brain, starting with genes and ending on whole brains. It should be stressed, however, that each chapter is a self-contained treatment of a topic. Each chapter in its own way, and to the extent possible for each data domain within neuroscience, discusses the promise of networked, dynamical thinking for epilepsy research and practice.

References

1. Holland, J. H. *Hidden Order: How Adaptation Builds Complexity*. New York: Basic Books. 1996.

2. Buck, J., and Buck, E. Synchronous fireflies. *Sci Am.*, 234(5), 74–9, 82–5 (1976). doi:10.1038/scientificamerican0576-74

3. Sanger, G. F. Beyond isolation: Preferred rates of oscillation, from fireflies to epilepsy. *Med Hypotheses*, 41(3), 211–14 (1993). doi:10.1016/0306-9877 (93)90232-f

4. Watts, D. J., and Strogatz, S. H. Collective dynamics of "small-world" networks. *Nature*, 393 (6684), 440–2 (1998). doi:10.1038/30918

5. Anderson, P. W. More is different: Broken symmetry and the nature of the hierarchical structure of science. *Science*, 177(4047), 393–6 (1972). www.science.org/doi/10.1126/science.177.4047.393

6. Kauffman, S. A. *The Origins of Order: Self Organization and Selection in Evolution*. New York: Oxford University Press. (1993).

7. Meadows, D. H. *Thinking in Systems: A Primer*. Vermont: Chelsea Green Publishing. (2008).

8. Bar-Tam, Y. *Dynamics of Complex Systems*. Boca Raton, FL: CRC Press. (1999). https://necsi.edu/dynamics-of-complex-systems

9. Wang, F., Xiong, S., Wu, L., et al. A novel TSC2 missense variant associated with a variable phenotype of tuberous sclerosis complex: case report of a Chinese family. *BMC Med Genet.*, 19(1), 90 (2018). Doi:10.1186/s12881-018-0611-z

10. Guerrini, R., Cellini, E., Mei, D., et al. Variable epilepsy phenotypes associated with a familial intragenic deletion of the SCN1A gene. *Epilepsia*, 51 (12), 2474–7 (2010). doi:10.1111/j.1528-1167.2010.02790.x

11. Forslund, M. V., Perrin, P. B., Røe, C., et al. Global outcome trajectories up to 10 years after moderate to severe traumatic brain injury. *Front Neurol.*, 10, 219, (2019). doi:10.3389/fneur.2019.00219

12. Easley, D., and Kleiburg, J. *Networks, Crowds, and Markets*. Cambridge: Cambridge University Press. 2021.

13. Althoen, S. C., King, L., and Schilling, K. How long is a game of snakes and ladders? *Math. Gaz.*, 77(478), 71–6, (1993). doi:10.2307/3619261

14. Brodie, M. J. Outcomes in newly diagnosed epilepsy in adolescents and adults: Insights across a generation in Scotland. *Seizure*, 44, 206–10, (2017). doi:10.1016/j.seizure.2016.08.010

15. Turvey, N. Everyone agreed: Cane toads would be a winner for Australia. The Conversation. November 7, 2013. http://theconversation.com/everyone-agreed-cane-toads-would-be-a-winner-for-australia-19881

16. Peterson, Christine. 25 years after returning to Yellowstone, wolves have helped stabilize the ecosystem. National Geographic. July 10, 2020. www.nationalgeographic.com/animals/article/yellowstone-wolves-reintroduction-helped-stabilize-ecosystem

17. Newman, M. E. J. *Networks: An Introduction*, Oxford: Oxford University Press. 2010.

Chapter 2

Systems Biology Approaches to the Genetic Complexity of Epilepsy

Jeffrey L. Brabec, Montana Kay Lara, Anna L. Tyler, and J. Matthew Mahoney

2.1 The Epilepsy Genetic Revolution

The genetic underpinnings of epilepsy have come into much clearer focus over the past two decades. Advances in high-throughput molecular techniques have markedly improved our ability to identify potential therapeutic targets in epilepsy. Many of the monogenic effects identified through these methods have resulted in effective therapeutic targets for seizure amelioration [1,2,3]. Currently, around 200 definitively annotated epilepsy genes causing a range of seizure disorders and phenotypes have been identified [4]. Many more genes with putative associations with epilepsy pathways require further study [5]. The expansion of known genetic mechanisms and risk factors presents us with several benefits, including an increased pool of possible drug targets [6], genetic subtyping of seizure disorders [7], and the possibility for integrative analysis across different disorders [8,9]. However, the increasingly rich collection of genetic associations has also revealed the complexity of seizure disorders. Many mutations in different genes can converge on a similar clinical presentation [10], while different mutations in the same gene can have radically divergent outcomes [11,12]. Moreover, while robust data from twin and family studies demonstrate that common epilepsies are highly heritable [13,14], association studies have only detected risk factors that account for a small fraction of risk [15]. Thus, the data on epilepsy suggests a dichotomy. On one side, genetics is critical for describing etiology [16]. On the other side, using this information for prognosis or therapeutic development is limited by our current understanding of the complex genetic underpinnings of the disease and our analytic tools [10,17]. As a response to this complexity, researchers have started to shift toward complex systems approaches to genetics, which changes the focus from individual mutations to interactions among many mutations. The purpose of this chapter is to elaborate this ethos and present examples of this approach.

It is important to stress that genetic associations in epilepsy come from two essentially distinct sources. One source is rare variant detection via whole-exome or whole-genome sequencing. In these studies, a patient's and family members' DNA is sequenced to identify putatively deleterious rare mutations [18]. These studies are typically undertaken in patients with epileptic encephalopathies for which no known genetic etiology is implicated. The other source of associations are genome-wide association studies (GWAS), in which large populations of cases and controls are genotyped at a set of common genetic variants, which are then statistically associated with disease status. The GWAS approach is used for common epilepsies such as temporal lobe epilepsy (TLE) and idiopathic generalized epilepsies (IGE). As will be discussed in the next section, these two approaches typically fall on two ends of a spectrum, on one end of which reside the monogenic disorders that are caused by mutation of a single gene and on the other end the polygenic disorders that arise through the combined effects of many genes.

The International League Against Epilepsy (ILAE) recently published a GWAS "mega-analysis" for several common epilepsies, including focal and generalized epilepsies [15]. Their analysis revealed 11 novel loci associated with common epilepsies, which implicated diverse biological mechanisms across epilepsy subtypes. Despite the statistical significance of these associations, the risk conferred by the newly associated variants was low (1.5–3.3 odds ratios). This is typical of GWAS for many complex diseases, and not a feature of epilepsy GWAS per se [19,20]. For monogenic epilepsies, there have been concerted bioinformatic efforts to collate rare variant data into searchable public databases. Resources such as the Online Mendelian Inheritance in Man (OMIM) database [21] collect validated mutations, while research databases such as ClinVar [22] enable investigators to share variants of unknown significance detected in their patients alongside corresponding clinical presentations.

Despite this wealth of publicly available information, we are still far from precision medicine for patients with epilepsy. Indeed, few new therapies have been developed for specific genetic targets. A notable exception is Everolimus, which targets overactivation of mTOR signaling caused by mutations in the mTOR pathway. Unfortunately, Everolimus has only modest effects on epilepsy symptoms and does not appear to be more efficacious than other, nontargeted anti-seizure drugs at controlling seizures [23]. Why has the genetic revolution not resulted in a treatment revolution? To begin to answer this question, it helps to take a theoretical perspective and survey the genetic architecture of complex traits.

2.2 The Genetic Architecture of Complex Traits

The goal of genetic analysis is to identify a mathematical function that predicts an individual's phenotype from their genotype: a *genotype–phenotype map*. A phenotype can be a quantitative measure, such as body mass index, or a discrete category, such as disease status. In the latter case, which is most common for GWAS, the genotype–phenotype map predicts a risk for belonging to a given category. Assuming such a function can be found, it would appear to accomplish multiple objectives simultaneously. First, it would allow rigorous prediction of an individual's phenotype. Second, it would establish the individual contributions of genetic variants to overall risk. This latter property, more than just quantifying risk, should aid in developing a mechanistic understanding of the disease. The idea of precision medicine is predicated, in part, on using such predictive models for prognosis and treatment selection [24]. Of course, how predictive the genome is for a given trait and just what mathematical form a genotype–phenotype map should take are nuanced questions that require careful consideration.

The space of all possible genotype–phenotype maps is truly vast. Across the human population, the number of genetic variants in the genome is so large – and our sample sizes so minuscule by comparison – that we must be guided by theoretical considerations and be willing to accept reasonable approximations to make any headway.

There are on the order of 10^7 single nucleotide polymorphisms (SNPs; i.e., common point mutations) in the human population. This is in addition to insertion-deletions (indels), structural variants, such as copy number variations, and so-called rare variants, which can be point mutations or larger structural variants [25–27]. A genotype–phenotype map would therefore include the effects of tens of millions of variables and all their possible interactions to predict a trait. To get a feel for the magnitude of combinatorial possibilities, note that for 10 million SNPs there are on the order of 100 trillion pairs of SNPs, to say nothing of higher-order interactions. This is colloquially known as combinatorial explosion. (To make a scale comparison, the number of possible SNP pairs is greater than the number of stars in the Milky Way.) To make matters yet more complicated, many genetic factors only become relevant through interactions with specific environments, such as an in utero exposure, so a generic genotype–phenotype map also requires terms for all possible interactions among genetic variants and variables representing environmental factors [28].

The above considerations paint a dire picture of our ability to estimate a genotype–phenotype map in general. Fortunately, the situation is not nearly so bleak in practice. For most diseases, we typically assume that only a tiny fraction of the putative predictors (e.g., SNPs) are in fact predictive. Thus, using an association study design we can statistically screen for a small number of relatively strong effects for further consideration. The association studies discussed in the previous section fit this pattern and have made significant advances in identifying genetic risk factors for common epilepsies.

It is worth noting, however, that the existence of a small number of relatively strong effects is not a biological imperative and is, in fact, quite rare for common diseases [25–27]. In principle, the variants influencing a trait could be diffuse throughout the genome, where a large number of extremely weak effects conspire to produce a given phenotype. Indeed, this was the model Ronald Fisher had in mind when developing the early tools of statistical genetics [29–31]. In that model, developed decades before the discovery of DNA as a store of heritable variation, Fisher conceptualized an infinite number of genes (operationally defined as units of inherence), each making an infinitesimal contribution to the overall trait. Fisher was motivated, in part, by the observation that many heritable traits are normally distributed, i.e., have bell curve distributions, which follows naturally from a theoretical analysis of his infinitesimal model. Fisher's model has had a strong influence on many fields of genetics, including selective breeding and evolutionary and population genetics [32], and has received modern resonance in Boyle *et al.*'s concept of omnigenic inheritance. In the omnigenic model, essentially every gene contributes to every phenotype [33].

Paradigmatic among polygenic traits is height. Height is highly heritable – you are roughly as tall as your parents – but there is far from only one "height gene." On the contrary, the most recent meta-analysis of height has identified tens of thousands of SNPs that significantly influence height, but each contributes only a tiny fraction of a millimeter one way or the other [34]. One's height is largely determined by the complement of these tiny nudges inherited from one's parents. For any phenotype of interest, however, the question of whether a small number of strong effects, a large number of weak effects, or some heterogeneous combination of both, is a question that will need to be resolved with experiments. The answer to this question is often referred to as the *genetic architecture* of the trait.

In the present case of epilepsy genetics, we see a spectrum of genetic architectures. In rare, sporadic epileptic encephalopathies, exome sequencing has revealed a relatively simple architecture of a small number of large effects [35]. (Note that the simplicity of the architecture does not imply the simplicity of identifying these effects!) In contrast, many common seizure disorders, e.g., TLE and IGE, are expected to have the latter kind of inheritance [36]. This has significant ramifications for how to identify and, more importantly, how to use genetic associations that arise from association studies. We will discuss strategies for coping with this genetic complexity in the next section.

Before discussing how to approach genetic complexity, it is worth asking why individual genetic effects are often so weak. Part of the answer is that in GWAS the associations are made to SNPs, which are by definition common variants. No SNP with minor allele frequency of, say, 20% can be a complete causal explanation of a disease that afflicts at most a few percent of the population.

At best, SNPs can reveal modifiers of an underlying pathology that alter disease risk. This is reflected in the odds ratios for disease risk for individuals SNPs, which are often in the range of 2 to 10. Alternatively, there could be cryptic causal variants that are not SNPs but are correlated with them (known as linkage disequilibrium). Finding a preponderance of SNP associations at some location, each with weak individual effects, can often signal the presence of a hidden strong variant. Thus, SNPs are a blunt instrument. However, this is unlikely to be the whole answer. Consider tuberous sclerosis complex (TSC), which is caused by loss-of-function mutations in either the TSC1 or the TSC2 genes. Despite the proximate cause of TSC being such a mutation, TSC is still highly heterogeneous. Indeed, even siblings who inherit identical mutations and have essentially identical environments can have markedly different outcomes [37]. While such case reports cannot rule out unmeasured environmental insults or rare mutations as second genetic hits, they do suggest hypothetical genetic modifiers of disease outcomes that interact with the primary mutation to push outcomes one way or another. This latter hypothesis implicates network-level effects even in putatively monogenic disorders, and all the more so in complex traits.

No gene operates in isolation. Indeed, genes are regulated by interconnected transcriptional networks and their products take part in overlapping signaling cascades and binding interactions [38–40]. There have been multiple attempts to organize our models of molecular networks that have variously emphasized the *computational* aspects, the *physical interactions*, and the *circuit-like* aspects of molecular systems (Fig. 2.1). In the 1990s, Denis Bray showed that the basic enzyme kinetics equations of signaling cascades in c ells are formally mathematically equivalent to multilayer perceptrons, a form of artificial neural network [41] (Fig. 2.1A). He posited that cells are biologically instantiated classification devices for transforming external stimuli into transcriptional responses [42]. Multilayer perceptrons have several appealing properties as computational architectures. They can implement highly nonlinear input–out relationships. Thus, signaling cascades in cells can make complex calculations on stimuli and respond with a vast repertoire of responses. Furthermore, multilayer perceptrons have a "graceful degradation" property that corrupted

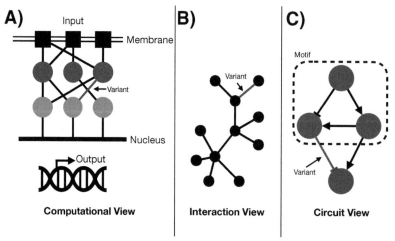

A) Computational View

Input
Membrane
Variant
Nucleus
Output

B) Interaction View

Variant
Variant

C) Circuit View

Motif
Variant

Figure 2.1 Schematic of network views common in systems biology. The mathematical language of networks is a useful tool in systems biology to capture the organization of molecular systems. A) An early view in systems biology was the *computational view* that used ideas from machine learning to analogize cell signaling interactions as a multilayer perceptron, which is a form of artificial neural network. In this view, the concentrations of molecules outside the cells are *input* and the transcriptional response is *output*. The signaling cascade itself instantiates a nonlinear relationship between input and output. B) As high-throughput data on molecular interactions, such as protein–protein interactions, became available, a purely topological *interaction view* became popular. In this view, one effectively ignores the dynamics of the system and studies the patterns of interactions and correlates them to other molecular properties, such as the effects of mutations. C) A *circuit view* of a molecular network attempts to decompose a topologically complex network into commonly repeated subunits, called motifs. The dynamics of motifs in isolation can provide some insight into how those motifs function within the full system. In each view, the effect of a genetic variant is to alter an interaction in the system, e.g., by altering the strength of a binding interaction.

networks have decreased performance in proportion to the amount of corruption, rather than catastrophic failure after a few components are removed [43]. This *computational view* hypothesized that it is the computational capabilities of cells that are positively selected by evolution, and these systems have converged on networks that are robust to mutations. Therefore, the convoluted interconnectivity of molecular networks appears as a property that mitigates the effects of individual mutations. Thus, the complex organization of signaling pathways is not a "bug" due to historical contingencies of evolution, but an essential "feature" of the computational architecture of cells.

Network-theoretic investigations have established that biological networks are indeed largely robust to random perturbations. For example, Barabási and collaborators have argued that protein–protein interaction networks, i.e., networks of physical binding between proteins, have evolved into so-called scale-free topologies that are robust to random mutations that knock out a random protein [44]. This *interaction view* abstracts away from the complexity of the dynamics of molecular systems and emphasizes the topology of those interactions. The scale-free network concept of Barabási & Albert has come under significant scrutiny [45]. However, the general point that protein–protein interaction networks have highly nonrandom structure that makes them robust to randomly deleting a node appears sound [46] (Fig. 2.1B). Likewise, Alon and collaborators have identified network motifs in transcriptional regulation networks, which confer robustness to transcription as a function of biophysical parameters that could be altered by mutations (Fig. 2.1C) [39,47]. In this *circuit view*, the complex interactions and dynamics of molecular systems can be approximately decomposed into subsystems, each themselves nonlinear components, that perform functions that are robust to perturbations of their parameters.

Through collecting these insights, a provisional explanation of the polygenic nature of many traits takes form. Common mutations provide small perturbations to the function of one component or interaction in a system, for example, the efficacy of a signaling protein (Fig. 2.1A), the binding affinity of a protein to a partner (Fig. 2.1B), or of a transcription factor to the binding site of another transcription factor (Fig. 2.1C). Network robustness attenuates the effect of these perturbations to maintain overall function. The tortuous path from any mutation to an observable phenotype is mediated through hundreds/thousands/millions of molecular interactions, many of which have been perturbed by other mutations, each contributing additional variance to the subpopulation carrying the first mutation. Hence, at the population level, most variants have a small effect.

So far, we have only considered the effect of one variant at a time within an association-analysis framework. This ignores the putative interaction terms described in the generic genotype–phenotype map. Given the preceding discussion of networks and interacting mutations, it seems reasonable to model these interactions. Statistical interactions among variants, i.e., deviation from additivity in a linear model, is called *statistical epistasis* [48,49]. Epistasis has a long history in genetics going back to Sewall Wright [50]. The existence of significant statistical epistasis in human populations is an ongoing point of controversy. Some argue that epistasis is both statistically detectable with reasonable sample sizes (despite the combinatorial explosion of the number of interactions) and identifies biologically relevant networks [51–54]. Others argue from theoretical evolutionary genetics models and empirical considerations that nearly all population-level genetic variance in humans is captured by additive models, despite the underlying nonlinear molecular interactions among gene products [55,56]. In model systems, where experimental crosses between evolutionarily diverged lines are possible, epistasis is not controversial. It has been observed in multiple model species that epistasis is particularly important for predicting extreme phenotypes [52,54,57], indicating the potential relevance of epistasis for predicting individual disease risk. With these caveats, the present authors are sympathetic to epistasis analysis in general and look to promising computational [58,59] and theoretical [60,61] advances that will potentially make epistasis modeling impactful for epilepsy GWAS.

2.3 Overcoming Genetic Complexity for New Insights

The discussion in Section 2.2 argued that it may be impossible to completely enumerate all genetic risk factors for epilepsy. Despite heritability, some amount of risk may be so diffusely embedded in molecular networks that we will never observe it in association analyses. This does not prevent our ability to make progress, but it does require that we modify our approach. In the following sections, we describe examples of approaches that confront this complexity directly.

2.3.1 Genetics of Gene Expression Networks: The Case of SESN3

One straightforward solution to the inadequacy of GWAS data to resolve all risk genes is to augment the genetic data with additional information. The most obvious choice is gene expression data, which provides a functional readout of the genome and can be measured in tissue from patients who undergo epilepsy surgery. Just as "omics" approaches, which study high-throughput cross-sections of molecular systems, are called *systems biology*, the combined analysis of genetics and gene expression is called *systems genetics*. Recently, Johnson *et al.* performed a systems genetic analysis of TLE [62]. Starting with gene expression data from resected hippocampal tissue from patients with TLE, they modeled gene co-expression using a gaussian graphical model, which captures the partial correlations among all gene pairs to estimate direct gene interactions. This allowed them to build a hippocampus-specific gene interaction network whose structure encodes the pathways that connect genes to each other. To ascertain whether this network was directly linked to underlying genetic risk for TLE, they performed a de novo analysis of TLE GWAS data and used a relatively liberal false discovery rate-based correction for multiple hypothesis testing. Within their hippocampus network, they identified two gene expression modules that were highly enriched for TLE GWAS risk genes. Each module was then run through pathway analysis to identify significantly enriched pathways. By accepting a certain amount of statistical noise in the gene associations, they were able to get a robust pathway-level signal for TLE risk genes.

One of the modules was highly enriched for pro-inflammatory cytokine signaling that was conserved across humans and mice. The expression of the genes in this module, therefore, represents an endophenotype for TLE risk, i.e., an intermediate phenotype with a clearer connection to genetics [63]. They then used the module expression as a phenotype for genetic mapping and identified one significant genomic locus

9

altering module expression. Through gene prioritization of the candidates within the locus, they were able to identify and validate the gene *SESN3* as a novel regulator of a proconvulsant gene network. Interestingly, *SESN3* was not present in the original module, suggesting that *SESN3* is a *trans*-acting regulator of expression.

The study by Johnson *et al.* highlights several key features of systems genetics analysis [62]. First, there is always a tension between false positives and false negatives in any high-throughput screen such as GWAS or transcriptomics. In this study, rather than requiring stringent evidence in each layer of data, evidence accumulated across multiple layers, ultimately implicating a novel gene that would have been missed by stringent statistical criteria. Second, by treating gene expression as a network phenomenon, they were able to resolve biologically specific co-expression modules, one of which was sufficiently genetically regulated to enable novel gene discovery. Third, the use of gene expression as an endophenotype is a powerful approach to resolving the complexity of genotype–phenotype maps. Gene expression more closely reflects the underlying genetic sequence than a subject-level outcome.

In follow-up work, Delahaye-Duriez *et al.* further elaborated the convergence of genes for rare and common epilepsies on shared functional networks [10]. Similarly, Johnson *et al.* showed that cognitive and neurodevelopmental disorders also share common genetic networks [64]. These studies suggest that, despite overt differences in genetic architecture and clinical presentation, there is some mechanistic convergence underlying epilepsy and comorbidities, and regulators of these networks, such as *SESN3*, can be identified through systems genetics and therapeutically targeted to improve outcomes.

2.3.2 Augmenting Statistical Genetics with Functional Networks

The empirical finding that genetic risk alleles for epilepsy are enriched in specific gene networks opens the possibility that we could search for those functional gene networks directly. In the systems biology field, several tools have been developed to combine genomic data with bioinformatic gene interaction networks to rigorously circumscribe disease gene networks [65–70]. For example, the Network-wide Association Study (NetWAS) tool uses GWAS summary statistics to identify tissue-specific disease gene networks that are enriched for risk alleles. In the original article on NetWAS, Greene *et al.* used NetWAS to reprioritize genes from a hypertension GWAS study using a blood vessel tissue-specific functional gene interaction network [68]. The top genes from their model were localized to an IL-1β inflammatory response network, a known disease pathway in hypertension. Moreover, the network-based gene rankings dramatically outperformed GWAS summary statistics at identifying drug targets for antihypertensive medications. Importantly, NetWAS and similar tools are designed to work with liberal statistical cutoffs for GWAS associations, using bioinformatic prior knowledge to "de-noise" the underlying signal. In their proof of concept on hypertension, Greene *et al.* were able to show that the network-based signals for hypertension were indeed highly enriched for biologically actionable information, including drug targets, despite using liberal GWAS cutoffs for gene associations.

Since the original publication, NetWAS has been cited 508 times, and applied to numerous complex diseases. While it has not yet been used for epilepsy, it has been applied to several neurological disorders, including Alzheimer's disease (AD) [71]. The present authors used a NetWAS-like approach to identify genes involved with amygdalar and hippocampal atrophy in AD, implicating genes involved in actin regulation whose dysfunction leads to the collapse of the tripartite synapse and excitotoxic neuron death [72]. Chang *et al.* applied similar network techniques to rank genes for association to schizophrenia, another heterogeneous and genetically complex neurological disorder [73]. Additionally, Krishnan *et al.* functionally characterized genes in autism spectrum disorder using network-based methods [74]. While AD, autism, schizophrenia, and hypertension are each biologically distinct, and different from epilepsy, they share many similar features in their genetic architecture. Bioinformatic network-based techniques are a promising avenue for detecting epilepsy risk gene pathways from faint genome-wide signals.

2.3.3 Model System Studies of Risk Factors and Modifiers

While genetic complexity is a hindrance to statistics in observational studies like GWAS, we can use complexity as an entry point for experimental studies of model organisms. For example, different genetic strains of mice have profoundly different phenotypes, including differential outcomes from specific mutations [75,76]. The neurophenotypic diversity of mice is particularly high, as some laboratory strains were systematically bred by "mouse fanciers" to have docile behavior [76], while recently wild-derived strains have much more typical behavior for wild mice [77]. These model systems allow the experimental dissection of risk and modifier genes for epilepsy. Below we describe studies that experimentally leverage genetic diversity to identify novel modifiers of seizure outcomes.

There is a long history of using panels of genetically diverse mice to probe for genetic modifiers of seizure outcomes. One of the oldest such panels is composed of the BXD recombinant inbred lines [78]. These mouse strains were generated by interbreeding the C57BL/6J (B) strain with the DBA/2J (D) strain. Each BXD strain is a genetic mosaic of the B and D genomes that is homozygous everywhere. Thus, each individual genome can be infinitely probed with different experimental challenges and each genome needs only to be sequenced once. Over the last three decades, there has been a broad accumulation of phenotypic data on the BXD mice including response to multiple seizure-induction modalities [79–82]. One durable genetic locus that has been identified for flurothyl- and kainic-acid-induced seizures is the seizure susceptibility 1 (*Szs1*) locus on mouse chromosome 1 [83,84]. Mice with the D allele at this locus are much more susceptible to seizures than those with the B allele [84]. By fine mapping with congenic strains, this region was narrowed to a small segment containing three compelling candidate genes, *Kcnj9*, *Kcnj10*, and *Atp1a2* [84]. *Kcnj10* has a missense mutation between the B and D alleles [84], while *Kcnj9*, has an expression quantitative trait locus (eQTL), where the D allele of the gene is expressed at a higher level than the B allele [85]. Together, these results implicate both *Kcnj9* and *Kcnj10*. Importantly, the human ortholog of *Kcnj10*, *KCNJ10*, is implicated in multiple forms of human epilepsy [86–88], demonstrating that the natural variation in seizure susceptibility across mouse strains at least partly overlaps the corresponding human risk gene networks.

The differences across mouse strains in seizure pathophysiology is not limited to one channelopathy in the DBA/2J strain. In a recent study, Ferland *et al.* used the Hybrid Mouse Diversity Panel (HMDP), a collection of inbred mouse strains including multiple BXDs [89,90], to identify genetic modifiers of generalized seizure threshold after flurothyl-induced kindling [91]. They identified a novel locus they termed epileptogenesis factor 1 (*Esf1*) that influences seizure threshold after multiple challenges. This chromosome 4 locus is distinct from the *Szs1* locus, demonstrating a distinct genetic modifier for response to repeated seizure challenges. Using a systems genetics approach, they nominated *Camta1* as a putative causative gene in this locus, along with three other possible candidates by expression (*Per3*, *Park7*, and *Vamp3*). Intriguingly, they also showed that the effect of the *Esf1* locus is dependent on the genotype at the *Szs1* locus, which is consistent with the D allele at the *Szs1* locus potentiating the effect of the *Esf1* locus. This epistatic effect is proof of concept that genetic interaction analysis in mice enables novel pathophysiological inferences for epilepsy.

In the last 15 years, a new recombinant inbred panel of mice called the Collaborative Cross (CC) has been developed by systematically interbreeding eight founder strains of mice representing three distinct subspecies [92]. The CC strains exhibit an even higher degree of phenotypic diversity than previous panels because of the inclusion of three recently wild-derived strains [93]. Gu *et al.* recently showed using CC mice challenged with flurothyl that some of these strains display extreme variation in multiple epilepsy associated phenomena, including seizure susceptibility, seizure propagation, epileptogenesis, and sudden unexplained death in epilepsy (SUDEP) [94]. Using a systems genetics approach, they mapped a high-confidence candidate gene for extreme seizure susceptibility, *Gabra2*. This is the first use of this modern mouse panel for systems genetics of epilepsy. Extrapolating from the results of Ferland *et al.* discussed above, it is likely that the CCs will be a critical platform for experimentally dissecting the interacting genetic factors driving different components of epilepsy pathophysiology.

The results in Ferland *et al.* showed that epistasis among loci can support pathophysiological inferences about gene function (in that case, that the *Szs1* locus potentiates the effect of the *Esf1* locus). However, their analysis was not designed to detect large networks of epistatic interactions;

11

rather, checking for an interaction with *Szs1* was natural given prior knowledge of that locus in their population. Tyler *et al.* recently published an epistasis network analysis of a combined population of multiple experimental crosses of mice carrying mutations associated with absence epilepsy (AE) [95]. In that study, they fixed one AE-causing mutation in three different genes (*Gabrg2*, *Scn8a*, and *Gria4*) on two genetic backgrounds, C57BL/6J (B6) and C3HeB/FeJ (C3H). The C3H strain had a uniformly worse phenotype across all mutations, with more frequent and longer lasting spike-and-wave discharges than the B6 strain, demonstrating the existence of genetic modifiers in the C3H background that exacerbate epilepsy across all three genetic insults. To map these modifiers, they crossed the B6 and C3H mice carrying one of these mutations and combined all three populations for mapping. Critically, they systematically modeled epistasis among all loci. They identified a large network of interactions among loci, demonstrating that epistasis is a significant feature of the genetic architecture of background modifier effects on spike-and-wave discharge in mice. In particular, they identified two strong modifiers that each exacerbated epilepsy on the C3H background, but when combined produced no worse phenotype, suggesting that the causal genes within these loci act in the same functional pathway, so that loss of both is no worse than loss of one. While this study was not powered to detect individual candidate genes, it demonstrates that epistatic interaction networks are a significant component of the genetic architecture of epilepsy traits in mice.

2.3.4 Targeting Gene Expression Instead of Gene Mutations

The human and model system studies discussed so far largely focus on the risk of particular outcomes. Implicitly, there is always hope that by cataloging risk genes we will also be developing lists of druggable targets. However, risk genes can have a wide variety of effects, including modifications of brain development, responses to insults, or active maintenance of a disease state. From a therapeutic perspective, it is much harder, for example, to restructure a malformed brain than disable an ion channel. Moreover, a priori there is no reason why a successful therapy needs to target the causal mutation. Instead, what is required is that ongoing molecular dynamics in brains with epilepsy be normalized to those of a brain without epilepsy.

One intriguing approach to normalizing gene expression in disease is called genome-based drug repurposing (GDR) [96,97]. The central idea of GDR is that any given drug can have a widespread influence on gene expression, independent of its physical molecular target. By matching disease gene expression signatures with anticorrelated drug-induced expression signatures from cell culture systems, GDR attempts to leverage these molecular network-mediated effects of a drug to reverse pathological gene expression. Recently, Mirza *et al.* applied GDR to gene expression signatures from TLE [98]. They identified multiple drug compounds that had predicted anti-seizure effects, including a novel finding of sitagliptin, a diabetes drug, which caused a dose-dependent reduction of seizures in a drug-resistant mouse model of epilepsy. This finding has been corroborated in multiple other rodent studies that have elucidated anti-oxidative stress and anti-neuroinflammatory effects [99] and suppressive effects on CXCR3/RAGE signaling by sitagliptin [100]. While this approach is still in the proof-of-concept stage, these early results suggest that strategies that specifically leverage the network effects of gene co-expression can extend "treat to target" approaches to provide actionable leads.

2.4 The Outlook of Systems Genetics in Epilepsy

Looking forward, we can see major trends in disease genetics that are likely to significantly influence the genetic analysis of epilepsy. With the ever-decreasing costs of "omics" technologies, it is now possible to combine information about epigenetics, protein abundance and post-translational modification, and metabolite abundance, with genotype data. These tools are further expanding as single-cell [101] and spatially resolved [102] technologies are developed. New analyses are also being developed to accommodate these multi-omic designs, such as multi-omic factor analysis (MOFA) [103]. These data give much more granular cross-sections of the molecular activity in biological samples and are poised to extend the inferences possible from systems genetics approaches to epilepsy.

Beyond molecular assays, there has been significant progress on novel phenotyping approaches.

In contrast to case-control designations alone, many modern GWAS for neurological disorders, such as the Alzheimer's Disease Neuroimaging Initiative and the IMAGEN consortium, are using imaging genetics approaches, where whole-brain scans and functional imaging are used as endophenotypes for genetic mapping. In parallel, the advent of deep learning over the last decade has fundamentally transformed image analysis [104], including in epilepsy [105]. Capitalizing on these trends for GWAS will likely require large national or international consortia, but the depth of the insights found in other diseases is likely to compel the epilepsy field in this direction. Systems approaches to electrophysiological data, such as those described in this book, are also likely to provide useful phenotypes for genetic analysis provided they can be collected and shared at scale using resources like the Children's Hospital Boston-MIT Scalp EEG database [106].

The treatment of seizures – and the genetic modeling of risk for seizures – is emphasized in epilepsy, although cognitive and behavioral impairments also have a major negative impact on quality of life [107,108]. Additionally, many anti-seizure medications have a wide range of efficacy and can have contradicting effects when used to treat different mutations of the same gene [109,110]. To successfully treat, and potentially cure, the range of symptoms in seizure disorders it will be essential to identify targets that impact both seizures and the associated morbidities. There has been significant recent interest in GWAS toward polygenic risk modeling of psychiatric and behavioral traits [111–113]. In addition to searching for individual genome-wide significant effects, polygenic risk scoring approaches aggregate noisy evidence across thousands, or even millions, of variants to define genetic propensity scores for large numbers of highly complex traits. Given that epilepsy commonly co-occurs with cognitive deficits and psychiatric comorbidities, we anticipate that polygenic risk modeling could improve outcome modeling, stratification to treatments, and possibly redefine clinical nosologies. Importantly, model systems phenotyping approaches have also innovated over the last several years, with deep learning systems being developed for ultrasonic vocalization detection [114], gait estimation [115], behavior classification [116,117], and many other complex phenotypes. Using systems genetics to model pleiotropy of mutations across a broad spectrum of seizure, cognitive, behavioral, and psychiatric phenotypes is now possible at a scale that has never existed before.

The next decades will see the genetic architecture of epilepsy come into clear focus not as a constellation of individual mutations with individual effects but as a network of interacting genetic components. The challenge is identifying those leverage points in the network in which we can intervene to improve patient outcomes. The network analytic perspective developed in systems genetics over the last 20 years will be critical to these efforts.

References

1. Kass, H. R., Winesett, S. P., Bessone, S. K., Turner, Z., and Kossoff, E. H. Use of dietary therapies amongst patients with GLUT1 deficiency syndrome. *Seizure*, 35, 83–7 (2016).

2. Mikati, M. A., Jiang, Y. H., Carboni, M., et al. Quinidine in the treatment of KCNT1-positive epilepsies. *Ann. Neurol.*, 78(6), 995–9 (2015).

3. Wilmshurst, J. M., Gaillard, W. D., Vinayan, K. P., et al. Summary of recommendations for the management of infantile seizures: Task Force Report for the ILAE Commission of Pediatrics. *Epilepsia*, 56(8), 1185–97 (2015).

4. Steward, C. A., Roovers, J., Suner, M.-M., et al. Re-annotation of 191 developmental and epileptic encephalopathy-associated genes unmasks de novo variants in SCN1A. *NPJ Genom. Med.*, 4(1), 31 (2019).

5. Wang, J., Lin, Z.-J., Liu, L., et al. Epilepsy-associated genes. *Seizure*, 44, 11–20 (2017).

6. King, E. A., Davis, J. W., and Degner, J. F. Are drug targets with genetic support twice as likely to be approved? Revised estimates of the impact of genetic support for drug mechanisms on the probability of drug approval. *PLoS Genet.*, 15(12), e1008489 (2019).

7. Anderson, V. E., Hauser, W. A., and Rich, S. S. Genetic heterogeneity in the epilepsies. *Adv. Neurolo.*, 44, 59–75 (1986).

8. Bachoo, R. M., Kim, R. S., Ligon, K. L., et al. Molecular diversity of astrocytes with implications for neurological disorders. *Proc. Natl. Acad. Sci. USA*, 101(22), 8384–9 (2004).

9. Baranzini, S. E. Gene expression profiling in

neurological disorders. *NeuroMolecular Med.*, 6(1), 31–51 (2004).

10. Delahaye-Duriez, A., Srivastava, P., Shkura, K., et al. Rare and common epilepsies converge on a shared gene regulatory network providing opportunities for novel antiepileptic drug discovery. *Genome Biol.*, 17(1), 245 (2016).

11. Ceulemans, B. P. G. M., Claes, L. R. F., and Lagae, L. G. Clinical correlations of mutations in the SCN1A gene: From febrile seizures to severe myoclonic epilepsy in infancy. *Pediatr. Neurol.*, 30(4), 236–43 (2004).

12. Northrup, H., Krueger, D. A., Northrup, H., et al. Tuberous sclerosis complex diagnostic criteria update: Recommendations of the 2012 international tuberous sclerosis complex consensus conference. *Pediatr. Neurol.*, 49 (4), 243–54 (2013).

13. Hemminki, K., Li, X., Johansson, S.-E., Sundquist, K., and Sundquist, J. Familial Risks for Epilepsy among Siblings Based on Hospitalizations in Sweden. *Neuroepidemiology*, 27 (2), 67–73 (2006).

14. Tsuboi, T., and Endo, S. Genetic studies of febrile convulsions: analysis of twin and family data. *Epilepsy Res. Suppl.*, 4, 119–28 (1991).

15. Abou-Khalil, B., Auce, P., Avbersek, A., et al. Genome-wide mega-analysis identifies 16 loci and highlights diverse biological mechanisms in the common epilepsies. *Nat. Commun.*, 9(1), 5269 (2018).

16. Kobow, K., Ziemann, M., Kaipananickal, H., et al. Genomic DNA methylation distinguishes subtypes of human focal cortical dysplasia. *Epilepsia*, 60(6), 1091–03 (2019).

17. Symonds, J. D., Zuberi, S. M., and Johnson, M. R. Advances in epilepsy gene discovery and implications for epilepsy diagnosis and treatment. *Curr. Opin. Neurol.*, 30(2), 193–99 (2017).

18. Bartha, Á., and Győrffy, B. Comprehensive outline of whole exome sequencing data analysis tools available in clinical oncology. *Cancers*, 11 (11), 1725 (2019).

19. Deming, Y., Li, Z., Kapoor, M., et al. Genome-wide association study identifies four novel loci associated with Alzheimer's endophenotypes and disease modifiers. *Acta Neuropathol.*, 133(5), 839–56 (2017).

20. Taylor, K. E., Chung, S. A., Graham, R. R., et al. Risk alleles for systemic lupus erythematosus in a large case-control collection and associations with clinical subphenotypes. *PLoS Genet.*, 7 (2), e1001311 (2011).

21. Amberger, J. S., Bocchini, C. A., Schiettecatte, F., Scott, A. F., and Hamosh, A. OMIM.org: Online Mendelian Inheritance in Man (OMIM®), an online catalog of human genes and genetic disorders. *Nucleic Acids Res.*, 43(Database issue), D789–98 (2015).

22. Landrum, M. J., Lee, J. M., Riley, G. R., et al. ClinVar: public archive of relationships among sequence variation and human phenotype. *Nucleic Acids Res.*, 42(Database issue), D980–5 (2014).

23. Brandt, C., Hillmann, P., Noack, A., et al. The novel, catalytic mTORC1/2 inhibitor PQR620 and the PI3K/mTORC1/2 inhibitor PQR530 effectively cross the blood-brain barrier and increase seizure threshold in a mouse model of chronic epilepsy. *Neuropharmacology*, 140, 107–20 (2018).

24. Ma, J., Yan, Z., Zhang, J., et al. A genetic predictive model for precision treatment of diffuse large B-cell lymphoma with early progression. *Biomark. Res.*, 8(1), 33 (2020).

25. Hernandez, C. C., Klassen, T. L., Jackson, L. G., et al. Deleterious rare variants reveal risk for loss of GABAA receptor function in patients with genetic epilepsy and in the general population. *PLoS One*, 11(9), e0162883 (2016).

26. Myers, K. A., Bennett, M. F., Grinton, B. E., et al. Contribution of rare genetic variants to drug response in absence epilepsy. *Epilepsy Res.*, 170, 106537 (2021).

27. Wolking, S., Moreau, C., McCormack, M., et al. Assessing the role of rare genetic variants in drug-resistant, non-lesional focal epilepsy. *Ann. Clin. Transl. Neurol.*, 8(7), 1376–87 (2021).

28. Todorova, M. T., Mantis, J. G., Le, M., Kim, C. Y., and Seyfried, T. N. Genetic and environmental interactions determine seizure susceptibility in epileptic EL mice. *Genes Brain Behav.*, 5(7), 518–27 (2006).

29. Fisher, R. Statistical methods in genetics. *Int. J. Epidemiol.*, 39 (2), 329–35 (2010).

30. Fisher, R. A. The resemblance between twins, a statistical examination of Lauterbach's measurements. *Genetics*, 10(6), 569–79 (1925).

31. Fisher, R. A., Immer, F. R., and Tedin, O. The genetical interpretation of statistics of the third degree in the study of quantitative inheritance. *Genetics*, 17(2), 107–24 (1932).

32. Thompson, E. A. R.A. Fisher's contributions to genetical statistics. *Biometrics*, 46(4), 905–14 (1990).

33. Boyle, E. A., Li, Y. I., and Pritchard, J. K. An expanded view of complex traits: From

polygenic to omnigenic. *Cell*, 169(7), 1177–86 (2017).

34. Wood, A. R., Esko, T., Yang, J., et al. Defining the role of common variation in the genomic and biological architecture of adult human height. *Nat. Genet.*, 46(11), 1173–86 (2014).

35. Veeramah, K. R., Johnstone, L., Karafet, T. M., et al. Exome sequencing reveals new causal mutations in children with epileptic encephalopathies. *Epilepsia*, 54(7), 1270–81 (2013).

36. Dibbens, L. M., Heron, S. E., and Mulley, J. C. A polygenic heterogeneity model for common epilepsies with complex genetics. *Genes Brain Behav.*, 6(7), 593–7 (2007).

37. Wang, F., Xiong, S., Wu, L., et al. A novel TSC2 missense variant associated with a variable phenotype of tuberous sclerosis complex: case report of a Chinese family. *BMC Med. Genet.*, 19(1), 90 (2018).

38. Kauffman, S. Gene regulation networks: A theory for their global structure and behaviors. *Curr. Top. Dev. Biol.*, 6(6), 145–82 (1971).

39. Shen-Orr, S. S., Milo, R., Mangan, S., and Alon, U. Network motifs in the transcriptional regulation network of Escherichia coli. *Nat. Genet.*, 31(1), 64–8 (2002).

40. Yook, S. H., Oltvai, Z. N., and Barabási, A. L. Functional and topological characterization of protein interaction networks. *Proteomics*, 4(4), 928–42 (2004).

41. Bray, D. Intracellular signalling as a parallel distributed process. *J. Theor. Biol.*, 143(2), 215–31 (1990).

42. Bray, D. (1995). Protein molecules as computational elements in living cells. *Nature*, 376(6538), 307–12.

43. Alon, U. *Introduction to Systems Biology: Design Principles of Biological Circuits*, 1st ed. New York: Chapman & Hall/CRC. 2006.

44. Barabási, A.-L., and Albert, R. Emergence of scaling in random networks. *Science*, 286 (5439), 509–12 (1999).

45. Broido, A. D., and Clauset, A. Scale-free networks are rare. *Nat. Commun.*, 10(1), 1017 (2019).

46. Smith, H. B., Kim, H., and Walker, S. I. Scarcity of scale-free topology is universal across biochemical networks. *Sci. Rep.*, 11(1), 6542 (2021).

47. Milo, R., Shen-Orr, S., Itzkovitz, S., et al. Network motifs: Simple building blocks of complex networks. *Science*, 298(5594), 824–7 (2002).

48. Moore, J. H., and Williams, S. M. Epistasis and its implications for personal genetics. *Am. J. Hum. Genet.*, 85(3), 309–20 (2009).

49. Visser, J. A. G. M. de, Cooper, T. F., and Elena, S. F. The causes of epistasis. *Proc. R. Soc. B*, 278(1725), 17–3624 (2011).

50. Kinghorn, B. P. The nature of 2-locus epistatic interactions in animals: evidence from Sewall Wright's guinea pig data. *Theor. Appl. Genet.*, 73(4), 595–604 (1987).

51. Avery, L., and Wasserman, S. Ordering gene function: The interpretation of epistasis in regulatory hierarchies. *Trends Genet.*, 8(9), 312–6 (1992).

52. Forsberg, S. K. G., Bloom, J. S., Sadhu, M. J., Kruglyak, L., and Carlborg, Ö. Accounting for genetic interactions improves modeling of individual quantitative trait phenotypes in yeast. *Nat. Genet.*, 49(4), 497–503 (2017).

53. Lehner, B. Molecular mechanisms of epistasis within and between genes. *Trends Genet.*, 27(8), 323–31 (2011).

54. Tyler, A. L., Donahue, L. R., Churchill, G. A., and Carter, G. W. Weak epistasis generally stabilizes phenotypes in a mouse intercross. *PLoS Genet.*, 12(2), e1005805 (2016).

55. Carter, A. J. R., Hermisson, J., and Hansen, T. F. The role of epistatic gene interactions in the response to selection and the evolution of evolvability. *Theor. Popul. Biol.*, 68(3), 179–96 (2005).

56. Hill, W. G., Goddard, M. E., and Visscher, P. M. Data and theory point to mainly additive genetic variance for complex traits. *PLoS Genet.*, 4(2), e1000008 (2008).

57. Campbell, R. F., McGrath, P. T., and Paaby, A. B. Analysis of epistasis in natural traits using model organisms. *Trends Genet.*, 34(11), 883–98 (2018).

58. Tyler, A. L., Lu, W., Hendrick, J. J., Philip, V. M., and Carter, G. W. CAPE: An R Package for Combined Analysis of Pleiotropy and Epistasis. *PLoS Comput. Biol.*, 9(10), e1003270 (2013).

59. Zhu, S., and Fang, G. MatrixEpistasis: Ultrafast, exhaustive epistasis scan for quantitative traits with covariate adjustment. *Bioinformatics*, 34(14), 2341–8 (2018).

60. Pedruzzi, G., and Rouzine, I. M. An evolution-based high-fidelity method of epistasis measurement: Theory and application to influenza. *PLoS Pathog.*, 17(6), e1009669 (2021).

61. Slim, L., Chatelain, C., Azencott, C.-A., and Vert, J.-P. Novel methods for epistasis detection in genome-wide association studies. *PLoS ONE*, 15(11), e0242927 (2020).

62. Johnson, M. R., Behmoaras, J., Bottolo, L., et al. Systems

genetics identifies Sestrin 3 as a regulator of a proconvulsant gene network in human epileptic hippocampus. *Nat. Commun.*, 6(1), 6031 (2015).

63. Preston, G. A., & Weinberger, D. R. (2005). Intermediate phenotypes in schizophrenia: a selective review. *Dialogues Clin. Neurosci.*, 7(2), 165–79.

64. Johnson, M. R., Shkura, K., Langley, S. R., et al. Systems genetics identifies a convergent gene network for cognition and neurodevelopmental disease. *Nat. Neurosci.*, 19(2), 223–32 (2016).

65. Califano, A., Butte, A. J., Friend, S., Ideker, T., and Schadt, E. Leveraging models of cell regulation and GWAS data in integrative network-based association studies. *Nat. Genet.*, 44(8), 841–7 (2012).

66. Carter, H., Hofree, M., and Ideker, T. Genotype to phenotype via network analysis. *Curr. Opin. Genet. Dev.*, 23(6), 611–21 (2013).

67. Cowen, L., Ideker, T., Raphael, B. J., and Sharan, R. Network propagation: A universal amplifier of genetic associations. *Nat. Rev. Genet.*, 18(9), 551–62 (2017).

68. Greene, C. S., Krishnan, A., Wong, A. K., et al. Understanding multicellular function and disease with human tissue-specific networks. *Nat. Genet.*, 47(6), 569–76 (2015).

69. Ideker, T., Ozier, O., Schwikowski, B., and Siegel, A. F. Discovering regulatory and signalling circuits in molecular interaction networks. *Bioinformatics*, 18(suppl 1), S233–40 (2002).

70. Mitra, K., Carvunis, A.-R., Ramesh, S. K., and Ideker, T. Integrative approaches for finding modular structure in biological networks. *Nat. Rev. Genet.*, 14(10), 719–32 (2013).

71. Yao, X., Jingwen, Y., Kefei, L., et al. Tissue-specific network-based genome wide study of amygdala imaging phenotypes to identify functional interaction modules. *Bioinformatics*, 33(20), 3250–7 (2017).

72. Brabec, J. L., Lara, M. K., Tyler, A. L., and Mahoney, J. M. System-level analysis of Alzheimer's disease prioritizes candidate genes for neurodegeneration. *Front. Genet.*, 12, 625246 (2021).

73. Chang, S., Fang, K., Zhang, K., and Wang, J. Network-based analysis of schizophrenia genome-wide association data to detect the joint functional association signals. *PLoS One*, 10(7), e0133404 (2015).

74. Krishnan, A., Zhang, R., Yao, V., et al. Genome-wide prediction and functional characterization of the genetic basis of autism spectrum disorder. *Nat. Neurosci.*, 19 (11), 1454–62 (2016).

75. Silver, L. M. *Mouse Genetics*, New York: Oxford University Press. 1995.

76. Yoshiki, A., and Moriwaki, K. Mouse phenome research: Implications of genetic background. *ILAR J.*, 47(2), 94–102 (2006).

77. Chesler, E. J. Out of the bottleneck: The diversity outcross and collaborative cross mouse populations in behavioral genetics research. *Mamm. Genome*, 25(1), 3–11 (2014).

78. Peirce, J. L., Lu, L., Gu, J., Silver, L. M., and Williams, R. W. A new set of BXD recombinant inbred lines from advanced intercross populations in mice. *BMC Genet.*, 5(1), 7 (2004).

79. Miner, L. L., and Marley, R. J. Chromosomal mapping of loci influencing sensitivity to cocaine-induced seizures in BXD recombinant inbred

strains of mice. *Psychopharmacology*, 117(1), 62–6 (1995).

80. Neumann, P. E., and Collins, R. L. Genetic dissection of susceptibility to audiogenic seizures in inbred mice. *Proc. Natl. Acad. Sci.*, 88(12), 5408–12 (1991).

81. Philip, V. M., Duvvuru, S., Gomero, B., et al. High-throughput behavioral phenotyping in the expanded panel of BXD recombinant inbred strains. *Genes Brain Behav.*, 9(2), 129–59 (2010).

82. Wakana, S., Sugaya, E., Naramoto, F., et al. Gene mapping of SEZ group genes and determination of pentylenetetrazol susceptible quantitative trait loci in the mouse chromosome. *Brain Res.*, 857(1–2), 286–90. (2000).

83. Ferraro, T. N., Golden, G. T., Smith, G. G., et al. Mapping murine loci for seizure response to kainic acid. *Mamm. Genome*, 8(3), 200–8 (1997).

84. Ferraro, T. N., Golden, G. T., Smith, G. G., et al. Fine mapping of a seizure susceptibility locus on mouse chromosome 1: Nomination of Kcnj10 as a causative gene. *Mamm. Genome*, 15(4), 239–51 (2004).

85. Mozhui, K., Ciobanu, D. C., Schikorski, T., et al. Dissection of a QTL hotspot on mouse distal chromosome 1 that modulates neurobehavioral phenotypes and gene expression. *PLoS Genet.*, 4(11), e1000260 (2008).

86. Buono, R. J., Lohoff, F. W., Sander, T., et al. Association between variation in the human KCNJ10 potassium ion channel gene and seizure susceptibility. *Epilepsy Res.*, 58 (2–3), 175–83 (2004).

87. Lenzen, K. P., Heils, A., Lorenz, S., et al. Supportive evidence

for an allelic association of the human KCNJ10 potassium channel gene with idiopathic generalized epilepsy. *Epilepsy Res.*, 63(2–3), 113–8 (2005).

88. Reichold, M., Zdebik, A. A., Lieberer, E., et al. KCNJ10 gene mutations causing EAST syndrome (epilepsy, ataxia, sensorineural deafness, and tubulopathy) disrupt channel function. *Proc. Natl. Acad. Sci.*, 107(32), 14490–5 (2010).

89. Bennett, B. J., Farber, C. R., Orozco, L., et al. A high-resolution association mapping panel for the dissection of complex traits in mice. *Genome Res.*, 20(2), 281–90 (2010).

90. Ghazalpour, A., Rau, C. D., Farber, C. R., et al. Hybrid mouse diversity panel: a panel of inbred mouse strains suitable for analysis of complex genetic traits. *Mamm. Genome*, 23(9–10), 680–92 (2012).

91. Ferland, R. J., Smith, J., Papandrea, D., et al. Multidimensional genetic analysis of repeated seizures in the hybrid mouse diversity panel reveals a novel epileptogenesis susceptibility locus. *G3 (Bethseda)*, 7(8), 2545–58 (2017).

92. Threadgill, D. W., Miller, D. R., Churchill, G. A., and Villena, F. P.-M. de. The collaborative cross: A recombinant inbred mouse population for the systems genetic era. *ILAR J.*, 52 (1), 24–31 (2011).

93. Srivastava, A., Morgan, A. P., Najarian, M. L., et al. Genomes of the mouse collaborative cross. *Genetics*, 206(2), 537–56 (2017).

94. Gu, B., Shorter, J. R., Williams, L. H., et al. Collaborative Cross mice reveal extreme epilepsy phenotypes and genetic loci for seizure susceptibility. *Epilepsia*, 61(9), 2010–21 (2020).

95. Tyler, A. L., McGarr, T. C., Beyer, B. J., Frankel, W. N., and Carter, G. W. A genetic

interaction network model of a complex neurological disease. *Genes Brain Behav.*, 13(8), 831–40 (2014).

96. Duan, Q., Flynn, C., Niepel, M., et al. LINCS Canvas Browser: Interactive web app to query, browse and interrogate LINCS L1000 gene expression signatures. *Nucleic Acids Res.*, 42(Web Server issue), W449–60 (2014).

97. Lamb, J., Crawford, E. D., Peck, D., et al. The connectivity map: Using gene-expression signatures to connect small molecules, genes, and disease. *Science*, 313(5795), 1929–35 (2006).

98. Mirza, N., Sills, G. J., Pirmohamed, M., and Marson, A. G. Identifying new antiepileptic drugs through genomics-based drug repurposing. *Hum. Mol. Genet.*, 26(3), 527–37 (2017).

99. Sun, Q., Zhang, Y., Huang, J., et al. DPP4 regulates the inflammatory response in a rat model of febrile seizures. *Biomed. Mater. Eng.*, 28(s1), S139–52 (2017).

100. Liu, Y., Hou, B., Zhang, Y., et al. Anticonvulsant agent DPP4 inhibitor sitagliptin downregulates CXCR3/RAGE pathway on seizure models. *Exp. Neurol.*, 307, 90–8 (2018).

101. Olsen, T. K., and Baryawno, N. Introduction to single-cell RNA sequencing. *Curr. Protoc. Mol. Biol.*, 122(1), e57 (2018).

102. Rusk, N. Spatial RNA mapping. *Nat. Methods*, 16(9), 803 (2019).

103. Argelaguet, R., Velten, B., Arnol, D., et al. Multi-omics factor analysis – A framework for unsupervised integration of multi-omics data sets. *Mol. Syst. Biol.*, 14(6), e8124 (2018).

104. Shen, D., Wu, G., and Suk, H.-I. Deep learning in medical image analysis. *Annu. Rev. Biomed. Eng.*, 19(1), 221–48 (2017).

105. Kubach, J., Muhlebner-Fahrngruber, A., Soylemezoglu, F., et al. Same same but different: A Web-based deep learning application revealed classifying features for the histopathologic distinction of cortical malformations. *Epilepsia*, 61(3), 421–32 (2020).

106. Shoeb, A., Edwards, H., Connolly, J., et al. Patient-specific seizure onset detection. *Epilepsy Behav.*, 5(4), 483–98 (2004).

107. Auriel, E., Landov, H., Blatt, I., et al. Quality of life in seizure-free patients with epilepsy on monotherapy. *Epilepsy Behav.*, 14(1), 130–3 (2009).

108. Meneses, R. F., Pais-Ribeiro, J. L., Silva, A. M. da, and Giovagnoli, A. R. Neuropsychological predictors of quality of life in focal epilepsy. *Seizure*, 18(5), 313–9 (2009).

109. Naimo, G. D., Guarnaccia, M., Sprovieri, T., et al. A systems biology approach for personalized medicine in refractory epilepsy. *Int.J. Mol. Sci.*, 20(15), 3717 (2019).

110. Perucca, P., and Perucca, E. Identifying mutations in epilepsy genes: Impact on treatment selection. *Epilepsy Res.*, 152, 18–30 (2019).

111. Ikeda, M., Saito, T., Kanazawa, T., and Iwata, N. Polygenic risk score as clinical utility in psychiatry: a clinical viewpoint. *J. Hum. Genet.*, 66(1), 53–60 (2021).

112. Martin, A. R., Daly, M. J., Robinson, E. B., Hyman, S. E., and Neale, B. M. Predicting polygenic risk of psychiatric disorders. *Biol. Psychiatry*, 86 (2), 97–109 (2018).

113. Neumann, A., Jolicoeur-Martineau, A., Szekely, E., et al. Combined polygenic risk scores of different psychiatric traits predict general and specific psychopathology in childhood. *J. Child Psychol.*

17

Psychiatry. (2021). doi:10.1111/jcpp.13501

114. Coffey, K. R., Marx, R. G., and Neumaier, J. F. DeepSqueak: A deep learning-based system for detection and analysis of ultrasonic vocalizations. *Neuropsychopharmacology*, 44 (5), 859–68 (2019).

115. Mathis, A., Mamidanna, P., Cury, K. M., et al. DeepLabCut: Markerless pose estimation of user-defined body parts with deep learning. *Nat. Neurosci.*, 21(9), 1281–9 (2018).

116. Geuther, B. Q., Peer, A., He, H., et al. Action detection using a neural network elucidates the genetics of mouse grooming behavior. *ELife*, 10, e63207 (2021).

117. Gharagozloo, M., Amrani, A., Wittingstall, K., Hamilton-Wright, A., and Gris, D. Machine learning in modeling of mouse behavior. *Front. Neurosci.*, 15, 700253 (2021).

Chapter

3

Transcriptomic and Epigenomic Approaches for Epilepsy

Anika Bongaarts, Jagoda Glowacka, Konrad Wojdan, Angelika Mühlebner, Eleonora Aronica, and James D. Mills

3.1 Introduction

In the mid-1980s a number of scientists and research bodies conceived the idea of determining the DNA sequence of the entire human genome. Initiated in 1990 and known as the Human Genome Project (HGP), this ambitious, publicly funded project relied on contributions from numerous international laboratories and remains the world's largest collaborative biological-based project to date. The completion of the HGP thirteen years later in 2003 allowed scientists to view the human genome in its entirety for the first time [1]. It was thought that this would usher in a new age for biological research, allowing for a more comprehensive understanding of complex human diseases and phenotypes. While this was true to an extent, completion of this project led to a series of new, more complicated questions, as is often the case in research.

Perhaps, one of the most interesting aspects of the HGP was the finding that there are approximately 23,000 protein-coding genes in the human genome. These genes are expressed in a myriad of different ways across approximately 1×10^{14} cells with 1×10^{10} neurons in the brain alone [2]. Conversely, the relatively simple nematode *Caenorhabditis elegans* has a similar number of protein-coding genes expressed across just 1,000 relatively homogenous cells[3]. Against intuition, this suggests that a similar set of genes used to produce a simple organism with a small number of differentiated cells can also produce the relatively complex human with a diverse range of specialized cells. Further, the protein-coding sequences of the human and chimpanzee genome share somewhere between 98–99% of their sequence identity [4]. Even with these similarities there exist marked phenotypic differences, including extensive differences in brain development, size, and rate of growth. These findings suggest that the pathway from DNA sequence to organism phenotype is not simply reliant on the genomic sequence, but on how the genome is expressed and regulated at different levels. Two important levels of regulation that influence the outcome can be found embedded at the level of the transcriptome and epigenome.

The transcriptome refers to the set of RNA molecules expressed in a cell. Unlike the genome, which remains relatively fixed throughout the lifetime of a cell, the transcriptome is dynamic, changing depending on environmental factors, disease state, and developmental stage [5]. The transcriptome of different cells is made up of a varied collection of RNA transcripts, transcribed pervasively across the genome. Indeed, the ENCODE project showed that up to 75% of the human genome is transcribed in a cell-type-specific manner [5]. Transcription can produce both protein-coding and non-coding RNAs (ncRNAs), including circular RNAs (circRNAs), microRNAs (miRNAs), and long non-coding RNAs (lncRNAs). Each of these can, in turn, be alternatively spliced, edited, or modified to produce functionally distinct RNA or protein molecules [6,7]. This means that the relationship between DNA locus and functional unit (RNA or protein) is far from one-to-one. Furthermore, gene expression, and thus the transcriptome, can be further controlled through regulation of the epigenome via epigenetic mechanisms such as DNA methylation [8]. DNA modifications, introduced by DNA methyltransferases, reversibly modify the structure of the DNA resulting in the silencing or switching on of target genes. Overall, each of these different elements add extra levels of regulation, whereby gene expression can be precisely controlled and modulated across different cell types or time points to achieve higher levels of complexity [9]. While these multiple levels of regulation allow for the construction of more heterogeneous tissue types with specialized cell-to-cell interactions and functions, it also creates a system in which there are numerous components that can be disrupted, leading to an abnormal phenotype.

Regulation of the transcriptome and epigenome are particularly pertinent to the most complex organ of all, the human brain, and the associated neurological diseases and disorders that inflict it, such as epilepsy. Epilepsy affects over 70 million people worldwide, making seizures one of the most prevalent symptoms of brain disease [10]. Clinically epilepsy is characterized by a lasting predisposition to generate spontaneous seizures and has a vast array of neurobiological, cognitive, and psychosocial consequences [11]. The causes and risk factors for epilepsy are wide and varied. In the pediatric population, perinatal insults, and congenital abnormalities (such as malformations of cortical development) with a genetic etiology are often associated with severe epilepsy and developmental delay. In older individuals, cerebrovascular disease is the most common risk factor. Epilepsy is also associated with traumatic brain injury, infections, and tumors that can occur at any age. Anti-seizure medication can be used to suppress seizures but do not alter the long-term prognosis of the underlying condition [12]. Surgical intervention is generally seen as the most effective way to achieve seizure freedom in patients with drug-resistant focal epilepsy but this comes with associated risks and is only viable for a highly selected group of patients. As such there is an urgent need to better understand the molecular mechanisms underlying the various forms of epilepsy to develop novel, molecular-targeting based therapies. It is possible that analysis of the transcriptome and the epigenome may achieve these goals and help unravel the complexity of epilepsy and other neurological diseases.

This chapter will discuss the array of different techniques available to investigate changes in the transcriptome and epigenome and give an overview of how to analyze the resultant data (Fig. 3.1). Further, examples of how these techniques have been applied to epilepsy-associated research will be discussed. Finally, machine learning techniques will be discussed along with the pitfalls and strengths of applying these algorithms to transcriptomic and epigenomic data.

3.2 Transcriptome Profiling

Since the early 2000s, the development of various next-generation (also known as second-generation) and third-generation sequencing techniques have transformed the landscape of research in molecular biology. One such sequencing technique known as RNA-sequencing (RNA-seq), has surpassed microarrays as the gold standard for gene expression studies [13]. Unlike microarrays, which use probe hybridization technology to quantify gene expression over a set of predefined probes, RNA-seq produces a digital signature from a cDNA input. Further, RNA-seq allows for the entire gene expression profile of a sample to be assessed in a high-throughput manner, giving a snapshot of the gene expression profile of a tissue or cell at a specific moment in time. As well as quantifying gene expression levels and detecting differentially expressed genes, RNA-seq can be leveraged to explore alternative splicing events, detect novel transcripts, discover gene fusion events, map transcription start sites, identify sequence variation in transcribed regions, and detect circRNAs [13–15]. Furthermore, modifications of the standard RNA-seq workflow have given rise to several different RNA-seq-based technologies, including small RNA-seq, single-cell RNA-seq (scRNA-seq), single-nuclei RNA-seq (snRNA-seq), and spatial transcriptomics.

3.2.1 Current Technologies
3.2.1.1 Next-Generation Sequencing: RNA-seq

Currently, the most commonly used and cost-effective RNA-seq technology makes use of short-read technology where millions of short reads (50–150 nucleotides(nts)) are produced in parallel per sample. This form of sequencing falls into the class of next-generation sequencing (also known as second-generation sequencing). A next-generation RNA-seq experiment can be divided into three distinct phases: sample or library preparation, sequencing, and data analysis (Fig. 3.2). Here, we will discuss library preparation and sequencing; in a later Section 3.2.2 data analysis techniques for all the different RNA-seq methods will be discussed.

Perhaps the most important component of any RNA-seq experiment is the library preparation step. Any biases or contamination introduced during this step will be enriched during the sequencing phase. Consequently, in order to produce high-quality sequencing results it is paramount that high-quality, pure RNA is utilized for the input [16]. While several different library preparations methods exist, each is conceptually similar. In brief, first RNA is isolated from a

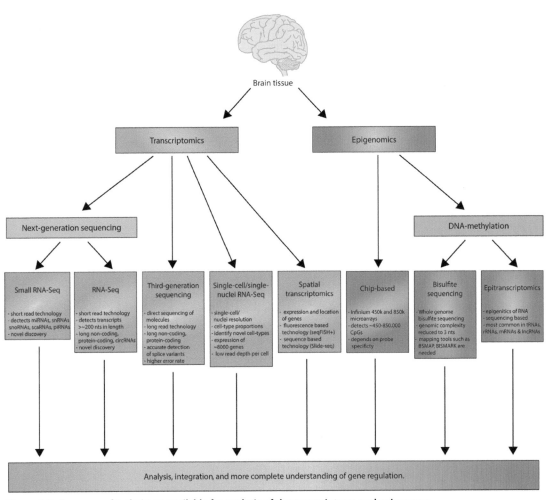

Figure 3.1 Summary of techniques available for analysis of the transcriptome and epigenome.

sample and reversed transcribed into cDNA. This is followed by ligation of adapters to the end of the ensuing molecules resulting in the generation of a cDNA library [14]. The ligation of adapters introduces a unique barcode to each sample allowing for multiplexing of samples during sequencing. Throughout the library preparation steps there are a number of options that can be chosen that will impact on the data produced [13,17]. RNA for RNA-seq can be poly-A selected or selected via ribosomal(ribo)-depletion; poly-A selection enriches for mRNAs and the polyadenylated fraction of ncRNAs, while ribo-depletion enriches for mRNA, pre-mRNA, and ncRNA, and also allows for the identification of circRNAs [18]. RNA-seq can also be strand specific, meaning that the strand of origin from which the transcript was transcribed is preserved, allowing for the detection of antisense transcripts [19]. The most common

strand-specific protocol in current use is the deoxy-UTP (dUTP) strand-marking protocol [20]. Here, the second strand of cDNA is synthesized by incorporating dUTP into the second strand. Prior to sequencing, the dUTP marked strand is selectively degraded by Uracil-DNA-Glycosylase. This leaves only one strand for sequencing and so strand information is retained. The modifications used will depend on the research question that is being addressed and the interest of the researcher.

The generated cDNA library is then subject to sequencing, utilizing the sequencing-by-synthesis strategy. While sequencing itself is a rather trivial process, there are a number of parameters or sequencing conformations that must be considered, including read length, single-end (SE) or paired-end (PE), and read depth [21]. A longer read length improves the accuracy at which the

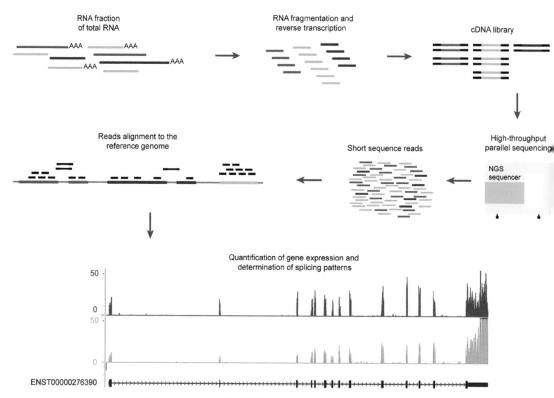

Figure 3.2 Next-generation RNA-seq workflow. The RNA fraction of interest is isolated, fragmented, and reverse transcribed into cDNA. Sequencing adapters are subsequently added to each cDNA fragment, and the generated cDNA library is subjected to high-throughput sequencing. The resulting short sequence reads are mapped to the reference genome. The resulting read alignments provide information about the levels of gene expression from the number of reads mapping to each exon. Moreover, through the detection and quantification of the sequence reads spanning exon/exon boundaries, the splicing patterns of individual transcripts can be reconstructed. Figure adapted with permission from Mills and Janitz 2012 [14].

reads can be mapped to the genome, as longer reads are more likely to be unique and map to only a single region of the genome. It also allows for more accurate transcript assembly. SE sequencing refers to the sequencing of only one end of the cDNA molecule, whereas in PE sequencing both ends of the molecule are sequenced. As with read length, PE sequencing allows for more accurate mapping of reads and is vastly superior for transcript discovery and is also preferable for the characterization of poorly annotated genomes and transcriptomes. Read depth is another important parameter that must be considered, the greater the read depth the greater the number of fragments that are sequenced per sample [22]. If a sample is sequenced to a deeper level more transcripts will be detected, including lowly expressed transcripts, and quantification will be more precise. As with sequencing length and SE versus PE sequencing, an increase in read depth will allow for much better transcript assembly and discovery of novel transcripts. It has been suggested that as few as 5 million reads are adequate for quantifying highly expressed genes, while other researchers will insist that as many as 100 million reads are required for quantification of lowly expressed genes and accurate transcript assembly [23]. Overall, shorter length SE reads to a minimal read depth are cheaper. However, longer read length with PE sequencing to a greater read depth will provide more reliable results. As such, it is often necessary to find the balance between sequencing parameters and overall cost. Finally, it must be noted that it is known that lane and flow cell biases exist during sequencing. Thus, it is important to make sure that samples are pooled and/or split across lanes, and when possible all sequenced in the same run and on the same flow-cell [24].

3.2.1.2 Next-Generation Sequencing: Small RNA-seq

One of the most interesting modifications of the RNA-seq short-read technology has seen the advent of what is known small RNA-seq [25]. Small RNA-seq library preparation is similar to the standard RNA-seq protocol. However, it requires a size selection step. Starting from total RNA, a polyacrylamide gel or magnetic beads can be used to select a fraction of the total RNA of interest; for small RNA-seq this means fragments usually 18–30 nucleotides in length. This size selection step will allow not only miRNAs to be captured, but also for a plethora of other small non-coding RNA species including small nucleolar RNAs (snoRNAs), small nuclear RNAs (snRNAs), small cajal body-specific RNAs (scaRNAs), piwi-interacting RNAs (piRNAs), and the even novel small RNAs [26,27]. Parameters such as read length, SE and PE reads, and read depth also apply to small RNA-seq. However, as the number of small RNAs is fewer than the number of long RNA species and alternative splicing is not as prevalent, most small RNA-seq experiments are SE to a read length of 50–75 nucleotides and to a read depth of 10–30 million reads.

Currently, among all small RNA species, miRNAs have received the most interest as a molecule for study. These short RNAs are crucial post-transcriptional regulators of gene expression; miRNAs work in concert with the RNA-inducing silencing complex (RISC) to direct post-transcriptional repression of target mature mRNA transcripts by binding to complementary 3' untranslated regions (UTR) [28]. Furthermore, each miRNA can regulate the expression of multiple target genes, and each transcript can be targeted by multiple miRNAs [29]. Thus, miRNAs can potentially regulate entire pathways or networks of genes and as such are immensely important regulators of the transcriptome. miRNAs appear to play pivotal roles in the regulation of cellular proliferation, differentiation, and apoptosis [30]. Further, the development of small RNA-seq approaches has also led to the appreciation that individual miRNAs can be heterogenous in length and/or sequence through both 5' and 3' sequence modifications to produce what are known as miRNA isoforms or isomiRs [31]. These miRNAs modifications can affect both the target genes of the miRNAs and also the localization of the miRNAs [31] adding yet another level of complexity to the regulation of the transcriptome.

3.2.1.3 Single-Cell and Single-Nuclei RNA-seq

Next-generation and third-generation RNA-seq techniques have played a pivotal role in shaping our understanding and appreciation of the complexity of the transcriptome. Currently, the majority of RNA-seq experiments are carried out on bulk tissue samples that consist of heterogeneous collections of different cell types. While performing RNA-seq on bulk tissue is useful for elucidating the overall trends in gene expression patterns, subtle and potential important gene expression changes from specific cell types may be obscured. Hence, RNA-seq lacks the ability to establish which cell types may be the major drivers of pathology. The development of scRNA-seq and snRNA-seq overcomes this issue and both have been applied to various tissue types to gain insights into the transcriptional landscape at the level of a single cell or nuclei. These innovative techniques are useful for understanding dynamic states, transcriptional networks, functional processes, and the discrete make-up of the cellular populations in heterogeneous bulk tissue. This is particularly applicable to the human brain, which has enormous cellular diversity. In fact snRNA-seq analysis of nuclei isolated from six distinct regions of the human cerebral cortex identified 16 neuronal subtypes, further underlying this point [32].

Currently, the most popular high-throughput and unbiased method used to isolate and capture cells for scRNA-seq or snRNA-seq are the droplet-based technologies. The three most commonly applied platforms are 10x Genomics Chromium, DropSeq, and inDrop [33]. While differences do exist between each of these droplet-based technologies, each can be generalized into five steps: sample preparation, encapsulation in droplets, library preparation, sequencing, and data analysis (for an in-depth review please see Salomon et al. [33]). In brief, sample preparation refers to the disassociation of the original sample into a single-cell suspension. The suspension is then passed through to one of the droplet-based technologies where each cell is encapsulated into a droplet. It is inside each of these droplet-based reactors that library preparation takes place. First the cell is lysed, releasing the RNA contents. The polyadenylated component of the RNA is captured and first-strand cDNA synthesis is carried out. At this stage a cell barcode and unique molecular identifier (UMI) are incorporated into the cDNA molecule. The cell barcode attaches a label to every amplified transcript belonging to a specific cell, allowing for the multiplexing of samples. The UMI individually tags each polyadenylated sequence captured from each cell and enables digital transcript counting and normalization of amplification artifacts. The first-strand cDNA is then amplified by different methods depending on the scRNA-seq platform being used. Regardless of the technique being used the final result is an Illumina-compatible cDNA library (see Section 3.2.1.1). Currently, at sequencing the expected outputs are of 500–10,000 cells (3,000 cells are considered optimal) with each cell sequenced to a depth of 10,000–50,000 reads. While lower depths (<10,000 reads) are sufficient for the classification of cell types in heterogenous tissues, approximately 50,000 reads appear to be necessary to pinpoint the finer distinctions within cell types and the set of genes explaining this variation. Increasing sequencing beyond this depth provides diminishing returns as single cells contain only a limited number of transcripts, of which many are lost during preparation and manipulation [34].

One of the major shortcomings of scRNA-seq is the requirement for fully intact cells. These can be challenging to isolate from frozen postmortem brain tissue or surgical resections as the cell membranes are easily damaged due to mechanical and physical stress during freeze thaw cycles [35]. Furthermore, the majority of the single-cell isolation and preparation methods make use of harsh enzymatic disassociation steps which can harm the fragile and heterogenous cells in brain tissue. The isolation of cell nuclei provides an alternative RNA source as nuclei are more resistant to both mechanical and physical stress. snRNA-seq has successfully been applied to postmortem human brain tissue along with mouse hippocampal tissue [35]. Several studies have compared scRNA-seq and snRNA-seq runs from matched tissue [36]. There, it was shown that snRNA-seq shared a high degree of similarity with scRNA-seq in terms of genes detected and resolved cell types, although snRNA-seq does show a higher level of intronic reads than scRNA-seq. The same droplet-based technologies and sequencing techniques used for scRNA-seq can also be applied to snRNA-seq. The major difference is that the sample preparation step involves the construction of a single-nuclei suspension rather than a single-cell suspension. As such, snRNA-seq is a feasible alternative to scRNA-seq for the study of epilepsy and conditions in which epilepsy is a comorbidity using human brain tissue.

3.2.1.4 Spatial Transcriptomics

For a complete molecular understanding of tissue, it is important to not only characterize gene expression profiles, but also to identify where across the tissue each gene is expressed. This spatial information is lost when performing RNA-seq on bulk tissue, and while it is possible to map cell types identified from snRNA-seq or scRNA-seq back to their original location, this is a time-consuming, and difficult process. Another option to garner spatial transcriptomic information is through the use of fluorescence in situ hybridization (FISH)-based methods. Here, individual transcripts are probed and their location down to the cell level or even subcellular level can be resolved. However, due to overlapping fluorescent signals it is only possible to visualize a few hundred transcripts in parallel [37]. Two new methodologies have been recently developed that allow for gene expression information to be gathered while retaining spatial information.

One such technique is known as sequential-FISH+ (seqFISH+) [38]. seqFISH+ is essentially a modified FISH assay where the transcript-specific primary probes are labeled with four barcode sequences that act as targets for fluorescently labeled secondary probes, rather than the primary probes themselves being fluorescently tagged. The key element to seqFISH+ is the expansion of a barcode base palette from 4 or 5 colors to 60 pseudo colors across three channels. Each round of barcoding is further subdivided into 20 serial hybridizations; this feature combined with three channels means that only one-sixtieth of the transcripts are visualized per image, thus overcoming the overcrowding problem commonly associated with FISH. seqFISH+ has been successfully used to quantify gene expression of 10,000 genes on cultured mouse cells and in slices of mouse brain [38]. These results were quantitively equivalent to RNA-seq data.

The second spatial transcriptomics method, known as Slide-seq, relies on spatial capture of genes with DropSeq beads [39]. DropSeq was originally developed for scRNA-seq (see Section 3.2.1.3); here single cells are encapsulated in droplets with a barcoded bead that labels transcripts with cell-specific barcodes. In Slide-seq these uniquely labeled barcoded beads are placed on a rubber-coated glass coverslip forming a mono-layer termed a "puck." Sequencing is used to uniquely determine the bead barcode sequences. A tissue section is placed on the puck and the RNA is released from the tissue and hybridize to the bead in its location. While each bead is not strictly capturing RNA from a single cell, the placement of the beads on the coverslip is packed in such a way that it matches the generalized cellular spacing of mammalian cells. RNA-seq libraries can then be produced that incorporate the position-specific barcode. After sequencing, the spatial gene expression information can be mapped back on to the coverslip. This Slide-seq technique has been used to successfully identify known tissue structures in mouse and human organs [39].

3.2.1.5 Third-Generation Sequencing

While the high-throughput ability and the reduction of the associated costs of next-generation RNA-seq has resulted in population scale transcriptomic analyses of many plant and animal species, there are inherent limitations to this technique, including poor or ambiguous mapping to repetitive elements, limited ability to span indels or structural variants, amplification of artifacts during library construction, and, most importantly, an inability to accurately resolve the structures of the most complex genes and splice variants [40,41]. Third-generation sequencing makes use of direct sequencing of RNA molecules, often producing reads over 10kb in length. This enables entire transcripts to be captured with a single read, thus allowing for the exact underlying exon structure to be determined, helping to resolve many of these issues. This is particularly important when analyzing the human transcriptome, where it is estimated that 95% of multi-exon genes are alternatively spliced [42]. This is further underlined by the fact that at least 15% and perhaps as many as 50% of human genetic diseases arise from mutations that impact on alternative splicing events [43].

Currently, the two most widely used third-generation sequencing technologies available on the market are the single-molecule real time (SMRT) sequencer from Pacific Bioscience (PacBio) and the nanopore based sequencer from Oxford Nanopore Technologies (ONT) [44]. PacBio adopts a similar sequencing-by-synthesis strategy to that used by Illumina sequencers, the most common next-generation sequencers

currently in use [44]. The major difference is that while Illumina next-generation sequencers detect an augmented signal from a clonal population of amplified cDNA fragments, PacBio captures the direct signal from a single cDNA molecule. The PacBio transcriptome sequencing method is known as Iso-Seq. As the signal-to-noise ratio from a single cDNA molecule is low, the error rate of PacBio data is relatively high at approximately 13–15% of the sequenced nucleotides [45]. To overcome this, the PacBio platform uses a circular DNA template by ligating hairpin adapters to both ends of the target template. The circular DNA sequence is sequenced multiple times. These multiple reads can then be joined together to generate a circular consensus sequence. ONT uses a different approach in which an RNA or cDNA molecule is directly sequenced by measuring current changes as the bases are threaded through the nanopore by a molecular motor protein [44]. As with PacBio, ONT also has higher error rates when compared to next-generation sequencing techniques. This has resulted in the development of hybrid sequencing techniques that utilize a combination of third-generation and next-generation sequencing, where next-generation sequencing is used to correct the inherent errors in third-generation sequencing, and third-generation sequencing is leveraged to accurately assemble splice variants [46].

3.2.2 Making Sense of the Data: Analysis Techniques

Although the production of RNA-seq data has become rather standardized, predominantly through the large market share held by Illumina (San Diego, CA, USA), no optimal or standard data analysis pipeline exists. This is further compounded by the existence of a large body of literature outlining different workflows and analysis techniques with each purporting to offer a superior, more "true" representation of the transcriptome. In reality there is not one optimal analysis technique, with each different tool having various strengths and weaknesses. The analysis techniques used are often dependent on the biological question being asked, the profiling technique used (e.g., RNA-seq or small RNA-seq) and the personal preference of the bioinformatician analyzing the data (for reviews and comparisons please see Conesa et al. [21], and Costa-Silva et al. [47]).

Regardless of the type (next-generation, third-generation, single-cell/nuclei RNA-seq) of RNA-seq carried out, the data analysis workflow is made up of the following steps: quality control (QC), mapping of reads, quantification of expression of genes or transcripts to generate a count (or expression) matrix. Once a gene or transcript count matrix has been constructed, differentially expressed genes can be identified, followed by a pathway or gene ontology enrichment analysis. More advanced analysis techniques can also be used, including weighted gene co-expression network analysis (WGCNA) or various machine learning techniques (discussed in Section 3.4). In this section, the idea is not to provide an in-depth analysis of each available method but instead provide a broad overview and references for analyzing RNA-seq data that the reader can utilize as a starting point for their analysis.

3.2.2.1 Read Alignment and Quantification of Expression

The first step of the analysis of the RNA-seq data involves the QC step. QC involves the assessment of raw sequencing reads for overall quality (the probability that the base called is correct), the presence of contaminating sequences and adapter-sequence artifacts. Commonly used QC software packages include RSeQC [48] and FastqQC [49]. After quality assessment, low-quality reads, or contaminating reads, can be removed using the software packages Trimmomatic [50] or Cutadapt [51].

After quality assessment and the removal of low-quality reads, the reads must be mapped or aligned. This process is normally done in line with a reference genome; however, aligners can be also directed to assemble reads de novo. This will often depend on the organism that the RNA was sourced from, for example, the mouse and human genomes have been annotated and repeatedly updated, and as such, in the majority of cases the reads can be aligned to the reference genome. For other less well studied organisms for which no reference genome exists, reads will have to be assembled de novo. The software used for mapping the reads will depend on the method of sequencing (next-generation or third generation). For next-generation sequencing, commonly used alignment software includes TopHat, Burrow-wheeler aligner (BWA), and STAR [21,47]. In the case of small RNA-seq where alternative splicing is not expected,

alignment software such as Bowtie2 can be utilized [47]. As third-generation sequencing techniques produce much longer read lengths than the next-generation sequencing technologies, specialized aligners such as BBMap can be utilized, as well as short-read aligners such as STAR and GMAP with modified settings [52]. After read alignment to the genome, the number of reads that align to each gene must be summed; commonly used tools for this include FeatureCounts and htseq-count [21]. After this process an unnormalized count matrix will be produced that is ready for further analysis.

3.2.2.2 Differential Expression Testing

The most common way in which genes of interest are identified for further study is via differential expression analysis to identify genes that are up- or down-regulated due to the treatment or disease state. Again, there are a variety of different methods and software packages available for this, many of which have been written in the R statistical programming language, including DESeq2, limma, and EdgeR [47]. One important requirement of differential expression testing is normalization of the RNA-seq count matrix before analysis, with sequencing depth being the most crucial variable to correct for. For example, if directly comparing a sample sequenced to a depth of 20 million reads to a sample sequenced to 40 million reads, almost all genes in the second sample will appear to be highly expressed when the second sample is compared to the first. A variety of different normalization methods for RNA-seq data exist, many of which are built into the differential expression software packages. For a more in-depth analysis, the reader is directed to the research article by Costa-Silva et al. [47].

It must also be noted here that there do exist entire tool suites, such as Tuxedo, Ballgown, and RSEM, that integrate all elements of the RNA-seq data analysis pipeline from read-mapping to quantification of reads, normalization, and differential expression testing [53–55]. Furthermore, these suites can calculate abundance at the gene or isoform level, allowing for the detection of differentially expressed isoforms and alterations in alternative splicing events. There also exist online tools such as the Galaxy Project which is a freely available, user-friendly web-based tool that allows research scientists with little to no informatics expertise to build workflows and perform data analysis [56].

Table 3.1. RNA-seq experiments in experimental models and human epilepsy

Technique	Main finding	Reference
RNA-seq and small RNA-seq	miR-34a family regulates neurogenesis and glutamate receptor signaling in TSC	[60]
RNA-seq	*Csfr1* is a potential therapeutic target for TLE	[61]
RNA-seq	The transcription factors Tp73, Cebpd, Pax6, and Spi1 regulate chronic transcriptional changes after TBI	[62]
Small RNA-seq	tRNA act as biomarkers for seizure development	[65]

3.2.2.3 Other Analysis Techniques

Outside of differential expression testing to identify genes of interest, there exist a number of more sophisticated techniques that can be used to make sense of RNA-seq data. These include pathway or gene ontology enrichment analysis [57], drug repurposing [58], WGCNA [59], and machine learning techniques (covered in depth in Section 3.4). Many of these analysis techniques utilize the freely available statistical programming language R.

3.2.3 Transcriptomics and Epilepsy

As it currently stands there has been a wealth of publications and research projects that have utilized different transcriptome profiling techniques, predominantly next-generation sequencing techniques, to study epilepsy and epilepsy related pathologies. As such, here the focus will be on publications that have been written since 2016 and have utilized RNA-seq technologies in a unique and interesting way (Table 3.1). Further, at the time of writing, snRNA-seq and scRNA-seq (Section 3.2.1.3), third-generation sequencing (Section 3.2.1.5), and spatial transcriptomics (Section 3.2.1.4) methods have not yet been applied in the context of epilepsy or epilepsy-associated diseases. Once these techniques become more well established, with an associated reduction in costs, they will become more common throughout the epilepsy research field.

3.2.3.1 Next-Generation Sequencing: Integration of Small RNA-seq and RNA-seq

A study by Mills et al. utilized both small RNA-seq and RNA-seq to investigate the transcriptional landscape of tuberous sclerosis complex (TSC) cortical tubers [60]. TSC is multisystem genetic disorder that causes abnormal growths throughout almost every organ in the body.

Approximately 90% of TSC patients present with complex structural brain abnormalities throughout the cortex, known as cortical tubers. These tubers cause devastating and therapeutically challenging neurological manifestations, including neurodevelopmental delay, autism, and epilepsy. These features, including the associated seizures, have a major impact on the quality of life of patients and the family members, who often act as primary caregivers. Current treatments for TSC associated seizures, such as medication or surgical resection of tubers, are often ineffective or only provide temporary relief. Thus, there is an urgent need to better understand the underlying molecular mechanisms of TSC so that novel treatment targets can be identified.

First, RNA-seq was performed on TSC cortical tubers and healthy cortex tissue. Here, 269 genes were identified as up-regulated and 169 were identified as down-regulated in TSC. Using the same sample set, small RNA-seq was then used to identify differentially expressed small RNAs. Overall, 932 and 59 small RNAs were identified as up-regulated and down-regulated in TSC, respectively. Interestingly, the differential expressed small RNAs included miRNAs, snoRNAs, scaRNAs, and snRNAs. Using the WGCNA technique, the two data sets were then integrated [59]. First, each of the genes were divided into modules based on their expression patterns; genes that were co-expressed were grouped together. This resulted in the formation of 11 distinct modules of co-expressed genes. Using gene ontology enrichment tools, each of the modules were assigned a function; this included innate immune response, extracellular matrix organization, neurogenesis, and glutamate receptor signaling. Next, the overall expression patterns of each module were summarized as the module eigengene. The eigengene is a value that can then be correlated with external traits, in this case miRNA expression. As the most well-known relationship between miRNAs and mRNAs involves inverse expression patterns, modules with strong inverse correlations were identified. The genes in the modules that were negatively correlated with miRNA expression patterns were then assessed for an enrichment of miRNA targets. Using this methodology, the miR-34 family (miR-34a, miR-34b, and miR-34c) was identified as a regulator of glutamate receptor signaling and neurogenesis. Based on these results, miR-34b-5p was selected for further in vitro investigation. miR-34b-5p was found to increase interleukin 1 beta (*IL1B*) in human fetal astrocytes suggesting that miR-34b-5p could activate an immune response, a process that is thought to play an important role in seizure development. Next, through transfection of hippocampal neurons, it was shown that miR-34b-5p can modulate neurite outgrowth in neurons. This paper [60] provides an example of using RNA-seq and small RNA-seq and bioinformatic analysis techniques to generate a hypothesis that can be validated in vitro or in vivo.

3.2.3.2 Next-Generation Sequencing: RNA-seq and Identification of a Novel Antiepileptic Drug Target

Developing drugs for epilepsy and central nervous system diseases in general, is arguably one of the greatest challenges in drug discovery. Overall, the success rate is very low, with less than 1% of candidate drugs ending up on the pharmaceutical market, driving the total cost of research and development for one drug up to 2 billion euros. Although there are over 25 approved antiepileptic drugs (AEDs) on the market, as many as 30% of patients are resistant to the effects of these drugs. Using RNA-seq data and a novel "Casual Reasoning Analytical Framework for Target discovery" (CRAFT), Srivastava et al. were able to address this problem [61].

This study was based around a post status epilepticus (SE) mouse model of acquired temporal lobe epilepsy (TLE). In this model, pilocarpine is injected intraperitoneally to induce seizures; approximately four weeks after the initial insult the mice develop spontaneous recurrent seizures. Aside from seizures, these mice also reflect several of the behavioral and cognitive disturbances associated with TLE in humans. Further, the response of these mice to AEDs has been shown to be predictive of drug efficacy in human epilepsy. First, RNA-seq was performed on whole hippocampus samples from 100 epileptic mice and 100 control mice. In total, 9013 genes were identified as differentially expressed between the two conditions.

Next, using a method similar to that described in the Section 3.2.3.1, the genes were assigned to co-expression modules in the epileptic and control mice. The modules were then prioritized based on the following criteria: differential expression of the module, correlation with seizures, and conservation in human epileptic hippocampi. This left seven modules for further analysis. Based on the signature reversion paradigm, i.e., if a module expression is related to disease, then the restoration of the disease modules expression toward the healthy state should provide therapeutic benefit and the high number of existing drugs targeting membrane receptors, the authors set out to identify membrane receptors that exerted a regulatory effect over one or more of the modules and reverted them toward a healthy state. The colony-stimulating factor receptor 1 gene (*Csf1R*) was predicted to regulate two of the seven prioritized modules through the activation of genes. Hence, a small molecule that blocks Csfr1R should be therapeutic. As such, the known inhibitor of Csf1R, PLX3397, was assayed in the pilocarpine model of TLE, a mouse intrahippocampal kainite model of TLE and an ex vivo organotypic hippocampal slice culture model of epilepsy. In all cases the blocking of Csf1R activity attenuated seizure activity.

3.2.3.3 Next-Generation Sequencing: RNA-seq and Identification of Transcription Factors

Traumatic brain injury (TBI), characterized by an insult to the brain, induces several cellular changes, including neurodegeneration, inflammation, oxidative stress, axonal and myelin injury, and vascular changes ultimately resulting in various levels of disability, epilepsy, and even death. It is thought that molecular changes at the transcriptomic level underlie many of these changes. Lipponen et al. used RNA-seq to investigate the transcriptional changes in a rat model of TBI across the perilesional cortex, ipsilateral thalamus, and ipsilateral hippocampus [62]. To identify transcription factors that could be regulators of the transcriptional changes identified in the perilesional cortex and ipsilateral thalamus, a transcription regulatory network (TRN) was extracted from the SignaLink 2.0 database [63]. Using the generated RNA-seq data, transcription factors (TFs) that were differentially expressed were identified and their downstream targets were extracted from the TRN. The TFs paired box 6 (*Pax6*), CCAAT enhancer binding protein delta (*Cebpd*), spi-1 proto-oncogene (*Spi1*), and tumor protein P73 (*TP73*) were differentially expressed across both the perilesional cortex ipsilateral thalamus and had target genes that were differentially expressed. Finally, using the library of integrated network-based cellular signature (LINCS) database analysis, 118 molecules that can regulate the aforementioned TFs were identified [64].

3.2.3.4 Next-Generation Sequencing: Small RNA-seq and Biomarker Detection

A biomarker is a biological characteristic that can be objectively measured and evaluated as an indicator of a biological process, or as a response to therapeutic intervention. An ideal biomarker should be noninvasive, easy to measure, and have short turnaround times. Circulating blood-based molecules fulfill these criteria. Through the application of small RNA-seq to the plasma of control individuals and 16 patients with refractory focal epilepsy, Hogg et al. identified tRNA fragments that could distinguish pre- from post-seizure patients [65]. Based on these results, custom TaqMan assays were constructed to validate the expression of the three tRNA fragments of interest and confirmed that they were indeed elevated in pre-seizure individuals. This study identified a new class of RNA molecule that may be involved in or reflect the development of seizures; such identification would not have been possible without the use of an unbiased approach such as small RNA-seq.

3.3 Epigenomic Profiling

Epigenetics refers to the process by which specific epigenetic marks can influence gene regulation and transposon activity without altering the actual sequence of the DNA. The most recognized epigenetic marker is DNA methylation, which is characterized by the addition of a methyl or hydroxymethyl by DNA methyltransferases (DNMTs) to cytosine residues in CG, CXG, and CXX DNA sequences (CpG sites; where X corresponds to A, T, or C), producing 5-methylcytosines (5-mC). When located in a gene promoter region, it is generally associated with silencing of gene expression [66]. DNA methylation is thought to play a role in several key processes, including genomic imprinting,

X-chromosome inactivation, repression of transposable elements, aging, and carcinogenesis.

3.3.1 Methylation Profiling Techniques

Currently there exist two major methods for identifying methylation differences on specific genes/regulatory regions. The gold standard method for identifying differentially methylated regions across the genome makes use of bisulfite sequencing. First, the DNA of interest undergoes a bisulfite treatment that converts cytosine to uracil while leaving the 5-mC sites intact. The treated DNA is then sequenced via Sanger sequencing or next-generation sequencing (see Section 3.2.1.1); here, the converted uracil will be read as thymine. Though aligning the sequencing reads to the consensus reference genome, it is then possible to calculate the level of methylation at each CpG-site [67,68]. Whole genome bisulfite sequencing (WGBS) is the most comprehensive method for analyzing DNA methylation patterns. However, WGBS can be bioinformatically challenging to analyze as after bisulfite treatment the genomic complexity is reduced to three nucleotides, meaning the data cannot be directly mapped to a reference genome using common alignment tools such as Bowtie2 [69]. However, novel tools such as BSMAP Segemehl, BISMARK., and BS-Seeker can overcome these issues [70–73].

The other widely utilized methylation analysis method uses specialized microarrays developed by Illumina known as the Infinium 450k microarray or the more recently developed Infinium 850k microarray [74]. Again, DNA is bisulfite-treated, but rather than sequencing, the specific CpG sites are detected through hybridization to complementary probes. For each potential methylation site of interest there are two probes, one that hybridizes with the converted CpG site and one that hybridizes with the original sequence. By calculating the ratio between the intensity of these two probes it is possible to calculate the methylation level at each site and compare across conditions. The 450K microarray is limited to 1.5% of the CpGs in the human genome, whereas the 850K microarray contains 90% of the CpGs on the 450K microarray plus an additional 350K CpGs, including CpGs in the promotor regions as well as gene body regions [74]. The array output data can be normalized using various packages in R, including minfi and methylumi,

Table 3.2. DNA methylation profiles in experimental models and human epilepsy

Tissue and species	Main finding	References
Mice cortical neurons	altered DNA promoter methylation of *Bdnf*	[84]
Mice hippocampal slices	inhibition of DNMTs decreased synaptic plasticity	[80]
Mice hippocampal neurons	inhibition of DNMTs decreased synaptic plasticity and neuronal excitability	[81]
Human TLE hippocampus	altered DNA promoter methylation of *RELN*	[88]
Conditional *Dnmt1* and *Dnmt3a* knockout mice	Knock down of *Dnmt1* and *Dnmt3a* decreased synaptic plasticity	[82]
Human TLE hippocampus	High expression of DNMT1 and DNMT3A in TLE	[83]
Human TLE hippocampus	altered DNA promoter methylation of *CPA6*	[90]
Mouse KA induced SE	Genome-wide DNA methylation analysis	[91]
Rat model of epilepsy (Pilocarpine)	Genome-wide DNA methylation and transcriptome analysis	[92]
Mouse hippocampal organotypic cultures and rat post-KA induced SE	altered DNA promoter methylation of *Gria2*	[86]
Rat post-KA Induced SE	altered DNA promoter methylation of *Grin2b*	[87]
Human TLE hippocampus	altered DNA promoter methylation of *CPA6*	[89]
Mouse hippocampus (control and KA) and mouse neuroblastoma N1E-115 cells	altered DNA promoter methylation of *Scn3a*	[85]
Human TLE hippocampus	Genome-wide DNA methylation analysis	[94]
Rat model of epilepsy (pilocarpine, amygdala stimulation, and TBI)	Genome-wide DNA methylation analysis	[93]
Human FCD	Subclassification of FCD types by methylation 450K	[95]
Human LEATs (GGs and DNTs)	New classification of LEATs by methylation 450K	[96]

TLE = temporal lobe epilepsy; KA = kainic acid; SE = status epilepticus; TBI = traumatic brain injury; FCD = focal cortical dysplasia; LEATs = low-grade epilepsy-associated brain tumors; GG = gangliogliomas; DNTs = dysembryoplastic neuroepithelial tumors

which include options for normalizing for probe intensity as well as background corrections using the control probes [75,76]. After normalization, either the β-values (which are equivalent to the absolute DNA methylation levels) or the M-Value (a Logit transformation of the β-values) can be used for further analysis [77]. However, despite all these normalization tools bias can occur due to batch effects, the presence of SNPs, and unspecific binding of probes [75,76].

3.3.2 Methylation Profiling and Epilepsy

Changes in DNA methylation patterns have been well studied in cancer but have also been found in neurological diseases such as autism spectrum disorders, schizophrenia, and epilepsy [78,79]. Table 3.2 provides a summary of findings to date. DNMTs are highly expressed in neurons of the adult brain, and inhibition of these DNMTs in mice hippocampal slices and mice hippocampal primary neurons decreased synaptic plasticity, neuronal excitability, and network activity, processes known to be involved with epilepsy [80,81]. Furthermore, a conditional knockout mice of *Dnmt1* and *Dnmt3a* in excitatory neurons of the forebrain showed decreased synaptic plasticity, learning, and memory [82]. Both *DNMT1* and *DNMT3A* are found to be highly expressed in the neocortex of patients with TLE [83]. Other studies have shown that expression of genes associated with seizures and epilepsy, including *bdnf*, *Scn3a*, *Gria2*, and *Grin2b*, can be regulated through the alteration of methylation patterns in the promotor region [84,85,86,87]. Furthermore, increased promoter methylation of *Reelin* (*RELN*) and *carboxypeptidase A6* (*CPA6*), and the subsequent downregulation in gene expression was shown in TLE patients with hippocampal sclerosis [88,89]. The downregulation of *RELN* is associated with the granule cell dispersion seen in TLE patients with hippocampal sclerosis whereas loss of function mutations of *CPA6* has been linked to seizures and epilepsy [88,90]. More comprehensive studies using genome-wide DNA methylation analysis in different rodent models of epilepsy showed distinct methylation patterns between injured and healthy control animals [91–93]. In the kainic acid (KA)-induced status epilepticus (SE) mouse model most genes were characterized by hypomethylation, while in the rat epilepsy models (pilocarpine induced, amygdala stimulation, or TBI model) hypermethylation was more pronounced [91–93]. Furthermore, the methylation patterns in a (pilocarpine induced) chronic rat epilepsy model inversely correlated with the gene expression changes identified using RNA-seq [92,93]. However, the pathophysiological differences between the different rat models were reflected in the DNA methylation patterns, but not necessarily at the level of RNA expression [93].

The first genome-wide DNA methylation analysis of the hippocampus of human TLE patients identified genes differentially methylated related to gene ontology terms associated with development, neuronal remodeling, and neuron maturation. However, only a few epilepsy related genes were found to be differentially methylated [94]. A more recent study performed whole genome DNA methylation on samples from focal cortical dysplasia (FCD) patients suffering from severe drug-resistant focal epilepsy and showed that the DNA methylation can be used to distinguish human FCD subtypes (FCDIa, IIa, and IIb) as well as from patients with TLE and non-epilepsy autopsy controls [95]. Also, for low-grade epilepsy-associated brain tumors (LEATs) methylation profiling using the 450K methylation array has been shown to be useful in classifying subtypes [96]. Classification of these glioneuronal tumors is based on histological criteria and the presence of *BRAF-V600E* mutations or *FGFR1* abnormalities.

However, the broad spectrum of LEATs makes classification using these systems very difficult [96]. The molecular classification based on the methylation profile for these glioneuronal tumors and FCD highlights the importance of DNA methylation in integrating molecular diagnostics and classification.

Taken together, these studies implicate the importance of aberrant DNA methylation patterns in epilepsy. However, many of these studies face difficulties with tissue heterogeneity resulting in a dilution effect, since different cell types may contribute differently to molecular signatures such as DNA methylation [97]. Therefore, novel techniques such as single cell DNA methylation may become the next step in DNA methylation analysis.

3.3.3 Epitranscriptomics

While epigenetic modifications of DNA and chromatin are well documented, less is known about similar modifications that take place at the level of RNA. The study of these modifications is known as epitranscriptomics. While more than 160 different RNA modifications have been identified, little is known about their abundance, distribution, and functional significance, and this field of research remains in its infancy [98]. Systematic mapping of RNA modifications across the transcriptome of different species and tissues by antibody pull-down or chemical labeling coupled with sequencing has only recently commenced. It appears that the most common modifications occur in tRNAs, rRNAs, mRNAs, and lncRNAs [98]. Currently, the three most well studied modifications are N6-methyladenosine (m6A), 5-methylcytosine (5mC), and 5-hydroxymethylcytosine (5hmC). As this field continues to grow, our understanding of the role of these epitranscriptomic modifications in diseases such as epilepsy will improve.

3.4 Machine Learning Techniques and Integration of Data

To date, the most common approach to data analysis is based on classical statistics (see Section 3.2.2). However, in recent years there has been growing interest in applying machine learning (ML) algorithms to -omics studies. ML is a field of computer science that combines computational statistics and data mining techniques to identify unobserved connections within data sets that are dependent on the manner in which the algorithm was trained. In contrast to classical statistic methods, prior knowledge of how the system behaves is not required in the process of selecting the candidates for model construction. ML algorithms look for patterns and informative features in high-dimensional data among all available features that may not be obvious or even feasible for a scientific researcher to detect.

There are two main categories of ML: supervised and unsupervised. In supervised methods, the category label of each sample is known. Given the outcome and the input data, the algorithm learns general rules for how to categorize a sample to a particular condition or group. Therefore, supervised learning is typically used for classification problems with a binary/multilabel output and for regression. The most popular supervised ML algorithms are: linear classifiers (such as Logistic regression, Naive Bayes, or Linear Discriminant Analysis (LDA)) and trees classifiers (e.g., decision or boosted trees, random forest). Unsupervised machine learning techniques are designed to work with unlabeled and unstructured sets of data. It is common to perform these by grouping the observations based on "similarities" within high-dimensional data sets. The predicted result is unknown a priori, therefore each iteration of the algorithm might produce different outcomes. Unsupervised learning approaches are useful for identifying novel or unknown relationships in data. Clustering (e.g., k-means or hierarchical) and neural networks are widely used unsupervised methods.

3.4.1 Machine Learning and Epilepsy

Although ML algorithms have been successfully applied in substantial number of -omics research fields (e.g., personalized cancer treatment) they still play only a marginal role in the field of epilepsy -omics research (Table 3.3). Among the approximately 360 results obtained by combining the phrases "machine learning" and "epilepsy" that can be found in PubMed database, the majority of papers investigate EEG and/or MRI features as predictors of epilepsy [99,100]. The use of data gathered from wearable devices has been gaining attention in the process of seizure occurrence predictions due to its widespread accessibility [101]. The major reasons that ML has not been

widely adopted across transcriptomic and epigenomic studies in epilepsy is due to limitations and problems that are inherent to the collection and shape of the data, including sample size, missing values, and the number of features being greater than the number of samples. Here, these limitation problems along with ways to overcome them will be discussed.

3.4.1.1 Sample Size

The main limitation of applying ML to -omics and, more generally, epilepsy studies is that of small sample size. This may be due to the rarity of the disease under investigation, ethical reasons, large dropout numbers, or financial aspects. Small sample size becomes a particular issue when attempting to evaluate the performance of ML algorithms. Adequate evaluation of a ML algorithm requires proof that the model works sufficiently well on an independent data set. If the number of samples is sufficient, then the best practice is to split the data into training and test sets and, if possible, to also include a validation set [102] (Fig. 3.3). Training and validation sets would be then used in the process of developing the model and optimizing hyperparameters, and the test set to assess the model's prediction error. However, when there are not enough samples to split the data into such sets, as is often the case with medical research, it is possible to use resampling methods. The most commonly used resampling techniques are various types of cross-validation (e.g., k-Fold, leave-one-out, Monte Carlo cross-validation) and bootstrap methods. The samplings are repeatedly pulled from the available training set and the model is refitted (Fig. 3.3). After multiple repetitions, the resulted metrics are averaged to give a broadened view on the model performance.

3.4.1.2 Missing Data

An important issue to address is missing data that might occur due to technical aspects of the experiment, such as low coverage sequencing or detection limit. Data imputation is not always possible because of the specificity of the study type and might be very challenging for qualitative variables due to an increased probability of bias introduction. However, quantitative variables such as Counts per Million (CPM), an often-used metric for RNA-seq data, might be inferred based on

Table 3.3. Examples of machine learning applied to -omics data sets.

Study	ML algorithm	Evaluation method	Dimensionality reduction	Included data sets	References
An integrative data mining and omics-based translational model for the identification and validation of oncogenic biomarkers of pancreatic cancer	Random forest	10-fold CV	PCA	Gene expression, miRNA, previously published compendium, and databases	[110]
Deep learning-based multi-omics data integration reveals two prognostic subtypes in high-risk neuroblastoma	Neural networks, k-means clustering in training set, SVM, naive Bayes, logistic regression, XGBoost in validation set	Training and validation set split, 10-fold CV in validation set	Autoencoder in training set, ANOVA in validation set	Gene expression, CNV	[111]
Global proteomics profiling improves drug sensitivity prediction: results from a multi-omics, pan-cancer modeling approach	Bayesian efficient multiple kernel learning	Leave-one-out CV	Rule based protein selection (RBPS)	Point mutations, CNV, gene and miRNA expression, proteomics profiles	[112]
Multi-omics integration for neuroblastoma clinical endpoint prediction	Integrative network fusion (linear SVM or random forest), autoencoder	Training and test set split, 5-fold CV	SVM weights, RF Gini index, ANOVA	Gene expression, CNV	[113]
Prediction of inherited genomic susceptibility to 20 common cancer types by a supervised machine learning method	k-nearest neighbors	Training and test set split	PCA	SNP with 21 phenotypes	[114]
Association of omics features with histopathology patterns in lung adenocarcinoma	Random forest, Lasso regression	Training and test set split	RF information gain, Lasso regression	Genetic variants, gene expression, protein expression, clinical variables, histopathology images	[115]

PCA = principal component analysis; CV = cross-validation; SVM = support vector machine; CNV = copy number variation; RF = random forest.

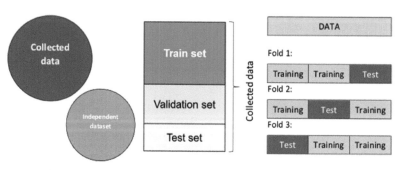

Figure 3.3 **Different methods of model performance evaluation.** (Left) Independent data set. (Center) Splitting data into training, validation, and test set. (Right) n-Fold (here, 3-fold) cross-validation.

non-missing values if the number of samples is sufficient. When concatenating multiple data sets, the problem spreads across the whole matrix as the probability of having missing data increases. One solution is to use only complete cases in the final analysis, but this may greatly reduce sample size, which as mentioned above, is hardly ever satisfactory. Simple numerical data imputation is possible only for data missing completely at random (MCAR), while for data missing at random (MAR) the process should be applied carefully, and for missing not at random (MNAR) it is necessary to model the mechanism of missing data [102]. Some learning algorithms are able to manage missing values in data, such as algorithms based on trees (such as Random Forest or XGBoost) and deep learning algorithms, as they allow multiple reasoning paths [103].

3.4.1.3 Solving the Problem of p >> n

One aspect inherent to the transcriptomics and epigenomics data collection techniques, is that for each sample there can be 1000s or 100,000s of features (genes or CpGs) assayed. Eventually, the obtained data set will have a number of features (p) many times greater than number of samples (n). This increases the risk of overfitting, i.e., finding the model that gives ideal prediction on training data but does not work on the test set. Moreover, as a large number of different models might be created in the search of the best fitting one, and each model performance is scored multiple times, this becomes a very computationally demanding task. Therefore, the recommendation is to perform feature selection, which enables reducing the number of variables used in modeling, or feature extraction, which scales down the dimensionality. Preselection of features will also facilitate the exploration of the underlying processes generating the data.

Feature selection techniques attempt to identify a subset of possible candidates that outperform other variables. The procedure of feature selection might be model-agnostic or model-based [104]. The model-agnostic approach, also called filter selection, is independent of a chosen classifier. Filters methods rely on statistical measures such as AUC, chi-square, or information gain, due to the lack of an underlying classification algorithm. Each variable is scored on its ability to separate the data set. An arbitrary threshold is defined as a cut-off point, so that a reasonable number of variables are retained. Model-agnostic feature selection is proven to work fast, and it is easy scalable depending on dimensions of the data set. However, it ignores relations between variables [105,106]. The second approach, model-based feature filtering, relies on the use of classification algorithms in the process of making a decision about the usefulness of a variable in further analyses [105]. The use of model-based algorithms is computationally intensive and increases the risk of overfitting, although in contrast to model-agnostic filtering it offers multivariate subset selection and has better capability to capture feature dependencies.

Feature extraction enables the reduction of high-dimensional space into lower dimensional set of features. As a result, the initial data set might be replaced by a reduced representation containing relevant and nonredundant information. This is particularly important in the fields of transcriptomics and epigenomics, where changes in expression of multiple genes or CpGs might come from the modification of one specific pathway. Principal Component Analysis (PCA) and its variations are commonly used tools for feature extraction that allow for a simplification of connections within data sets and an overall reduction of the noise [107]. The measure of variability explained represents the variance in the data records and might help in the search of both the general principle hidden in the data as well as small but substantial relations. Moreover, PCA is a powerful instrument to explore and visualize the data and should often be the first step in any data analysis pipeline.

3.4.2 Integration of Data

To fully comprehend the complexity of the molecular mechanisms underlying diseases such as epilepsy researchers are required to take advantage of all possible sources of molecular data. Therefore, it is valuable to concatenate multiple types of -omics data sets such as transcriptomics and epigenomics in the search of possible biomarkers or novel molecules involved in disease pathology. Multi-omics approaches have the potential to outperform a single-type analysis due to the increased ability to capture relations between different layers of information. ML sits as an attractive way to analyze multiple levels of -omics data. Two main approaches for joining the data are model-based integration and concatenation-based integration [108]. The principle of model-based integration is to generate various models from single data types in the training process and then to combine them into one model obtained from previous models in the later phase. The second technique unites data from multiple sources into one large matrix before the modeling process begins [108]. Joining several sets of data requires data normalization which allows for the transformation of variables from different sources to be on a similar scale. To date, no such -omics studies in the field of epilepsy have been presented. Among other disciplines, the most common source of -omics and easy to produce data is from transcriptomics and epigenomics [109]. As such, the data collection techniques discussed in this chapter are ideal methods for the collection of data for ML analysis.

3.5 Conclusions and Perspectives

Transcriptomics and epigenomics are two rapidly growing, technologically based fields that allow for an in-depth understanding of the complex processes that are involved in the regulation of DNA as it is transcribed and eventually translated into protein. As the techniques described here assay the whole transcriptome and epigenome, they are perfectly suited for understanding epilepsy as a systems-based disease. However, many are yet to be adopted in the field of epilepsy research. As the associated costs of each technique decrease and the relevant skill sets required for data analysis become more common, whole transcriptomic and epigenomic analysis will become much more widely used. Finally, ML approaches, as outlined in Section 3.4, have great potential for understanding the swathes of data produced by these techniques and sits poised to be a useful tool for the integration of not only transcriptomic and epigenomic data, but many other levels of data captured by researchers as they seek to understand the underlying pathogenesis of epilepsy.

References

1. International Human Genome Sequencing Consortium. Finishing the euchromatic sequence of the human genome. *Nature*, 431, 931–45 (2004).

2. Azevedo, F. A. C., Carvalho, L. R. B., Grinberg, L. T., et al. Equal numbers of neuronal and nonneuronal cells make the human brain an isometrically scaled-up primate brain. *J. Comp. Neurol.*, 513(5), 532–41 (2009).

3. Hillier, L. W., Coulson, A., Murray, J. I., et al. Genomics in C. elegans: So many genes, such a little worm. *Genome Res.*, 15(12), 1651–60 (2005).

4. Varki, A., and Altheide, T. K. Comparing the human and chimpanzee genomes: Searching for needles in a haystack. *Genome Res.*, 15(12), 1746-58 (2009).

5. Djebali, S., Davis, C. A., Merkel, A., et al. Landscape of transcription in human cells. *Nature*, 489(7414), 101–8 (2012).

6. Blencowe, B. J. Alternative splicing: New insights from global analyses. *Cell*, 126(1), 37–47 (2006).

7. Peng, Z., Cheng, Y., Tan, B. C., et al. Comprehensive analysis of RNA-Seq data reveals extensive RNA editing in a human transcriptome. *Nat. Biotechnol.*, 30(3), 253–60 (2012).

8. Keshet, I., Yisraeli, J., and Cedar, H. Effect of regional DNA methylation on gene expression. *Proc. Natl. Acad. Sci. USA*, 82(9), 2560–4 (2006).

9. Mattick, J. S., and Makunin, I. V. Non-coding RNA. *Hum.*

Mol. Genet., 15 Spec No 1, R17–29 (2006).

10. Thijs, R. D., Surges, R., O'Brien, T. J., and Sander, J. W. Epilepsy in adults. *Lancet*, 393 (10172), 689–701 (2019).

11. Fisher, R. S., Acevedo, C., Arzimanoglou, A., et al. ILAE official report: A practical clinical definition of epilepsy. *Epilepsia*, 55(4), 475–82 (2014).

12. Blumcke, I., Spreafico, R., Haaker, G., et al. Histopathological findings in brain tissue obtained during epilepsy surgery. *N. Engl. J. Med.*, 377, 1648–56 (2017).

13. Wang, Z., Gerstein, M., and Snyder, M. RNA-Seq: A revolutionary tool for transcriptomics. *Nat. Rev. Genet.*, 10(1), 57–63 (2009).

14. Mills, J. D., and Janitz, M. Alternative splicing of mRNA in the molecular pathology of neurodegenerative diseases. *Neurobiol. Aging*, 33(5), 1012. e11–24 (2012).

15. Jeck, W. R., and Sharpless, N. E. Detecting and characterizing circular RNAs. *Nat. Biotechnol.*, 32(5), 453–61 (2014).

16. van Dijk, E. L., Jaszczyszyn, Y., and Thermes, C. Library preparation methods for next-generation sequencing: Tone down the bias. *Exp. Cell Res.*, 322(1), 12–20 (2014).

17. Kukurba, K. R., and Montgomery, S. B. RNA sequencing and analysis. *Cold Spring Harb. Protoc.*, 2015(11), 951–69 (2015).

18. Szabo, L., and Salzman, J. Detecting circular RNAs: Bioinformatic and experimental challenges. *Nat. Rev. Genet.*, 17(11), 679–92 (2016).

19. Mills, J. D., Kawahara, Y., and Janitz, M. Strand-specific RNA-Seq provides greater resolution of transcriptome profiling. *Curr. Genomics*, 14 (3), 173–81 (2013).

20. Parkhomchuk, D., Borodina, T., Amstislavskiy, V., et al. Transcriptome analysis by strand-specific sequencing of complementary DNA. *Nucleic Acids Res.*, 37(18), e123 (2009).

21. Conesa, A., Madrigal, P., Tarazona, S., et al. A survey of best practices for RNA-seq data analysis. *Genome Biol.*, 17, 13 (2016).

22. Mortazavi, A., Williams, B. A., McCue,K., Schaeffer, L., and Wold, B. Mapping and quantifying mammalian transcriptomes by RNA-Seq. *Nat. Methods*, 5(7), 621–8 (2008).

23. Sims, D., Sudbery, I., Ilott, N.E., Heger, A., and Ponting, C.P. Sequencing depth and coverage: Key considerations in genomic analyses. *Nat. Rev. Genet.*, 15 (2), 121–32 (2014).

24. Gilad, Y.,and Mizrahi-Man, O. A reanalysis of mouse ENCODE comparative gene expression data. *F1000Research*, 4, 121 (2015).

25. Buschmann, D., Haberberger, A., Kirchner, B., et al. Toward reliable biomarker signatures in the age of liquid biopsies – How to standardize the small RNA-Seq workflow. *Nucleic Acids Res.*, 44(13), 5995–6018 (2016).

26. Amaral, P. P., Dinger, M. E., Mercer, T. R., and Mattick, J. S. The eukaryotic genome as an RNA machine. *Science*, 319 (5871), 1787–9 (2008).

27. Martens-Uzunova, E. S., Olvedy, M., and Jenster, G. Beyond microRNA – Novel RNAs derived from small non-coding RNA and their implication in cancer. *Cancer Lett.*, 340(2), 201–11 (2013).

28. Bartel, D. P. MicroRNAs: Target recognition and regulatory functions. *Cell*, 136 (2), 215–33 (2009).

29. Lewis, B. P., Burge, C. B., and Bartel, D. P. Conserved seed pairing, often flanked by adenosines, indicates that thousands of human genes are microRNA targets. *Cell*, 120(1), 15–20 (2005).

30. Zhao, Y., and Srivastava, D. A developmental view of microRNA function. *Trends Biochem. Sci.*, 32(4), 189–97 (2007).

31. Koppers-Lalic, D., Hackenberg, M., Bijnsdorp, I. V., et al. Nontemplated nucleotide additions distinguish the small RNA composition in cells from exosomes. *Cell Rep.*, 8(6), 1649–58 (2014).

32. Lake, B. B., Ai, R., Kaeser, G. E., et al. Neuronal subtypes and diversity revealed by single-nucleus RNA sequencing of the human brain. *Science*, 352 (6293), 1586–90 (2016).

33. Salomon, R., Kaczorowski, D., Valdes-Mora, F., et al. Droplet-based single cell RNAseq tools: A practical guide. *Lab Chip*, 19 (10), 1706–27 (2019).

34. Pollen, A. A., Nowakowski, T. J., Shuga, J., et al. Low-coverage single-cell mRNA sequencing reveals cellular heterogeneity and activated signaling pathways in developing cerebral cortex. *Nat. Biotechnol.*, 32(10), 1053–8 (2014).

35. Kulkarni, A., Anderson, A. G., Merullo, D. P., and Konopka, G. Beyond bulk: A review of single cell transcriptomics methodologies and applications. *Curr. Opin. Biotechnol.*, 58, 129–136 (2019).

36. Lake, B. B., Codeluppi, S., Yung, Y. C., et al. A comparative strategy for single-nucleus and single-cell transcriptomes confirms accuracy in predicted cell-type

expression from nuclear RNA. *Sci. Rep.*, 7, 6031 (2017).

37. Burgess, D. J. Spatial transcriptomics coming of age. *Nat. Rev. Genet.*, 20(6), 317 (2019).

38. Eng, C. L., Lawson, M., Zhu, Q., et al. Transcriptome-scale super-resolved imaging in tissues by RNA seqFISH. *Nature*, 568(7751), 235–9 (2019).

39. Rodriques, S. G., Stickels, R. R., Goeva, A., et al. Slide-seq: A scalable technology for measuring genome-wide expression at high spatial resolution. *Science*, 363(6434), 1463–7 (2019).

40. Sedlazeck, F. J., Lee, H., Darby, C. A., and Schatz, M. C. Piercing the dark matter: Bioinformatics of long-range sequencing and mapping. *Nat. Rev. Genet.*, 19(6), 329–46 (2018).

41. Chaisson, M. J. P., Huddleston, J., Dennis, M. Y., et al. Resolving the complexity of the human genome using single-molecule sequencing. *Nature*, 517(7536), 608–11 (2015).

42. Pan, Q., Shai, O., Lee, L. J., Frey, B. J., and Blencowe, B. J. Deep surveying of alternative splicing complexity in the human transcriptome by high-throughput sequencing. *Nat. Genet.*, 40(12), 1413–5 (2008).

43. Matlin, A. J., Clark, F., Smith, C. W. J. Understanding alternative splicing: Towards a cellular code. *Nat. Rev. Mol. Cell Biol.*, 6(5), 386–98 (2005).

44. Weirather, J. L., de Cesare, M., Wang, Y., et al. Comprehensive comparison of Pacific Biosciences and Oxford Nanopore Technologies and their applications to transcriptome analysis. *F1000Research*, 6, 100 (2017).

45. Rhoads, A., Au, K. F. PacBio Sequencing and its applications. *Genomics,*

Proteomics Bioinformatics, 13 (5), 278–89 (2015).

46. Koren, S., Schatz, M. C., Walenz, B. P., et al. Hybrid error correction and de novo assembly of single-molecule sequencing reads. *Nat. Biotechnol.*, 30(7), 693–700 (2012).

47. Costa-Silva, J., Domingues, D., and Lopes, F. M. RNA-Seq differential expression analysis: An extended review and a software tool. *PLoS ONE*, 12 (12), e0190152 (2017).

48. Wang, L., Wang, S., and Li, W. RSeQC: Quality control of RNA-seq experiments. *Bioinformatics*, 28(16), 2184–5 (2012).

49. Brown, J., Pirrung, M., and McCue, L. A. FQC Dashboard: Integrates FastQC results into a web-based, interactive, and extensible FASTQ quality control tool. *Bioinformatics*, 33 (19), 3137–9 (2017).

50. Bolger, A. M., Lohse, M., and Usadel, B. Trimmomatic: A flexible trimmer for Illumina sequence data. *Bioinformatics* 30(15), 2114–2120 (2014).

51. Martin, M. Cutadapt removes adapter sequences from high-throughput sequencing reads. *EMBnet.journal*, 1(1), 10–2 (2011).

52. Križanović, K., Echchiki, A., Roux, J., and Šikić, M. Evaluation of tools for long read RNA-seq splice-aware alignment. *Bioinformatics*, 34 (5), 748–54 (2018).

53. Pertea, M., Kim, D., Pertea, G. M., Leek, J. T., and Salzburg, S.L. Transcript-level expression analysis of RNA-seq experiments with HISAT, StringTie and Ballgown. *Nat. Protoc.*, 11(9), 1650–67 (2016).

54. Trapnell, C., Roberts, A., Goff, L., et al. Differential gene and transcript expression analysis of RNA-seq experiments with

TopHat and Cufflinks. *Nat. Protoc.*, 7(3), 562–78 (2012).

55. Li, B., and Dewey, C. N. RSEM: Accurate transcript quantification from RNA-seq data with or without a reference genome. *BMC Bioinformatics*, 12, 323 (2011).

56. Afgan, E., Baker, D., Batut, B., et al. The Galaxy platform for accessible, reproducible and collaborative biomedical analyses: 2018 update. *Nucleic Acids Res.*, 46(W1), W537–44 (2018).

57. Khatri, P., Sirota, M., and Butte, A. J. Ten years of pathway analysis: Current approaches and outstanding challenges. *PLoS Comput. Biol.*, 8(2), e1002375 (2012).

58. Chan, J., Wang, X., Turner, J. A., Baldwin, N. E., and Gu, J. Breaking the paradigm: Dr Insight empowers signature-free, enhanced drug repurposing. *Bioinformatics*, 35 (16), 2818–26 (2019).

59. Langfelder, P., and Horvath, S. WGCNA: An R package for weighted correlation network analysis. *BMC Bioinformatics*, 9, 559 (2008).

60. Mills, J. D., Iyer, A. M., van Scheppingen, J., et al. Coding and small non-coding transcriptional landscape of tuberous sclerosis complex cortical tubers: Implications for pathophysiology and treatment. *Sci. Rep.*, 7(1), 8089 (2017).

61. Srivastava, P. K., van Eyll, J., Godard, P., et al. A systems-level framework for drug discovery identifies Csf1R as an anti-epileptic drug target. *Nat. Commun.*, 9, 3561 (2018).

62. Lipponen, A., El-Osta, A., Kaspi, A., et al. Transcription factors Tp73, Cebpd, Pax6, and Spi1 rather than DNA methylation regulate chronic transcriptomics changes after experimental traumatic brain

37

injury. *Acta Neuropathol. Commun.*, 6(1), 17 (2018).

63. Fazekas, D., Koltai, M., Türei, D., et al. SignaLink 2 – a signaling pathway resource with multi-layered regulatory networks. *BMC Syst. Biol.*, 7, 7 (2013).

64. Duan, Q., Flynn, C., Niepel, M., et al. LINCS Canvas Browser: Interactive web app to query, browse and interrogate LINCS L1000 gene expression signatures. *Nucleic Acids Res.*, 42, W449–60 (2014).

65. Hogg, M. C., Raoof, R., El Naggar, H., et al. Elevation in plasma tRNA fragments precede seizures in human epilepsy. *J. Clin. Invest.*, 129(7), 2946–51 (2019).

66. Law, J. A., and Jacobsen, S. E. Establishing, maintaining and modifying DNA methylation patterns in plants and animals. *Nat. Rev. Genet.*, 11(3), 204–20 (2010).

67. Lister, R., O'Malley, R. C., Tonti-Filippini, J., et al. Highly integrated single-base resolution maps of the epigenome in Arabidopsis. *Cell*, 133(3), 523–36 (2008).

68. Cokus, S. J., Feng, S., Zhang, X., et al. Shotgun bisulphite sequencing of the Arabidopsis genome reveals DNA methylation patterning. *Nature*, 452(7184), 215–9 (2008).

69. Kurdyukov, S., and Bullock, M. DNA methylation analysis: Choosing the right method. *Biology (Basel)*, 5(1), 3 (2016).

70. Xi, Y., and Li, W. BSMAP: Whole genome bisulfite sequence MAPping program. *BMC Bioinformatics*, 10, 232 (2009).

71. Hoffmann, S., Otto, C., Kurtz, S., et al. Fast mapping of short sequences with mismatches, insertions and deletions using index structures. *PLoS*

Comput. Biol., 5(9), e1000502 (2009).

72. Krueger, F., Andrews, S. R. Bismark: A flexible aligner and methylation caller for Bisulfite-Seq applications. *Bioinformatics*, 27(11), 1571–2 (2011).

73. Guo, W., Fiziev, P., Yan, W., et al. BS-Seeker2: A versatile aligning pipeline for bisulfite sequencing data. *BMC Genomics*, 14, 774 (2013).

74. Moran, S., Arribas, C., and Esteller, M. Validation of a DNA methylation microarray for 850,000 CpG sites of the human genome enriched in enhancer sequences. *Epigenomics*, 8(3), 389–99 (2016).

75. Bock, C. Analysing and interpreting DNA methylation data. *Nat. Rev. Genet.*, 13(10), 705–19 (2012).

76. Morris, T. J., Beck, S. Analysis pipelines and packages for Infinium HumanMethylation450 BeadChip (450k) data. *Methods*, 72, 3–8 (2015).

77. Kodandapani, R., Pio, F., Ni, C. Z., et al. A new pattern for helix-turn-helix recognition revealed by the PU.1 ETS-domain-DNA complex. *Nature*, 380(6573):456–460 (1996).

78. Jin, Z., and Liu, Y. DNA methylation in human diseases. *Genes Dis.*, 5(1), 1–8 (2018).

79. Kobow, K., and Blümcke, I. Epigenetics in epilepsy. *Neurosci. Lett.*, 667, 40–6 (2018).

80. Levenson, J. M., Roth, T. L., Lubin, F. D., et al. Evidence that DNA (cytosine-5) methyltransferase regulates synaptic plasticity in the hippocampus. *J. Biol. Chem.*, 281(23), 15763–73 (2006).

81. Nelson, E. D., Kavalali, E. T., and Monteggia, L. M. Activity-dependent suppression of miniature neurotransmission through the regulation of DNA methylation. *J. Neurosci.*, 28(2), 395–406 (2008).

82. Feng, J., Zhou, Y., Campbell, S. L., et al. Dnmt1 and Dnmt3a maintain DNA methylation and regulate synaptic function in adult forebrain neurons. *Nat. Neurosci.*, 113(4), 423–30 (2010).

83. Zhu, Q., Wang, L., Zhang, Y., et al. Increased expression of DNA methyltransferase 1 and 3a in human temporal lobe epilepsy. *J. Mol. Neurosci.*, 46(2), 420–6 (2012).

84. Martinowich, K., Hattori, D., Wu, H., et al. DNA methylation-related chromatin remodeling in activity-dependent BDNF gene regulation. *Science*, 302(5646), 890–3 (2003).

85. Li, H. J., Wan, R. P., Tang, L. J., et al. Alteration of Scn3a expression is mediated via CpG methylation and MBD2 in mouse hippocampus during postnatal development and seizure condition. *Biochim. Biophys. Acta*, 1849(1), 1–9 (2015).

86. Machnes, Z. M., Huang, T. C. T., Chang, P. K. Y., et al. DNA methylation mediates persistent epileptiform activity in vitro and in vivo. *PLoS ONE*, 8(10), e76299 (2013).

87. Ryley Parrish, R., Albertson, A. J., Buckingham, S. C., et al. Status epilepticus triggers early and late alterations in brain-derived neurotrophic factor and NMDA glutamate receptor Grin2b DNA methylation levels in the hippocampus. *Neuroscience*, 248, 602–19 (2013).

88. Kobow, K., Jeske, I., Hildebrandt, M., et al. Increased reelin promoter

methylation is associated with granule cell dispersion in human temporal lobe epilepsy. *J. Neuropathol. Exp. Neurol.*, 68 (4), 356–64 (2009).

89. Belhedi, N., Perroud, N., Karege, F., et al. Increased CPA6 promoter methylation in focal epilepsy and in febrile seizures. *Epilepsy Res.*, 108(1), 144–8 (2014).

90. Sapio, M. R., Salzmann, A., Vessaz, M., et al. Naturally occurring carboxypeptidase A6 mutations: Effect on enzyme function and association with epilepsy. *J. Biol. Chem.*, 287(51), 42900–9 (2012).

91. Miller-Delaney, S. F. C., Das, S., Sano, T., et al. Differential DNA methylation patterns define status epilepticus and epileptic tolerance. *J. Neurosci.*, 32(5), 1577–88 (2012).

92. Kobow, K., Kaspi, A., Harikrishnan, K. N., et al. Deep sequencing reveals increased DNA methylation in chronic rat epilepsy. *Acta Neuropathol.*, 126(5), 741–56 (2013).

93. Debski, K. J., Pitkanen, A., Puhakka, N., et al. Etiology matters – genomic DNA methylation patterns in three rat models of acquired epilepsy. *Sci. Rep.*, 6, 25668 (2016).

94. Miller-Delaney, S. F. C., Bryan, K., Das, S., et al. Differential DNA methylation profiles of coding and non-coding genes define hippocampal sclerosis in human temporal lobe epilepsy. *Brain*, 138(Pt 3), 616–31 (2015).

95. Kobow, K., Ziemann, M., Kaipananickal, H., et al. Genomic DNA methylation distinguishes subtypes of human focal cortical dysplasia. *Epilepsia*, 60(6), 1091–1103 (2019).

96. Stone, T. J., Keeley, A., Virasami, A., et al.

Comprehensive molecular characterisation of epilepsy-associated glioneuronal tumours. *Acta Neuropathol.*, 135(1), 115–29 (2018).

97. Guintivano, J., Aryee, M. J., and Kaminsky, Z. A. A cell epigenotype specific model for the correction of brain cellular heterogeneity bias and its application to age, brain region and major depression. *Epigenetics*, 8(3), 290–302 (2013).

98. Noack, F., and Calegari, F. Epitranscriptomics: A new regulatory mechanism of brain development and function. *Front. Neurosci.*, 12, 85 (2018).

99. Chen, S., Zhang, J., Ruan, X., et al. Voxel-based morphometry analysis and machine learning based classification in pediatric mesial temporal lobe epilepsy with hippocampal sclerosis. *Brain Imaging Behav.*, 14(5), 1945–54 (2019).

100. Bharath, R. D., Panda, R., Raj, J., and Bhardwaj, S. Machine learning identifies "rsfMRI epilepsy networks" in temporal lobe epilepsy. *Eur. Radiol.*, 29 (7), 3496–505 (2019).

101. Regalia, G., Onorati, F., Lai, M., Caborni, C., Pocard, R. W. Multimodal wrist-worn devices for seizure detection and advancing research: Focus on the Empatica wristbands. *Epilepsy Res.*, 153, 79–82 (2019).

102. Mirza, B., Wang, W., Wang, J., et al. Machine learning and integrative analysis of biomedical big data. *Genes (Basel)*, 10(2), 87 (2019).

103. Bertsimas, D., Pawlowski, C., and Zhuo, Y. D. From predictive methods to missing data imputation: An optimization approach. *J. Mach. Learn. Res.*, 18(196), 1–39 (2018).

104. Saeys, Y., Inza, I., and Larrañaga, P. A review of feature selection techniques in bioinformatics. *Bioinformatics*, 23(19), 2507–17 (2007).

105. Hira, Z. M., and Gillies, D. F. A review of feature selection and feature extraction methods applied on microarray data. *Adv. Bioinformatics*, 2015, 198363 (2015).

106. Chandrashekar, G., and Sahin, F. A survey on feature selection methods. *Comput. Electr. Eng.*, 40(1), 16–28 (2014).

107. Meng, C., Zeleznik, O. A., Thallinger, G. G., et al. Dimension reduction techniques for the integrative analysis of multi-omics data. *Brief. Bioinform.*, 17(4), 628–41 (2016).

108. Lin, E., and Lane, H. Y. Machine learning and systems genomics approaches for multi-omics data. *Biomark. Res.*, 5, 2 (2017).

109. Lopez de Maturana, E., Alonso, L., Alarcón, P., et al. Challenges in the integration of omics and non-omics data. *Genes (Basel)*, 10(3), 238 (2019).

110. Long, N. P., Jung, K. H., Anh, N. H., et al. An integrative data mining and omics-based translational model for the identification and validation of oncogenic biomarkers of pancreatic cancer. *Cancers (Basel)*, 11(2), 155 (2019).

111. Zhang, L., Lv, C., Jin, Y., et al. Deep learning-based multi-omics data integration reveals two prognostic subtypes in high-risk neuroblastoma. *Front. Genet.*, 9, 477 (2018).

112. Ali, M., Khan, S. A., Wennerberg, K., and Aittokallio, T. Global proteomics profiling improves drug sensitivity prediction: Results from a

multi-omics, pan-cancer modeling approach. *Bioinformatics*, 34(8), 1353–62 (2018).

113. Francescatto, M., Chierici, M., Rezvan Dezfooli, S., et al. Multi-omics integration for neuroblastoma

clinical endpoint prediction. *Biol. Direct*, 13(1), 5 (2018).

114. Kim, B. J., and Kim, S. H. Prediction of inherited genomic susceptibility to 20 common cancer types by a supervised machine-learning method. *Proc. Natl. Acad.*

Sci. USA, 115(6), 1322–7 (2018).

115. Yu, K. H., Berry, G. J., Rubin, D. L., et al. Association of omics features with histopathology patterns in lung adenocarcinoma. *Cell Syst.*, 5 (6), 620–7 (2017).

Phenomenological Mesoscopic Models for Seizure Activity

Maria Luisa Saggio and Viktor K. Jirsa

4.1 Introduction

Epilepsy is the most common of the chronic and severe neurological diseases. It affects 65 million people worldwide and is characterized by an augmented susceptibility to seizures. Seizures are "transient occurrence of signs and/or symptoms due to abnormal excessive or synchronous neuronal activity in the brain" [1]. Current therapeutic strategies have the goal of suppressing or reducing the occurrence of seizures, thus being symptomatic rather than curative. There are no known therapies able to modify the evolution of acquired epilepsy, or to prevent its development. Furthermore, 25–40% of patients do not respond to pharmacological treatment, and this number stays unchanged when using new generation antiepileptic drugs as compared to established ones. For drug-resistant patients with focal epilepsy (an epilepsy in which seizures start in one hemisphere) there exists an alternative to medication: surgical resection of the brain regions involved in the generation of seizures, the epileptogenic zone, under the constraints of limiting postsurgical neurological impairments. Rates of success of brain surgery for epilepsy treatment vary between 34% and 74% as a function of the type of epilepsy. Outcomes are very variable, depend on the patient condition, and can change in time.

Focal epilepsies involve widespread networks, so they are considered a network disorder [2]. From a network perspective, seizures depend on the interaction between the excitability of the single nodes of the network and the connections among them. What defines a node depends on the spatial scale of the problem we are dealing with, so that nodes can be neurons at the microscopic scale or brain regions at the mesoscopic one. While we have a better understanding of phenomena acting at the neuronal scale rather than mesoscopic one, clinicians have to base their hypothesis and decisions on mesoscopic observables when planning surgical strategies for drug-resistant patients. Efforts toward the understanding of mechanisms of seizure generation and propagation at this scale could provide clinicians with additional tools in their evaluation.

The spatial component is not enough to understand seizures: epilepsy is also a dynamic disease [3] and seizures exhibit a complex temporal evolution, as observed for example through electroencephalography (EEG) or stereotactic EEG (SEEG) recordings. These measurements reflect the global electrical activity generated by a huge number of neurons. While the degree of spike synchronization among neurons has a heterogeneous, highly variable and complex pattern, seizures are characterized by synchronized activity at the level of EEG and local field potential, especially during seizure evolution and termination. This implies a decrease in the degrees of freedom necessary to describe the activity of the underlying system, which may be amenable to mathematical modeling through the use of mesoscopic collective variables for the activity of a single brain region (i.e., a node in the network).

Large-scale mathematical and computational models have the potential to merge networks and dynamics to generate nontrivial predictions, which can push our understanding of the meso- and macroscopic mechanisms of seizure generation and evolution. In addition, they can provide a platform to perform in silico experiments, such as testing hypotheses on where the seizure starts (EZ) and where it propagates (propagation zone, PZ) and perform systematic virtual resections to establish the best surgical strategy, as well as proposing new approaches to prevent seizures by manipulations of quantities represented by other parameters of the network or of the dynamics [4–8]. Models can be informed with detailed patient-specific information, in terms of large-scale connectivity, presence of lesions and functional information, along the lines of personalized medicine [5].

At the level of a single node, there are different approaches to model the activity of a brain region. One possibility is to create a model that attempts to mimic physiologically realistic mechanisms and variables. The large number and non-identifiability of parameters poses one of the big challenges in model inference and the estimation of correlated parameters from empirical data is notoriously difficult. Errors, even small ones, in the values of these parameters and the fact that some parameter values may be context dependent (e.g., they may depend on the specific patient) or that they can evolve in time, may dramatically alter the dynamics of the model. While physiological models can foster our understanding of such specific mechanisms, they are often computationally expensive and may not be well suited to perform extensive simulations and parameter sweeps. Complementary approaches focus on the development of lower-dimensional models aiming at a faithful reproduction of data features, often rooted in principles derived from statistics or mathematics and linked to data structure rather than physiology. Such a *phenomenological* approach decreases the computational cost of the model and renders it a prime candidate for routine investigations in the clinics. Moreover, this focus on the essential dynamics provides a more tractable model amenable to mathematical investigation of its properties. Investigations that rely on realism in terms of dynamics, such as the study of the pattern of seizure propagation or of the reaction of a brain region to stimulation, can thus benefit from the use of phenomenological models. Furthermore, while phenomenological variables lack a clear correlate with the physical substrate, they allow modeling of observed phenomena for which the underlying physiology is not sufficiently clear or for which multiple physiological mechanisms may produce the same outcome, as for epileptic seizures. Despite the large range of seizure mechanisms acting on different time and spatial scales, electrographic signatures of these events are relatively stereotyped across different pathologies, and even among different species and primitive laboratory models. Seizures can also be induced in any otherwise healthy brain, from flies to humans and both in vivo and in vitro, and the electrographic signatures of these induced seizures are similar despite the variety of provoking conditions that may be used [9]. Such similarity among seizures points toward the existence of invariant dynamical properties in their underlying mechanisms across brain scales, regions, and across species [9] and phenomenological models are ideal to capture and study such key invariant properties.

In this chapter we will review meso- and macroscopic phenomenological models for seizure activity. We will start with a brief introduction to how the brain can be conceptualized as a complex system and how this allows the building of large-scale brain models. We will then show how this framework can be applied to the study of epilepsy, focusing on the description of mesoscopic phenomenological models for a brain region able to generate seizures. To conclude, we will discuss applications and insights coming from these models.

4.1.1 Network Approach to the Brain

Complex systems are ubiquitous in our universe. From the macroscopic world of galaxies and stars to the microscopic systems of cells, molecules, and atoms and even further. The surprising fact is that heterogeneous complex systems often show similar organizational properties when analyzed as networks. To build a network out of a complex system we need to identify two kinds of entities: nodes, which are the elements of the network, and links, which express some kind of connection between those elements, such as physical wiring or functional relationship. The same complex system can be conceptualized as a network in many different ways: the particular choice of which elements constitute the nodes and of which characteristics of their connections entail a link will depend on the specific goals of the investigation undertaken. Links can be summarized in the connectivity matrix, a squared matrix having the same dimension as the number of nodes in the system and whose entries express the pairwise value of the link between any two nodes.

The brain is among the most complex of systems, with approximatley 10^{11} neurons and 10^{14} synaptic connections, not counting the further degrees of freedom within each single neuron (dendritic branching, neurotransmitters, and so on) or the fact that the brain is constituted by cell types other than neurons, such as glia. Despite this astonishing number of elements and the intricacies of the wiring, the brain exhibits an impressive level of organization and network approaches are well suited to investigate these characteristics.

At the microscale, the building block of our brain is the neuron, at least for the purposes of this chapter. Molecular dynamics, especially in synapses, plays an increasingly important role in translational neuroscience and drug design [10] but shall not be further reviewed here. We can describe a neural network considering each neuron as a node and each synaptic connection between a pair of them as a link. In addition, we need to consider the dynamics of the single units and of the couplings to describe the temporal evolution of the network. The number of neurons that can be simulated with current technology depends on the level of details of the model used ranging from a million neurons with detailed morphology (e.g., the Human Brain Project) to 500 million highly simplified neurons (for instance, the DARPA Synapse project) [11]. These simulations, even with simple neurons, require enormous computational power and are currently not feasible to be performed routinely and in a personalized fashion in clinical settings. In addition, while such detailed microscopic simulations contribute to our understanding of some physiological brain mechanisms, there are questions that need a different, mesoscopic level of description. This level allows a comparison between simulation output and measures from noninvasive functional brain imaging techniques, such as EEG, functional magnetic resonance imaging (fMRI), and magnetoencephalography (MEG), as well as intracranial recordings such as SEEG used in the clinical exploration of epilepsy. A trade-off between large coverage and microscopic details can be reached through a mesoscopic level of description, which is able to reduce the degrees of freedom of a whole brain region to just a few variables [12]. Such a representation is more tractable and less computationally expensive. In addition, it puts emphasis on behaviors that may emerge at the mesoscopic scale and are not present in the microscopic description.

In large-scale brain models, the brain is usually parcellated into several mesoscopic cortical and subcortical interconnected regions. While the first large-scale network brain models used homogeneous connectivities, developments in diffusion imaging techniques over the last two decades provide subject-specific information on the brain's large-scale connectivity established by the white matter and may provide more sophisticated and personalized network constraints. Diffusion imaging is an MRI-based technique that tracks the diffusion of water molecules, which in the brain is maximally oriented along the axonal fibers. These data can be used to build a structural connectivity matrix, called a connectome, reflecting the presence and weight of anatomical connections. The connectome has recently been extended to also include the matrix of estimated tract lengths, which determine the time delays of signal propagation due to finite velocity along white matter fibers, as this can strongly affect the network behavior. The connectome has been used as a basis to build large-scale brain models for resting state activity and to understand the role of noise and time delays in the generation of resting state fluctuations [13]. Since 2009, when this study was published, the use of connectomes in network models has been followed up by many studies and connectome-based modeling has become a mature field.

Brain regions serve as network nodes in connectome-based brain models. At the level of a single node, the dynamics of a brain region is described using a small number of collective variables accounting for the global activity of the underlying networks of neurons. There exist formal approaches to perform this huge reduction of degrees of freedom, such as mean-field approximations, that benefit from results of statistical physics. Such approaches are widely used in physics. For example, under specific assumptions, we can describe the behavior of particles in a gas using collective variables such as temperature or pressure. In a brain region, neurons having similar or identical statistical properties and receiving similar or identical inputs are grouped into neural populations. The activity of each population is described by a probability density function for relevant neuronal states (e.g., the firing rate). In the presence of strong coherence among the neural states within a population, it is possible to restrict the model to the mean of the distribution, further reducing the degrees of freedom of the problem and allowing the study of several interacting populations within a single brain region. This provides the so-called neural mass model (NMM) [13]. The dynamics of a neural population can mirror that of each single neuron composing it, or the NMM can be informed using empirical observations of how a system responds to its inputs, to account for the fact that different levels of organization of complex system (micro- vs. meso- or macroscopic) may obey different

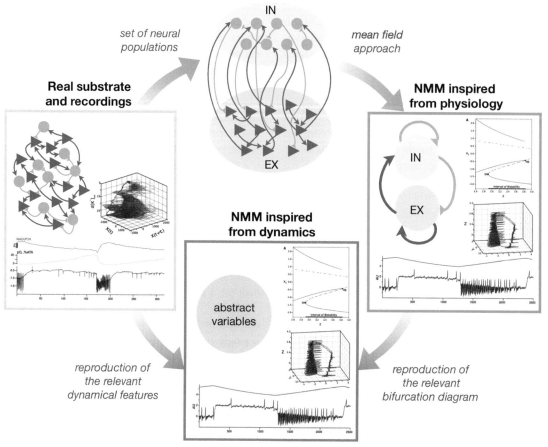

Figure 4.1 **Building Neural Mass Models (NMMs).** NMMs reproduce the mesoscopic global activity of underlying networks of neurons. Common steps for the construction of physiologically inspired NMMs (green arrows) include: the identification of clusters of neurons sharing similar statistical properties and connectivity – neural populations; the application of mean-field reduction techniques to obtain the dynamics of the collective variables describing each neural population and connections among them. In the figure we have schematically represented only two types of neurons (and thus neural populations), excitatory (red) and inhibitory (blue), but NMMs can include several types. The model obtained can be used to reproduce the observed time series. In addition, one could study the role of parameters and produce bifurcation diagrams to describe the dynamical repertoire of the model. Phenomenological models (lavender arrows), can be obtained in two ways: directly from data by identifying relevant features and reproducing them; or by building simpler models with an equivalent bifurcation diagram to that of physiological NMMs. Phenomenological models inspired by physiological ones do not aim at reproducing the full dynamical repertoire of the latter, but a subset of the dynamics which is judged relevant for a certain scope.

rules [14]. A well-known example of the latter approach is the Wilson–Cowan model, which includes an excitatory population of pyramidal neurons interacting with an inhibitory population of interneurons. Typically, NMMs are inspired from physiology, comprise different neural populations, and exhibit nonlinear dynamics. As already mentioned, another possibility is to model specific dynamical properties of the brain region, without attempting a realistic physiological implementation (Fig. 4.1). In some cases, a direct link can be drawn among the variables of these phenomenological models and neural populations

activities [15–17], so that the separation between NMMs and phenomenological ones is fuzzy. For this reason, we will refer to any model for the global activity of a brain region as a NMM, and will distinguish whether it is inspired from the neurophysiology or whether the model is phenomenological, i.e., inspired from the dynamics.

NMMs use differential equations to model the activity of a single node of the network and lack a spatial component. This limitation can be overcome, for example, by the use of neural field models. They can produce different spatiotemporal patterns of brain activity, including traveling waves, which seem to have an important role in the spreading of the ictal wavefront on the cortical surface [18,19].

In a large-scale brain model, connectivity, time delays, and node dynamics can be combined, together with the addition of the dynamics of the couplings between nodes. A generic mathematical formulation for such a computational model, referred to as brain network model (BNM) [15], or graph-based brain anatomical network [20], includes other elements, such as the local connectivity within a brain region. The dynamics of the full BNM can be implemented with limited computational resources provided that the number of nodes in the parcellation is not too high. Many studies use parcellations in the order of 100 regions, even though smaller or larger parcellations are possible (see [21] for the effect of parcellation size on simulation outcomes). BNMs have found applications in the study of both healthy and pathological conditions. There are studies on resting state, development, and aging, but also on the effects of brain lesions, stroke, schizophrenia, and dementia. Note that these works usually rely on results based on generic or average connectomes with some notable exceptions [6].

4.1.2 Large-Scale Patient-Specific Brain Models

BNMs based on the connectome can be extended to study the generation and propagation of epileptic seizures [8] and have been applied to the study of absence seizures [22,23], temporal lobe epilepsy [4], and in a general framework for focal seizures, the virtual epileptic patient (VEP) [5].

The first steps in the construction of a VEP model rely on the same elements described for a generic BNM, that is reconstruction of the connectome and choice of the NMM and coupling functions (Fig. 4.2). It is important that the reconstruction of structural connections is performed using state of the art methods to ensure that patient-specific features are captured [5]. Under this requirement, there are reliable and reproducible differences in individual connectomes and the patient-specific connectome gives the best outcome for the VEP, where the biggest role is played by the topology of connections rather than by the weights [6]. Together with large-scale models for epilepsy based on the connectome [4,5], there are other models that rely on functional connectivity (i.e., links represent temporal correlations among the activities of brain regions), as computed either from ictal or interictal recorded activity [7,24,25]. NMMs currently used in large-scale models for epilepsy are often phenomenological [4,5,7]. However, physiologically inspired (but still low-dimensional) NMMs have also been successfully used within this framework [25]. All these models contain a parameter for the excitability (or epileptogenicity), which describes how prone the brain region is to generate seizures. This is the key parameter that, together with the effect of the connectivity, marks the difference between healthy and epileptic brain tissue. The presence of brain lesions and clinical hypothesis on EZ and PZ, when available, can be included in the VEP by appropriate parameters modifications (Fig. 4.2). A hypothalamic hamartoma, for example, has been included by altering the local connectivity of the thalamus [5]. Clinical hypothesis on whether a brain region belongs to EZ, PZ or is healthy, can be set by tuning the value of the excitability parameter. The key feature of the model is the high degree of patient specificity.

4.2 Modeling Seizures Phenomenologically: NMMs

What model should be used for the node dynamics? A large variety of models have been proposed in the context of epilepsy and seizures [26]. They have been designed to investigate different types of epileptiform activity, including high frequency oscillations, spike-wave complexes, interictal spikes, fast oscillations at seizure onset, and status epilepticus. As previously motivated, we focus here on phenomenological NMMs able to generate seizure activity. We will start by introducing some of the language of dynamical system theory useful to describe those models.

4.2.1 The Language of Dynamical System Theory

In dynamical system theory, the activity of a system, for example a neuron or a brain region, is described by a few variables, called *state* variables, such as the membrane potential, the mean firing rates of a set of neural populations, or synaptic currents. The space spanned by the state variables is called state space, and the state of the system at a given time can be represented as a point in this space (Fig. 4.3A, left).

45

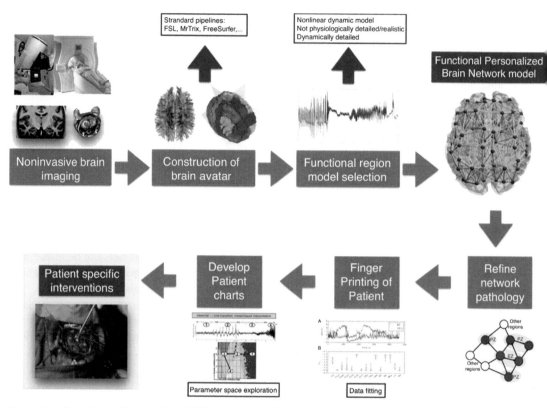

Strandard pipelines:
FSL, MrTrix, FreeSurfer,...

Nonlinear dynamic model
Not physiologically detailed/realistic
Dynamically detailed

Functional Personalized
Brain Network model

Noninvasive brain imaging

Construction of brain avatar

Functional region model selection

Refine network pathology

Finger Printing of Patient

Develop Patient charts

Patient specific interventions

Parameter space exploration

Data fitting

Figure 4.2 The virtual epileptic patient (VEP) approach. A VEP model starts from the construction of the patient's brain avatar, based on non-invasive imaging. The second step is to choose the model for the dynamics of a single brain region. Currently, this choice does not depend on patient-specific seizure characteristics. These steps result in the functional characterization of the BNM, after which the model can be further refined to consider differences in the excitability among regions, the presence of lesions, or clinical hypothesis on the location of EZ and PZ. The model can be estimated through extensive data fitting to produce patient charts containing information about the effects of specific modifications. These charts can be used to improve presurgical evaluation. Reprinted from Drug Discovery Today: Disease Models, 19, C. Bernard and V. Jirsa, Virtual Brain for neurological disease modeling, 5-10, Copyright (2016), with permission from Elsevier [52].

Differential equations encode the way in which state variables change over time, given a certain initial state of the system. They thus impose a vector field on state space (Fig. 4.3A, middle, right) and describe a movement in the state space, called a *trajectory* (Fig. 4.3B, left). After an initial transient, the system may settle in a specific behavior, such as steady or oscillatory, or even chaotic activities. In these cases, a portion of the state space, called an *attractor* (Fig. 4.3B), attracts trajectories passing from a specific region of the state space, the *basin of attraction*. An attractor can be a point in state space, as in the case of steady activity. This is called a stable *fixed point* (Fig. 4.3B, left). Oscillatory activity is exhibited by the system when the attractor is a closed trajectory, known as a stable *limit cycle* (Fig. 4.3B, right). *Strange attractors* are responsible for

chaotic behaviors. Portions of the state space are called *repellors* when they repel trajectories and comprise unstable fixed point and unstable limit cycles.

Differential equations can depend on some parameters, which are assumed to maintain a constant value while state variables evolve. In a neuron or NMM model they could encode, for example, the external applied current. When an attractor remains qualitatively the same for small changes of the parameter values, it is said to be *structurally stable*. When, instead, these variations cause a change in the type and/or number of attractors, the system has undergone a *bifurcation* (Fig. 4.3B–D). The parameter(s) that one needs to modify to cause a bifurcation is called a *bifurcation parameter(s)*. In the example of the neuron, this corresponds to the fact that applying an

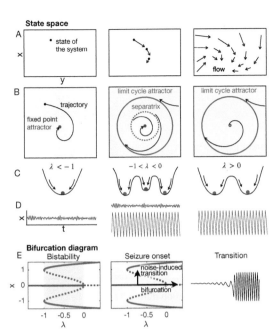

Figure 4.3 Concepts from dynamical system theory. If a system can be described using a few state variables (here two, (x,y)), its state can be described as a point in the (x,y) space, which is called state space (A, left). Differential equations describe how the system evolves in time starting form a given point, this imposes a flow (A, right) in state space. Following the flow from a given point, we obtain a trajectory (B, left). Trajectories can be attracted to specific regions of state space, called attractors (B). An attractor can be a fixed point (B, left). For easier visualization we can imagine a valley, where gravity pushes the system down to the lowest point of the valley (C, left). If we slightly displace the system, this will move again down to the fixed point. An example of timeseries in the presence of small level of noise is shown (D, left). Trajectories can converge to a closed orbit, a limit cycle attractor (C–D, right). This produces oscillatory activity. C, right should be visualized as a section of a Mexican hat, so that the two blue points are two points of the limit cycle. Attractors can also coexist (B-D middle). The basin of attraction of the limit cycle (shaded in blue) is separated from that of the fixed point (shaded in red) by a separatrix. A single system can display different attractors in a landscape when parameters (here lambda) are varied. When this occurs, the system has undergone a bifurcation. All the information in B can be represented in a compact form with a bifurcation diagram (E), where we plot one state variable versus the bifurcation parameter. The plot contains the attractors (solid lines) and the repellers, which are regions of state space that repel trajectories (dashed lines). The coexistence of a limit cycle and a fixed point, called bistability (shaded in gray in E, left), is particularly relevant for models of seizure onset and offset. Starting from the interictal state (red fixed point), we can cross the separatrix changing the value of the state variable or that of the parameter (E, middle). An example of transition due to the latter mechanism is shown in E, right.

changes its state to an oscillatory one. We can make a plot of state variables versus bifurcation parameters containing all the possible attractors and repellers of a system. This is a *bifurcation diagram* (Fig. 4.3E, left, middle) and is a powerful compact description of the dynamic repertoire of the system and how this depends on the values of parameters and initial conditions.

The use of collective variables is particularly justified when modeling epileptic seizures. During seizures, the firing activity of billions of neurons becomes highly organized, which greatly reduces the degrees of freedom, hence the number of differential equations necessary to describe the observed activity (Fig. 4.4) [27]. Phenomenological models aim at identifying the essential mechanisms able to produce the activity as observed, for example, in EEG recordings of seizures. They thus need to be able to generate sustained oscillatory activity, which requires the use of at least two state variables so that a limit cycle attractor can exist. Since large-scale brain models for epilepsy aim at studying seizure onset and propagation patterns, most of these phenomenological models focus on the possible mechanisms to start a seizure, as predicted by dynamic system theory. Of note, multi(-spatial) scales recordings in epileptic patients point to different dynamical mechanisms for seizure onset acting at the population level as compared to the single neuron scale [28], further highlighting the importance of investigating and modeling emergent mesoscopic behaviors. Other features that have been modeled phenomenologically include seizure termination, spike and wave complexes, preictal spikes, and status epilepticus. In the following sections we will review models for the mentioned phenomena in more details.

4.2.2 Mechanisms for Seizure Onset and Offset

Onset/offset mechanisms imply the transition between interictal to ictal states and vice versa. The interictal state is usually modeled as low amplitude fluctuations around a stable fixed point (or equilibrium), even though there exist models considering a non-quiescent interictal condition [29]. During the ictal state the system is usually in a stable limit cycle, but we will see an example where this does not occur. There are several possible onset dynamical mechanisms that have been identified in the literature [3,9,30,31], some act at

external current to a resting neuron does not trigger oscillations (the resting state is structurally stable) for a whole range of the current values. However, beyond the bifurcation point the system

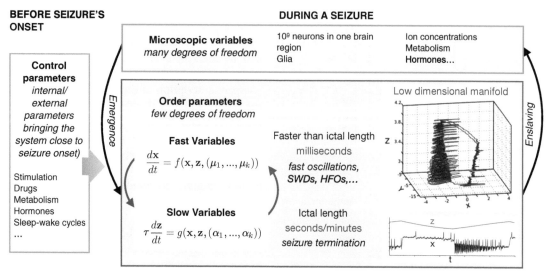

Figure 4.4 Emergence of a low-dimensional space with intrinsic timescale separation during a seizure. Before a seizure, some (control) parameters of the brain change and bring the system close to seizure onset. During the seizure, the microscopic variables, which compose a brain region, organize so that the emergent global activity can be described by a few collective variables. We have thus a collapse of the many degrees of freedom of the system to a few emergent variables. These collective variables, on the other hand, act on the microscopic variables, "enslaving" them. Some potential microscopic variables, which act as control parameters or on the slow timescale, are shown. The collective variables used to describe a seizure can be separated into at least two groups depending on the timescale at which they operate. Fast variables are responsible for the generation of a healthy "rest" state and for an oscillatory "seizure" state. Slow variables modulate the transition between these two states.

the level of a single node, while others rely on network effects (Fig. 4.5).

We will start with the single node. When the interictal (fixed point) and ictal (limit cycle) states coexists, as shown for example in (Fig. 4.3B–D, middle), we say we are in the presence of *bistability*. Looking at the bifurcation diagram of the bistable regime (Fig. 4.3E, left), we can identify at least two ways in which the system can leave the basin of attraction of the fixed point (shaded in red) and enter that of the limit cycle (shaded in blue), i.e., for a seizure to start (Fig. 4.3E, middle). In the first scenario, a change in the value of the state variable(s) (vertical axis) due to noise or to an internal/external stimulus can cause the system to cross the separatrix. We will refer to this for simplicity as *noise-induced transition*. In the second scenario a change in the value of the parameter (horizontal axis) can bring the system to a condition where the fixed point is no longer stable, i.e., a *bifurcation* has occurred. Onset via a bifurcation can occur also without bistability. These are the most common mechanisms at the level of a single brain region, even though other theoretically possible ones have been proposed (e.g., attractor deformation [3], see Fig. 4.5).

Proposed mechanisms that depend on the effect of spatially extended networks are *excitability* and *intermittency* [30]. In the first case, single nodes are not able to oscillate when isolated, but noise or internal/external stimuli can induce a single spike. When the nodes are coupled, the network can sustain oscillatory activity and a seizure is able to start and self-terminate. In the case of intermittency, heterogeneities in the network can create a new dynamical state at the level of the whole network that spontaneously produces brief seizures without the need of noise. Intermittency has only been observed in models for generalized seizures. More details are discussed in the following sections.

4.2.2.1 Noise-Induced Transitions

Models in which transitions are due to movements in state space (a change in the value of the state variable(s)) usually rely on noise fluctuations to trigger seizures, but transitions can also be caused by an internal or external stimulus.

Bistable models. The simplest possible system with a bistability between a fixed point and a limit cycle shows the bifurcation diagram described in (Fig. 4.3E, left). For the readers familiar with

SINGLE NODE

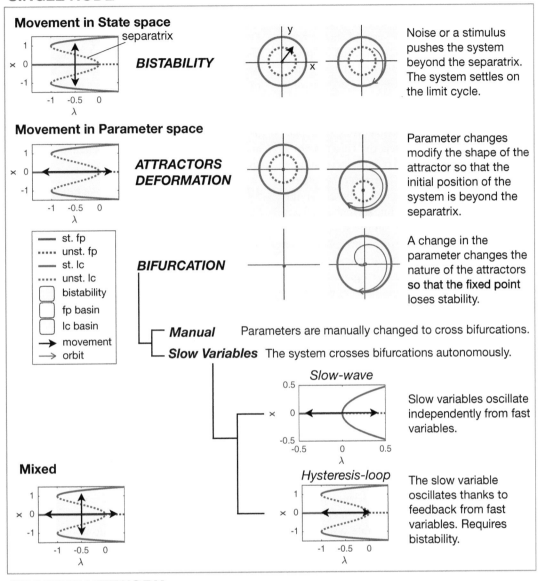

Movement in State space

separatrix

BISTABILITY

Noise or a stimulus pushes the system beyond the separatrix. The system settles on the limit cycle.

Movement in Parameter space

ATTRACTORS DEFORMATION

Parameter changes modify the shape of the attractor so that the initial position of the system is beyond the separatrix.

- st. fp
- unst. fp
- st. lc
- unst. lc
- bistability
- fp basin
- lc basin
- movement
- orbit

BIFURCATION

A change in the parameter changes the nature of the attractors so that the fixed point loses stability.

Manual Parameters are manually changed to cross bifurcations.

Slow Variables The system crosses bifurcations autonomously.

Slow-wave

Slow variables oscillate independently from fast variables.

Mixed

Hysteresis-loop

The slow variable oscillates thanks to feedback from fast variables. Requires bistability.

REQUIRE NETWORK

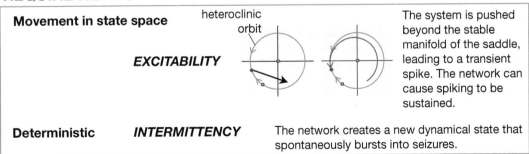

Movement in state space

heteroclinic orbit

EXCITABILITY

The system is pushed beyond the stable manifold of the saddle, leading to a transient spike. The network can cause spiking to be sustained.

Deterministic   **INTERMITTENCY**   The network creates a new dynamical state that spontaneously bursts into seizures.

Figure 4.5 Onset dynamical mechanisms. The upper panel shows mechanisms acting at the level of a single node, the lower panel those relying on the network effect. In the bifurcation diagrams, x is a variable and λ the bifurcation parameter. For each mechanism, two plots of the state space (x, y) are portrayed: in the first we assume that the system is at rest in the stable fixed point (fp) and draw an arrow to show the movement in state space when it applies; in the second plot we show the orbit followed by the system to settle in the limit cycle (lc) or back on the fp. When movements in parameter space are performed, the two state space plots are for different values of the parameter.

49

bifurcations, this diagram arises in the normal form of the unfolding of the codimension-2 Bautin (or generalized Hopf) singularity. A model based on a modification of this normal form, called the Z^6 model [32], has been proposed as a phenomenological model for seizure generation that reproduced the relevant dynamics of a biophysically inspired NMM. In this family of models, seizures arise abruptly when noise fluctuations or inputs bring the system beyond the separatrix. The parameter λ reflects the closeness to a bifurcation at which the fixed point loses stability, a subcritical Hopf bifurcation. The closer the value of λ is to the bifurcation (i.e., to 0), the closer the separatrix is to the fixed point, so that λ reflects the excitability of the system, in the sense of susceptibility to the generation of seizures. A greater excitability here translates in an average shorter escape time, that is the time employed by the system to make the transition due to noise fluctuations. Healthy brain regions can be modeled setting values of λ further away from the bifurcation. If λ is small enough ($<$-1) to be outside the bistability region, then the only possible attractor is the fixed point and seizures cannot be induced no matter how strong the input is. Seizure offset relies on the same noise-induced mechanism. However, for values of λ that make a node more susceptible to generate seizures by making the separatrix closer to the fixed point, the distance from the separatrix to the limit cycle is high (see Fig. 4.3E, left). This implies large escape times for seizure offset, i.e., very long seizures, so that often seizure offset is not observed in simulations. Phenomenological models based on this simple bistable system have been used to build networks [2,7,24,33], including a large-scale connectome-based model [4].

Excitable models. A system close to a bifurcation, i.e., an excitable system [34], can produce one or more oscillations if a stimulus is applied or as a consequence of noise fluctuations, before going back to the fixed point. In particular, a large amplitude oscillation can be produced by excitable systems close to what is called a saddle node on an invariant circle (SNIC) bifurcation. When several nodes close to a SNIC bifurcation are coupled together, this transient oscillation triggered by noise can become sustained so that spontaneous seizures occur in the network. This was observed, for example, by using a physiologically inspired NMM as a node in a large-scale brain model [25]. The NMM includes the activity

of four neural populations: one population of pyramidal neurons, one of excitatory interneurons and two of GABAergic interneurons. Depending on the values of its parameters it can also generate discharges through other mechanisms such as bistability, bifurcations, and intermittency. Even though this model is not phenomenological, we include it here for two reasons: this physiologically inspired NMM is being used in large-scale patient-specific models, and excitability as an onset mechanism is amenable to phenomenological modeling.

4.2.2.2 Slow Variable Dynamics and Bifurcations

Seizures can be generated by changes in the parameters of the model that cause the disappearance of the fixed point in favor of a limit cycle. In this case we talk about bifurcations. Changes in the parameters can also cause the opposite transition, leading to seizure termination, or to transitions among different oscillatory states during a single seizure. Earlier physiologically inspired models exploiting this mechanism aimed at reproducing relevant features of the EEG as observed during seizure evolution, such as the appearance of spike and wave complexes [35]. This was done by manually changing the parameters to mimic the observed EEG patterns or by estimating them automatically from real data [36]. While this type of model, thanks to their explicit link to physiology, can offer powerful insights on the mechanisms underlying different electrographic patterns and the relations among them, they cannot spontaneously produce a seizure.

To create models able to autonomously generate/terminate seizures through bifurcations, we can consider that the bifurcation parameter(s) is itself a state variable(s) changing on a much slower timescale than that of the variables responsible for the limit cycle representing the ictal state. These latter variables will be called *fast variables* as opposed to the *slow variable* that brings the system across onset and offset bifurcations (Fig. 4.4). The timescale of the fast variables would be that of the oscillations within a seizure, while the slow timescale is that of the duration of a seizure. Slow variables can change in time following their own dynamics or their variation can depend on the activity of the fast variables (Fig. 4.5) [34]. While it is not clear which of these processes is more suitable to describe seizure onset, the distribution of the ictal length's duration points to a negative feedback mechanism for seizure offset [27]. This implies that the ongoing seizure acts on the slow variables promoting a movement toward the offset bifurcation, as proposed in [9] within a phenomenological NMM for seizure activity, the Epileptor. Such a feedback mechanism requires the fast subsystem to exhibit bistability between the ictal and interictal states and can be implemented with the use of a single slow variable. The slow variable, called in [9] the permittivity variable, is likely to encompass all the autoregulatory mechanisms triggered by the seizure, such as changes in extracellular ion concentrations or in variables related to energy metabolism, which eventually bring seizure termination.

4.2.2.3 Mixed Scenario with Slow Dynamics

The advantage of the permittivity variable approach is to provide a mechanism through which seizures can both start and terminate autonomously in the system. However, as mentioned before, while such a mechanism seems well justified for seizure offset, it is less clear whether it suits seizure onset. With regards to the latter, evidence from the analysis of the distribution of interictal lengths brings mixed results [27]: seizures in in vitro hippocampal preparation are highly periodic, and thus point to a permittivity variable approach for onset; seizures in rat models for absence seizures and in patients with focal or absence seizures have heterogeneous distributions, some of which are more consistent with noise-induced transitions. It is possible that deterministic (slow variables) and stochastic (noise-induced transitions) mechanisms coexist, with some being more prevalent in some patients than in others. Some types of epilepsies have a clear cyclicity, such as catamenial epilepsy, in which the occurrence of seizures is linked to the menstrual cycle, or awakening seizures, in which seizures occur at a precise stage of the sleep-wake cycle. In general, though, such an evident cyclicity is lacking. Recently, however, it has been shown how the presence of circadian rhythms and clustering of seizures might be more ubiquitous than previously thought [37]. The analysis of long recordings (of the order of years) from patients with an implanted device for brain stimulation, showed that interictal epileptiform activity oscillates with both circadian and multi-diem rhythms, and that seizures preferentially occurred during specific phases of these cycles in a patient-specific fashion [37]. The

authors suggested that such rhythms are co-modulated by different elements acting on several timescales, such as hormonal, genetic, environmental, sleep-wake cycle, and behavior factors. These factors may act ultra-slowly (i.e., slower than ictal length) to periodically bring the system through the onset bifurcation or to alter brain excitability or circuitry, so that the separatrix gets closer to the fixed point and noise-induced transitions are facilitated. Interestingly, in models with a permittivity variable, the parameters can be set so that the onset can be noise-induced in a bistable regime and the offset due to slow movement in parameter space [9,38,39]. With the mathematical description proposed in [39], after seizure termination the system settles back to the fixed point with a value of the excitability much lower than it was at the beginning. In Fig. 4.3E (left) this would be a value close to -1. These settings are thus compatible with the intriguing possibility that seizures serve as an emergency rescue mechanism that the system uses to restore a better working point.

4.2.2.4 Patient-Specific Onset/Offset Bifurcations

While the slow variable mechanism can be applied to the bifurcation diagram described in the previous section (Fig. 4.3E, left), the Epileptor model differs in the type of bifurcations through which the fixed point/limit cycle loses stability (onset/offset bifurcation). There exist several bifurcations that can cause these transitions and they have different dynamical properties. Systems close to different bifurcations can react differently to an external stimulation or can have different synchronization properties which may affect seizure propagation (see [34] and references therein). Given the clinical relevance of these properties, it is important to inform a seizure model with the best pair of onset/offset bifurcations able to describe data. This is made feasible by the fact that bifurcations may have specific signatures that can be identified in data, such as the behavior of the frequency or amplitude, or the presence of a jump in the signal baseline. In systems with two fast variables, there are only four possible onset bifurcations and four offset ones. This gives a taxonomy containing sixteen theoretically possible classes. Jirsa et al. [9] analyzed data from different species (zebrafish, mouse, and human) and in vitro preparations and found that one specific class, having saddle-node onset and saddle-homoclinic offset, was

51

predominant. This class is characterized by a jump in the baseline in direct current (DC) recordings and logarithmically decreasing frequency toward seizure offset. Interestingly, a jump in subdural EEG recordings has previously been found to be predictive of the seizure focus and patient outcomes [40]. The Epileptor model reproduces these dynamics. However, 20% of the patients analyzed showed different dynamics, which justified the creation of a model able to account for the other classes to improve the patient specificity of the VEP [31]. This model predicted that seizures belonging to different classes could be produced by the same system. We have recently demonstrated, using a larger cohort of patients, that several classes are indeed necessary to describe the seizures analyzed and, furthermore, patients could have seizures of different types in time [39].

4.2.2.5 Excitability

In all the onset mechanisms described, the presence of a parameter that plays the role of excitability emerges. This excitability parameter reflects the distance to the bifurcation that destabilizes the interictal state, and this holds both for mechanisms based on movement on state space, and on the crossing of the bifurcation point. While, from a biological point of view, seizures can be accompanied by both increased neuronal excitation and/or inhibition, in models both processes can contribute to an increased excitability, in the sense of closeness to instability point. This makes the brain region more susceptible to generating seizures. In large-scale brain models for epilepsy, fixing the values of this parameter allows for alterations in the local dynamics of the different brain regions involved in the network. In practice this can be done in different ways. For example, an increased excitability can reflect anatomical abnormalities of the brain region (such as atrophy [4]) or can reflect clinical hypothesis on the location of EZ and PZ [5].

4.2.2.6 When a Seizure Fails to Terminate: Status Epilepticus

A failure in the mechanisms leading to seizure offset may result in a prolonged seizure (more than five minutes). This is a condition known as status epilepticus. We are not aware of phenomenological models designed specifically to reproduce status epilepticus. Interestingly, though, dynamical states and mechanisms consistent with

this condition have been found when investigating in greater detail some models for seizure onset and offset. Given their tractability, phenomenological models are amenable to a full exploration of the effects that changes in parameter values have on the landscape of attractors. This may uncover novel behaviors that were not intentionally included in the model. The more canonical the model, the likelier such "unintentional" behaviors are to survive the empirical test and their presence can foster our understanding of the full potential of the system we are studying.

With regards to status epilepticus, two hypotheses have emerged: (i) status epilepticus as an additional attractor coexisting with the ictal one, or (ii) as a consequence of a failure in the slow variable mechanisms. The first hypothesis arises from a detailed exploration of the bifurcation diagram of the Epileptor model, which led to the discovery of other attractors that are reminiscent of clinically relevant behaviors, including status epilepticus [41]. The authors provided the first experimental support for the existence of these attractors by performing experiments which trace out the paths in parameter space through experimental manipulations, in particular forcing the hippocampus (rodent, in vivo) through a sequence of different behaviors as predicted from the bifurcation diagram. Another phenomenological model instead found a behavior resembling status epilepticus when, in a specific region of the bifurcation diagram, the slow variable's attempts at bringing the system toward seizure termination were overridden by excessive noise [39]. This is in line with a dynamical hypothesis for status epilepticus previously formulated in the context of a physiologically inspired NMM [28], in which the system repeatedly approaches the critical transition without crossing it and retreats to the ictal attractor. In vivo data (EEG and intracranial EEG) in the latter study showed changes in the frequency, mean power, and mean autocorrelation similar to those predicted by the model for this dynamical mechanism.

4.2.3 Seizure Evolution: A Dictionary of EEG Patterns

4.2.3.1 Navigating the Parameter Space

The presence of multiple timescales within the variables responsible for the oscillatory activities observed during a seizure is at the heart of the generation of a variety of rhythms in physiologically inspired NMMs [42]. In particular, at least three variables with two timescales are necessary to produce complex activity such as spike and wave complexes or polyspike waves.

Wang and colleagues [42] proposed a minimal model of three generic neural processes acting on two timescales to reproduce different prototypical EEG patterns, as observed during seizure evolution, when the model's parameters vary. The model exhibits interictal activity as fixed-point dynamics. Bifurcations can cause the appearance of fast sinusoidal oscillations and spike trains, which are represented in the model in terms of simple limit cycles in the fast subsystem. Interaction with the slower variable produces slow waves, with different numbers of spikes riding on it. Note that this slower variable is still much faster than that leading to seizure offset. The authors suggest that it could be related to processes such as the regulation of extracellular potassium, glial processes, or the effect of subcortical input. Manually changing the parameters of the model allows navigation of the map of possible attractors of the system (i.e., the bifurcation diagram), mimicking the action of slow variables and reproducing the realistic successions of EEG patterns observed during a seizure. The model offers a variety of behaviors that can be used as a dynamic "dictionary" to help identifying relevant activities, and relationships among them, in more complex physiologically inspired NMMs or in data [43].

4.2.3.2 A Single Mechanism for Spike and Waves Discharges and Interictal Spikes

The addition of an intermediate timescale between fast and slow ones is also responsible for the generation of spike and wave complexes in another phenomenological model, the Epileptor. Here, the same mechanism is also responsible for the generation of preictal spikes. When the fast variables approach seizure onset, the intermediate system approaches a SNIC bifurcation: the average of the fast variables plays the role of bifurcation parameter for the intermediate system. Interestingly, this implies that the closer the fast variables are to seizure onset, the more likely the intermediate variables are to show isolated spikes due to noise fluctuations, consistent with the experimental observation of preictal spikes. In contrast to the fast subsystem of the model, this mechanism is ad hoc and needs to be

rooted in empirical data [9]. It accounts for the fact that the slow variable is stochastic and allows for phenomena such that the increase of the number of interictal spikes is not necessarily followed by a seizure. During the seizure, the intermediate variables produce a sharp oscillatory activity that interacts with the fast oscillations of the fast variables to create spikes and wave complexes, in a similar fashion to Wang et al. [42], but involving different bifurcations. These complexes are particularly evident as the seizure progress.

This modeling work allows us to discuss two further points. The first is about the interpretation of the groups of variables composing a phenomenological model, that in biophysically inspired NMMs are typically related to different neural populations, each composed of similar neurons. Experimental results from whole cell hippocampi recordings aimed at identifying the biophysical correlates of fast and intermediate Epileptor variables showed that, while the activity of the intermediate variables was more representative of GABAergic cells, pyramidal cells contributed as well. The interpretation of these sets of collective variables may be more complex than linking each of them to either an excitatory or inhibitory cells population and phenomenological NMMs can encode the activity of nonhomogeneous neural populations.

Second, this provides an example of how specific dynamical features can sometimes be modeled in isolation. While the intermediate subsystem contributes to our understanding of seizure related phenomena and makes the simulated timeseries more realistic, it was shown by the authors that this subsystem does not contribute to seizure onset and offset mechanisms. Successive work could thus be simplified by omitting the modeling of interictal spikes and spike and wave complexes, without losing any understanding of the mechanisms underlying seizure initiation and termination.

4.3 Applications and Future Directions

4.3.1 In Silico Experiments to Improve Treatment

4.3.1.1 Virtual Surgeries and Stimulations

Large-scale models for epilepsy can be used to find several important applications to improve treatment (Fig. 4.2). A first promising use is a better delineation of the epileptogenic zone (EZ) and propagation zone (PZ). This can be achieved by testing whether the clinical hypothesis brings simulated functional data that match the empirical ones, for example in terms of seizure onset and propagation pattern. Parameters in models can be changed iteratively to reduce the mismatch [5]. When several clinical hypotheses have been formulated, the large-scale patient model can be used to help to choose among them. In addition, it can be used to estimate EZ and PZ through Bayesian approaches, without prior hypothesis [5]. Of note, all these approaches to the delineation of EZ and PZ can be applied starting from noninvasive recordings and can be used to improve the placement of SEEG electrodes.

Large-scale models for epilepsy also provide a platform to perform in silico surgeries. Once the EZ has been delineated, one could test if resection would stop seizure propagation. Results could help improving the resection strategy [4,5,25] or could help understanding when the outcome of surgery will be unsatisfactory [7]. Even though these models have only been evaluated retrospectively, a mismatch between the resection predicted by the model and real resection correlates with poor surgical outcome [5,25]. These models can also help when proposing innovative surgical approaches that fully exploit the network nature of this disease, such as micro lesions or multiple lesions at different locations that could make use of recent stereotactic-guided laser technology [5]. This would provide a less invasive approach for network control [44]. Finally, a minimal resection is not necessarily the best strategy, as it may involve eloquent brain areas leading to post-surgery neurological complications. An exciting possibility is to use large-scale simulations to identify, among the possible efficient resections, those that are safest in terms of normal brain function [45].

In silico experiments could include the design of patient-specific stimulation protocols to prevent or abort seizures (see [46] for a review). Stimulation could be designed, for example, to force the system out of the basin of attraction of the limit cycle (the seizure) in a bistable regime, where the timing and amplitude of the stimulus necessary to abort the seizure would depend on the shape of the basin of attraction of the healthy state. Stimulations can also modify the bifurcation structure of the system or modulate its excitability to prevent seizure onset. Combining the local node dynamics with large-scale connectivity could result, again, in a less focal and more distributed intervention approach.

As reviewed in Section 4.2, the dynamics of a single brain region in current large-scale patient-specific models can rely on different dynamical mechanisms: (i) noise-induced transitions in a bistable regime created by a subcritical Hopf bifurcation in phenomenological models of the Bautin family (normal form of the Bautin singularity, Z6 model); (ii) slow variable induced bifurcations in phenomenological models (Epileptor); or (iii) excitability close to a SNIC bifurcation in a physiologically inspired model, in which the mechanism for seizure onset relies on the interplay between the node's excitability and the whole network activity (an isolated node cannot sustain oscillations). The way in which different brain regions influence each other varies in the literature, including linear and diffusive couplings, with or without time delays [4,7,24] and couplings across timescales [5,6,47]. The large-scale models also differ in the way the connectivity among brain regions is assessed (from structural or functional data, and in the latter case using ictal or interictal recordings), on the coverage (some brain regions or the whole brain), and in how the best treatment strategy is evaluated. Patient-specific resections can be suggested based entirely on brain network simulations or mathematical analysis. The most ictogenic nodes can be identified, for example, as those with shorter escape times (i.e., those generating a seizure more easily) [7], or those that, when removed from the network, decrease the occurrence of seizures [25]. Linear stability analysis applied to a combination of structural and dynamical information can be used to estimate the propagation zone and suggest minimal ablations in the connectivity to stop seizure recruiting [44]. In addition to connectivity and dynamics, one can also take advantage of the availability of functional data (EEG, SEEG, MEG, etc.) to apply data fitting techniques for the estimation of the excitability of each network node through model inversion [5].

Despite their differences, all these studies have brought positive results, while showing that network measures alone are not predictive and that dynamical models are essential [4,44]. The large-scale patient-specific model approach thus holds potential to help clinicians in their decisions about electrode placement and surgical interventions. Currently, positive results do not seem to strictly depend on the specific choices in terms of modeled dynamics and connections. This may be due to the use of different metrics to assess the predictive power of the approach. Future work may address under which circumstances the model's choice will affect the propagation pattern of seizures and what are the best domains of applications of the different models; open to the possibility that patient specificity may express itself also with the need of choosing one model over another.

For example, we have recently shown in a large cohort of patients that different bifurcations are needed to explain the variability at onset and offset among patients, and even in the seizures of a single patient. There is evidence in the literature that different bifurcations may greatly affect the synchronization properties of the nodes. A more systematic investigation of these properties, their effects on seizure recruitment, and their dependence on the type of coupling, would help to understand how much dynamical realism is necessary to include in the phenomenological model for a specific study. As for physiologically inspired models, for which one has to decide, depending on the specific question addressed and data available, what is the degree of biological realism needed (single neurons? dendritic branches? ion channels properties? etc.). Similarly, for phenomenological models one has to choose the level of dynamical realism. Further studies may address, for instance, when bistability is enough, when the specific bifurcations giving origin to the bistability or being directly responsible for seizure onset and offset matter, whether different mechanisms (noise-induced transitions, bifurcations with slow dynamics, excitability, intermittency, etc.) coexist, what is the interplay among them, and when one should choose one over the other. An explicit example is the coexistence between the slow variable mechanism, which can increase the excitability of a brain region by bringing it closer to an onset bifurcation, and noise-induced transitions that are facilitated with the increased excitability. This interplay has been suggested by several authors and, under some assumptions (e.g., timescales separation), can be used to justify the use of noise-induced transitions at seizure onset, while the slow dynamics is approximated by giving different excitability values to the nodes of the system.

Finally, beyond applications that can be directly used to improve patient-specific clinical care, these large-scale simulations can foster our understanding of the link between structure and function in epilepsy and seizure propagation [5] or of the conditions that facilitate seizure genesis and propagation. A complex system approach can help to advance counterintuitive hypotheses. For example, it is generally taught that, for a seizure to occur, we need: (i) an altered excitability of the single units involved (neurons, brain regions, etc.) and (ii) an altered network connectivity that promotes propagation and/or synchronization among units. However, it has been shown, on the basis of computational studies, that a pathological connectivity can even provoke seizures in networks composed only of "healthy" units [2]. It is then possible that the two requirements, of pathological units and pathological connectivity, need not necessarily be satisfied independently, but that it is the interplay between them that can result in a pathological condition.

4.3.1.2 New Strategies Out of Seizures

Virtual surgeries and stimulations are the most straightforward, although highly nontrivial, applications of meso- and large-scale phenomenological models in epilepsy. Another intriguing possibility is to use the bifurcation diagrams of mesoscopic models (both physiologically inspired and phenomenological) as a map to guide the system out of "dangerous" regions. A dangerous region would be any portion of the diagram in which the landscape of attractors facilitates seizures, as, for example, when the system gets very close to an onset bifurcation or to status epilepticus. A safer region would be far from such bifurcations, ideally outside the bistability region so that the interictal state is the only existing attractor.

However, this requires acting on the variables and parameters of the bifurcation diagram, which poses at least two challenges: identifying what these variables and parameters are in the real system and finding tools to manipulate them. This task may be particularly difficult when dealing with phenomenological models, since the link between the model's variables and the real biological substrate

55

is not evident. At the same time, this same type of model is particularly powerful in providing tractable bifurcation diagrams.

Strategies to find correlates also depend on how the phenomenological model was created. As shown in Fig. 4.1, one possible way to build such a model is to start from a biophysical inspired one, identify the relevant dynamics one wants to study (as represented, for example, in the bifurcation diagram), and create a simpler model (possibly the simplest) able to reproduce it. A classic example in neural modeling is the FitzHugh–Nagumo model, created to isolate the essential mechanisms underlying the dynamics of action potentials in the Hodgkin–Huxley model and to have a more tractable description. In the context of mesoscopic seizure models, we mentioned the Z6 model as an easier version of a physiologically inspired one. When a formal mathematical reduction is available, this provides a link between variables in the physiologically inspired and phenomenological models, where variables in the latter are typically a function of one or more physiological ones. Moreover, in general, a link can also be suggested by comparing variables and parameters appearing in the bifurcation diagrams.

Another class of phenomenological models (Fig. 4.1) instead aims at reproducing directly specific features of the activity observed in experimental data. The Epileptor model is an example of this approach. In these cases, one could make hypotheses on the physiological correlates of the variables based, for example, on the timescale at which the process acts, and try to test them experimentally. Another possibility is to compare the model with physiologically inspired ones that exhibit a similar bifurcation diagram a posteriori. However, it is important to bear in mind that a phenomenological model could have a variety of physiological implementations. In the case of seizures, Jirsa and colleagues [9] have shown how the specific dynamics they modeled in the Epileptor were conserved at different scales, from small networks of neurons to brain regions, and across species, from flies and zebra fish to mice and humans. This suggests that there are several substrates that can support the modeled activity. This could hold also for patients, given the considerable diversity of causes and conditions that can bring to epilepsy.

4.3.2 Dynamics as a Criterion to Classify Seizures

Keeping with the idea that there is not a single dynamical mechanism that can fully explain all seizures observed in patients, details about this mechanism could contribute to the classification of electrographic seizures. And in this, phenomenological models would help to isolate the essential dynamics. Current seizure classifications are based on a description of the empirical data: clinical manifestations (e.g., partial vs. generalized) together with visual descriptions of EEG signal and identification of the regions of the brain involved. In one of its position papers, the International League Against Epilepsy (ILAE) explains that, while several ways of classifying seizures could be possible, due to the lack of fundamental knowledge, the current classification is practical and based on previous classifications. Among the criteria mentioned that could be used to classify seizures are: pathophysiology, anatomy, networks involved, and practical criteria such as response to antiepileptic drugs, EEG patterns, and level of related cognitive and physical impairment. An additional criterion has been recently proposed [9,48], that distinguishes electrographic seizures based on the dynamical mechanisms leading to onset and, possibly, offset. One of the advantages of this approach is that it highlights differences in the underlying mechanisms of seizure generation, evolution, and termination that could contribute to our understanding of this phenomenon. Another advantage is that models for the different dynamics could be used to make useful predictions with applications in the clinical setting [49], as described in previous sections. There are currently two main proposals that are highly complementary. One focuses on spatial heterogeneities in the excitability within a single brain region [48], which can produce either low amplitude fast activity or high amplitude slow activity at seizure onset through different dynamical mechanisms (involving local and global bistability, monostability, stimulus induced transitions, and bifurcations). This modeling approach is powerful when capturing the contribution of the local spatiotemporal dynamics within a brain region and the authors show how the latter onset type is linked to worse surgical outcomes when a portion of the brain region is removed, in accordance with clinical results [50]. The second proposal focuses on the possible bifurcation scenarios at the level of a NMM [9], where different seizure classes have different onset/offset bifurcation pairs. Both approaches have the potential to result in useful predictions for the clinics, and future work could be done to propose a multi-scale classification. In general, we could say that a taxonomy of seizures based on dynamics could include the specification of any type of dynamical process leading to seizure onset, evolution, and offset. This would powerfully complement current operational classifications based on clinical information.

This could be applied also to different brain regions in a single patient. Is the difference between those in EZ, PZ, or healthy tissue just a matter of altered excitability as it is usually assumed, or are there deeper differences in terms of dynamical mechanisms? The latter hypothesis would translate into the need for different models for the various region types.

4.4 Conclusions

Epilepsy is a complex network and dynamic disease, involving several interacting spatial and timescales. Efforts to understand the mechanisms underlying the generation, evolution, and termination of epileptic seizures and to improve the life of epileptic patients benefit from the use of diverse complementary approaches. In this chapter we have reviewed phenomenological models of seizure-like activity. We have highlighted the advantages of this modeling approach, the types of questions it can be used to address, and how it has been applied in the investigation of epileptic seizures. Efforts in the field have focused mainly on identifying dynamical mechanisms responsible for seizure onset and offset. Systems able to autonomously generate, and possibly terminate, a seizure are at the heart of large-scale patient-specific brain models, which have the potential of improving clinical care for drug-resistant epileptic patients. These virtual epileptic patient models can be used not only as an additional tool to delineate the best treatment strategy within the realm of current clinical practice but can suggest innovative scenarios. Examples are distributed and minimally invasive ablations or stimulations that fully exploit the network and dynamical

properties of the system, or even modulation of the slow variables and parameters to force the system in safer regions of the bifurcation diagram. Applications are currently validated at best retrospectively on data from patients who have already undergone surgery, to help explain the surgical outcomes and propose better interventions. The target is to obtain a set of tools that could routinely help clinicians in making the best choice for each patient.

Beyond these applications of more immediate translational value, phenomenological models can help to foster our understanding of the mechanisms underlying epileptic seizures. The characterization of their essential dynamics could promote a taxonomy of seizures that bears predictive values for issues relevant for treatment.

All the phenomenological models considered in this review have the same spatial scale – a brain region. At the level of a single brain region there are three main ingredients that characterize the dynamics of the model and allow understanding of the relationship among different models.

The first is the bifurcation structure of the model, which determines the range of possible behaviors of the system. This is a key ingredient even when bifurcations do not occur in the model, since it nevertheless determines the excitability properties of the system.

The second ingredient is the role of what we here generically called "noise," which can include both internal and external fluctuations and stimulations. Noise can cause transitions among coexisting attractors, bringing to seizure onset or offset, also in the presence of slow variable mechanisms; it can cause preictal spiking when the system gets closer to an onset bifurcation; combined with the network effect, it can sustain oscillations in excitable systems that are not able to oscillate in isolation; and excessive noise might prevent seizure termination.

The third ingredient is the existence of several timescales having distinct roles in seizure dynamics (Fig. 4.4). A fast timescale is responsible for the oscillatory activity observed during a seizure. It groups phenomena acting on different timescales themselves, such as fast oscillations or spike and wave complexes. Despite this heterogeneity, all of them are much faster than the typical seizure duration. This fast timescale is typically linked to the electrical activity of neural populations, which produces oscillatory mesoscopic activity, but slower processes such as regulation of extracellular potassium, glial processes, or the effect of subcortical input contribute to shaping the different waveforms. These oscillations trigger slow microscopic processes that cooperate to terminate the seizure. The slow timescale is thus comparable to the ictal length. Interestingly, these processes can also be described by a collective variable, the permittivity, which emerges from the balance (or imbalance) of pro- and anti-seizure mechanisms pushing the fast system toward seizure offset. We thus have emergent collective variables exhibiting intrinsic timescales separation, with different scales influencing each other. This thinking is novel from the theoretical point of view. We can thus say that during an epileptic seizure the activities of billions of neurons, but also that of extracellular ion concentrations, glia, variables related to metabolism, and so on, become organized so that a few collective variables emerge that capture the system dynamics. This implies a collapse of the degrees of freedom of the system, and the repertoire of possible activities can be summarized using a low-dimensional manifold and the flow on it as induced by the landscape of attractors/repellers. Processes promoting the collapse on this "seizure manifold," typically acting on an ultra-slow timescale such as neuromodulators, hormones,

variables linked to the sleep-wake cycle, and so on, are those responsible for bringing the fast system close to the onset bifurcation. These processes would also be responsible for the expression of one seizure class over another, as described in previous sections.

It has been proposed that the ultra-slow and slow dynamics identified in the context of seizure modeling exist and play an equally important role in the healthy brain [51]. This hypothesis comes from the physiological evidence that any brain can exhibit seizures under the right conditions, so that they might be part of the dynamical repertoire of any brain together with other brain rhythms. The above description about the emergence of two-tiered order parameters (collective variables) is, in fact, reminiscent of the structured flows on manifold framework proposed as a formal description of behavioral and brain organization, characterized by the existence of at least two coevolving timescales in the order parameters linked to the emergence of behavior [51]. In particular, fast variables express the execution of cognitive and action tasks, while slow variables modulate the creation and annihilation of the specific low-dimensional space, and attractor landscape therein, in which a task can occur, in a similar fashion to the mechanism causing the collapse on the low-dimensional space on which seizure activity takes place.

References

1. Fisher, R. S., Boas, W. van E., Blume, W., et al. Epileptic seizures and epilepsy: Definitions proposed by the International League Against Epilepsy (ILAE) and the International Bureau for Epilepsy (IBE). *Epilepsia*, 46(4), 470–2 (2005).

2. Terry, J. R., Benjamin, O., and Richardson, M. P. Seizure generation: The role of nodes and networks. *Epilepsia*, 53(9), e166–9 (2012).

3. da Silva, F. L., Blanes, W., Kalitzin, S. N., et al. Epilepsies as dynamical diseases of brain systems: Basic models of the transition between normal and epileptic activity. *Epilepsia*, 44 (s12), 72–83 (2003).

4. Hutchings, F., Han, C. E., Keller, S. S., et al. Predicting surgery targets in temporal lobe epilepsy through structural connectome based simulations. *PLoS Comput. Biol.*, 11(12), e1004642 (2015).

5. Jirsa, V. K., Proix, T., Perdikis, D., et al. The virtual epileptic patient: Individualized whole-brain models of epilepsy spread. *Neuroimage*, 145, 377–88 (2017).

6. Proix, T., Bartolomei, F., Guye, M., and Jirsa, V. K. Individual brain structure and modelling predict seizure propagation. *Brain*, 140(3), 641–54 (2017).

7. Sinha, N., Dauwels, J., Kaiser, M., et al. Predicting neurosurgical outcomes in focal epilepsy patients using computational modelling. *Brain*, 140(2), 319–32 (2016).

8. Taylor, P. N., Kaiser, M., and Dauwels, J. Structural connectivity based whole brain modelling in epilepsy. *J. Neurosci. Methods.*, 236, 51–7, (2014).

9. Jirsa, V. K., Stacey, W. C., Quilichini, P. P., Ivanov, A. I., and Bernard, C. On the nature of seizure dynamics. *Brain*, 137 (8), 2210–30 (2014).

10. Südhof, T. C. Molecular neuroscience in the 21st century: A personal

perspective. *Neuron*, 96(3), 536–41 (2017).

11. Eliasmith, C., and Trujillo, O. The use and abuse of large-scale brain models. *Curr. Opin. Neurobiol.*, 25, 1–6 (2014).

12. Jirsa, V. K., and McIntosh, A. R. (Eds) *Handbook of Brain Connectivity*, Berlin, Germany: Springer. 2007.

13. Deco, G., Jirsa, V., McIntosh, A. R., Sporns, O., and Kötter, R. Key role of coupling, delay, and noise in resting brain fluctuations. *Proc. Natl. Acad. Sci.*, 106(25), 10302–7, (2009).

14. Breakspear, M. Dynamic models of large-scale brain activity. *Nat. Neurosci.*, 20(3), 340–52 (2017).

15. Sanz-Leon, P., Knock, S. A., Spiegler, A., and Jirsa, V. K. Mathematical framework for large-scale brain network modeling in The Virtual Brain. *Neuroimage*, 111, 385–430 (2015).

16. Kalitzin, S., Koppert, M., Petkov, G., and da Silva, F. L. Multiple oscillatory states in models of collective neuronal dynamics. *Int. J. Neural Syst.*, 24(6), 1450020, (2014).

17. Naze, S., Bernard, C., and Jirsa, V. Computational modeling of seizure dynamics using coupled neuronal networks: factors shaping epileptiform activity. *PLoS Comput. Biol.*, 11(5), e1004209 (2015).

18. Eissa, T. L., Dijkstra, K., Brune, C., et al. Cross-scale effects of neural interactions during human neocortical seizure activity. *Proc. Natl. Acad. Sci.*, 114(40), 10761–6 (2017).

19. Proix, T., Jirsa, V. K., Bartolomei, F., Guye, M., and Truccolo, W. Predicting the spatiotemporal diversity of seizure propagation and termination in human focal epilepsy. *Nat. Commun.*, 2018; 9(1):1088.

20. Iturria-Medina, Y. Anatomical brain networks on the prediction of abnormal brain states. *Brain Connect.*, 2013; 3 (1):1–21.

21. Proix, T, Spiegler, A, Schirner, M, et al. How do parcellation size and short-range connectivity affect dynamics in large-scale brain network models? *Neuroimage.*, 142, 135–49, (2016).

22. Taylor, P. N., Goodfellow, M., Wang, Y., and Baier, G. Towards a large-scale model of patient-specific epileptic spike-wave discharges. *Biol. Cybern.*, 107(1), 83–94 (2013).

23. Yan, B., and Li, P. The emergence of abnormal hypersynchronization in the anatomical structural network of human brain. *Neuroimage.*, 65, 34–51 (2013).

24. Benjamin, O., Fitzgerald, T. H. B., Ashwin, P., et al. A phenomenological model of seizure initiation suggests network structure may explain seizure frequency in idiopathic generalised epilepsy. *J. Math. Neurosci.*, 2(1), 1 (2012).

25. Goodfellow, M., Rummel, C., Abela, E., et al. Estimation of brain network ictogenicity predicts outcome from epilepsy surgery. *Sci. Rep.*, 6, 29215 (2016).

26. Wendling, F., Benquet, P., Bartolomei, F., and Jirsa, V. Computational models of epileptiform activity. *J. Neurosci. Methods.*, 260, 233–51 (2016).

27. Suffczynski, P., Da Silva, F. H. L., Parra, J., et al. Dynamics of epileptic phenomena determined from statistics of ictal transitions. *IEEE Trans. Biomed. E.ng.*, 53(3), 524–32 (2006).

28. Kramer, M. A., Truccolo, W., Eden, U. T., et al. Human seizures self-terminate across spatial scales via a critical transition. *Proc. Natl. Acad. Sci.*, 109(51), 21116–21 (2012).

29. Goodfellow, M., Schindler, K., and Baier, G. Intermittent spike – wave dynamics in a heterogeneous, spatially extended neural mass model. *Neuroimage.*, 55(3), 920–32 (2011).

30. Baier, G., Goodfellow, M., Taylor, P. N., Wang, Y., and Garry, D. J. The importance of modeling epileptic seizure dynamics as spatio-temporal patterns. *Front. Physiol.*, 3, 281 (2012).

31. Saggio, M. L., Spiegler, A., Bernard, C., and Jirsa, V. K. Fast–slow bursters in the unfolding of a high codimension singularity and the ultra-slow transitions of classes. *J. Math. Neurosci.*, 7(1), 7 (2017).

32. Kalitzin, S., Koppert, M., Petkov, G., Velis, D., and da Silva, F. L. Computational model prospective on the observation of proictal states in epileptic neuronal systems. *Epilepsy Behav.*, 22, S102–9 (2011).

33. Goodfellow, M., Taylor, P. N., Wang, Y., Garry, D. G., and Baier, G. Modelling the role of tissue heterogeneity in epileptic rhythms. *Eur. J. Neurosci.*, 36 (2), 2178–87 (2012).

34. Izhikevich, E. M. Neural excitability, spiking and bursting. *Int. J. Bifurc. Chaos.*, 10(06), 1171–266 (2000).

35. Wendling, F., Bartolomei, F., Bellanger, J. J., and Chauvel, P. Epileptic fast activity can be explained by a model of impaired GABAergic dendritic inhibition. *Eur. J. Neurosci.*, 15 (9), 1499–508 (2002).

36. Wendling, F., Hernandez, A., Bellanger, J.-J., Chauvel, P., and Bartolomei, F. Interictal to ictal transition in human temporal

lobe epilepsy: insights from a computational model of intracerebral EEG. *J. Clin. Neurophysiol.*, 22(5), 343 (2005).

37. Baud, M. O., Kleen, J. K., Mirro, E. A., et al. Multi-day rhythms modulate seizure risk in epilepsy. *Nat. Commun.*, 9 (1), 88 (2018).

38. Meisel, C., and Kuehn, C. Scaling effects and spatio-temporal multilevel dynamics in epileptic seizures. *PLoS ONE*, 7(2), e30371 (2012).

39. Saggio, M. L., Crisp, D., Scott, J., et al. A taxonomy of seizure dynamotypes. 2020. bioRxiv. doi: 10.1101/2020.02.08.940072

40. Ikeda, A., Taki, W., Kunieda, T., et al. Focal ictal direct current shifts in human epilepsy as studied by subdural and scalp recording. *Brain*, 122 (5), 827–38 (1999).

41. El Houssaini, K., Ivanov, A. I., Bernard, C., and Jirsa, V. K. Seizures, refractory status epilepticus, and depolarization block as endogenous brain activities. *Phys. Rev. E Stat. Nonlin. Soft Matter Phys.*, 91 (1), 010701 (2015).

42. Wang, Y., Goodfellow, M., Taylor, P. N., and Baier, G. Phase space approach for modeling of epileptic dynamics. *Phys Rev E.*, 85(6), 61918 (2012).

43. Touboul, J., Wendling, F., Chauvel, P., and Faugeras, O. Neural mass activity, bifurcations, and epilepsy. *Neural Comput.*, 23(12), 3232–86 (2011).

44. Olmi, S., Petkoski, S., Guye, M., Bartolomei, F., and Jirsa, V. Controlling seizure propagation in large-scale brain networks. *PLoS Comput. Biol.*, 15(2), e1006805 (2019).

45. An, S., Bartolomei, F., Guye, M., and Jirsa, V. Optimization of surgical intervention outside the epileptogenic zone in the Virtual Epileptic Patient (VEP). *PLoS Comput. Biol.*, 15(6), e1007051 (2019).

46. Wang, Y., Hutchings, F., and Kaiser, M. Computational modeling of neurostimulation in brain diseases. *Prog. Brain Res.*, 222, 191–228 (2015).

47. Proix, T., Bartolomei, F., Chauvel, P., Bernard, C., and Jirsa, V. Permittivity coupling across brain regions

determines seizure recruitment in partial epilepsy. *J. Neurosci.*, 34(45), 15009–21 (2014).

48. Wang, Y., Goodfellow, M., Taylor, P. N., and Baier, G. Dynamic mechanisms of neocortical focal seizure onset. *PLoS Comput. Biol.*, 10(8), e1003787 (2014).

49. Wang, Y., Trevelyan, A. J., Valentin, A., et al. Mechanisms underlying different onset patterns of focal seizures. *PLoS Comput. Biol.*, 13(5), e1005475 (2017).

50. Doležalová, I., Brázdil, M., Hermanová, M., et al. Intracranial EEG seizure onset patterns in unilateral temporal lobe epilepsy and their relationship to other variables. *Clin. Neurophysiol.*, 124(6), 1079–88 (2013).

51. McIntosh, R., and Jirsa, V. The hidden repertoire of brain dynamics and dysfunction. *Netw. Neurosci.*, 3(4), 994–1108 (2019).

52. Bernard, C, and Jirsa, V. Virtual brain for neurological disease modeling. *Drug Discov. Today Dis. Model.*, 19, 5–10 (2016).

Personalized Network Modeling in Epilepsy

Yujiang Wang, Gabrielle Marie Schroeder, Nishant Sinha, and Peter Neal Taylor

5.1 Introduction

Epilepsy is a family of neurological disorders in which patients experience unprovoked spontaneous seizures. Unfortunately, there is currently no cure for epilepsy, and seizure management is the target of most therapies. The first-line treatment of epilepsy is usually antiepileptic drugs. However, depending on the subtype of epilepsy and the individual, drug treatments fail to control the seizures in around one-third of patients. One challenge in the treatment of epilepsy is its heterogeneity. In each patient, seizures are thought to be generated by different mechanisms, processes, and parameters, and treatment outcomes will also depend on these.

Fortunately, epilepsy is one of the disorders that can be captured and measured on many spatial and temporal scales, even in human patients. For example, at the microscale, it is possible to infer single neuron firing patterns in patients using microelectrodes [1,2]. At a coarser spatial scale, scalp EEG and intracranial EEG allow long-term recording of spatiotemporal electrical signals [3]. Concurrent measurement of electrical signals with blood oxygenation at the whole-brain scale using functional MRI are also possible [4], even during seizures [5], and structural measurements of white matter integrity and connectivity can also be made using diffusion MRI [6]. High prevalence rates additionally enable recruitment of large cohorts for studies, and the lifetime impact of the disease facilitates longitudinal analyses [7]. This wealth of data enables the development of data-driven approaches to understanding patient-specific disease mechanisms, and designing patient-specific treatment strategies.

A key component in achieving data-driven and patient-specific treatments are personalized models of the epileptic dynamics in each patient. Models are generally useful in situations where we wish to predict something that is unknown, such as a treatment outcome, an impending seizure, or a parameter that cannot be directly measured. Personalized models usually make use of a general model structure (e.g., reflecting some basic assumptions on the structure and function of the brain), and additionally use patient-specific data to parameterize and validate it. Such personalized models can then be used to make predictions about disease mechanisms or treatment outcomes in individual patients.

5.1.1 Dynamical Systems Models and Incorporation of Personalized Brain Connectivity

Many types of models exist, including conceptual models based on a preconceived hypothesis, machine learning models built on data-driven features, and dynamical systems models consisting of parameters and variables. Dynamical systems models are particularly useful for simulating time-varying systems, especially when some prior knowledge of the mechanisms of the system are known. They have recently shown promise for making personalized predictions in epilepsy, and are the focus of this chapter.

A dynamical systems model is composed of a set of equations that usually describe how a property of interest changes with respect to time. A classic example in the neurosciences is the neural population model of Wilson and Cowan [8], where the equations describe how neural population firing rates change over time. In that model, two equations (variables) are used to represent excitatory and inhibitory neural populations. The assumption of the excitatory and inhibitory populations represents a prior knowledge of the system. A set of parameters and nonlinear functions govern all of the ways in which the two populations can

61

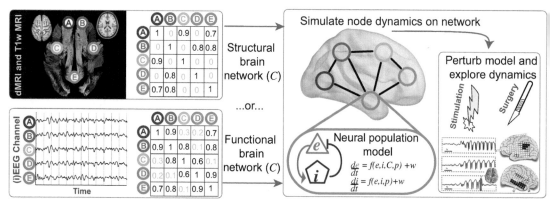

Figure 5.1 Schematic of processing and analysis pipeline for personalized brain network simulations. First, a personalized brain network is generated, which in this example contains nodes (A–E) and connections between them (entries in the matrix). Connections can be inferred from diffusion weighted MRI tractography (upper left panel), or from associations between time series recordings (lower left panel). This personalized brain network is then used for simulations, by placing a neural population unit in each node. The coupling between the nodes is dictated by the personalized brain network. Simulations result in time series for each variable (typically at least two per node, e.g., one excitatory and one inhibitory). The simulated time series can be analyzed to make inferences about the influence of the personalized connectivity on the dynamics. Perturbations or experiments can also be performed, e.g., by stimulating the model (through a simulated injection of current to one or more variables and nodes), or simulating surgery (by disconnecting nodes and re-simulating the dynamics). Insets show examples of simulated personalized stimulation and surgery [16,17].

possibly interact. More complex models can also be designed, incorporating additional, more specific populations of neurons, such as the Jansen–Rit model [9]. The additional complexity enables the model to have different types of dynamics, but at the cost of requiring more assumptions about the populations' behaviors and interactions.

Dynamical systems models of seizures usually use such neural population models to simulate the brain dynamics seen on EEG, as the EEG is thought to capture brain dynamics arising from populations of neurons. In the model, high amplitude oscillatory activity is commonly used to represent seizure (ictal) dynamics, while low amplitude irregular dynamics are understood as the non-seizure (interictal) state. Most earlier work investigated mechanisms of seizure onset in the model [10]. Seizure onset mechanisms have typically been modeled either as a parameter change through a bifurcation or as a noisy process in a bistable system, although other mechanisms are possible [11]. Parameter-induced seizure transitions work by simulating a slow change in a parameter such that the non-seizure state ceases to exist and the only stable attractor is a seizure state. The parameter value for which the state change occurs is known as a bifurcation point. The alternative approach uses bistability, where the seizure and non-seizure states both coexist, and external input drives seizure transitions.

Excitability parameters can then be defined as the proximity to the bifurcation [12], or likelihood of transition in a bistable system [13].

Traditionally, most previous epilepsy modeling work at the macroscopic spatial scale has not incorporated complex spatial interactions or personalized patient data [14]. This approach has only happened relatively recently, and has partly been driven by the increased understanding of how network interactions contribute to epileptic processes, even in focal epilepsies [15]. To incorporate patient networks into the model parameters, a set of equations that captures one of the above seizure-transition mechanisms is then coupled to another set of equations. The coupling typically takes the form of a connectivity matrix inferred from patient data. Simulated seizures can then occur in the model, and their spatiotemporal appearance is dependent on the model and its (patient-specific) connectivity parameters. Figure 5.1 shows a schematic of the approach.

In this chapter, we will discuss some recent examples that incorporate patient-specific connectivity into computational models for predictive value. This chapter is structured as follows: In Section 5.2 we discuss how subject-specific structural connectivity has been used to constrain model parameters. In Section 5.3 we discuss examples where patient-specific EEG functional connectivity has been used to constrain model parameters. Finally, we suggest some possible future directions in Section 5.4.

5.2 Structural Connectivity-Based Modeling

Structural whole-brain networks (connectomes) represent different brain regions that are interconnected by white matter fiber tracts. These networks are typically reconstructed from diffusion weighted magnetic resonance imaging (dMRI). From these images, white matter tracts reflecting the connectivity between different brain regions can be inferred using a fiber tracking algorithm. A network formulation is then possible by parcellating gray matter into predefined regions of interest, also referred to as nodes, with the fiber tracts connecting them becoming the edges (see [18] for an early example). Though dMRI tractography is not usually routinely analyzed clinically in epilepsy, recent studies have illustrated that it allows clinically useful predictions [19–21] and may improve understanding of the pathophysiology of epilepsy. For example, diffusion MRI has revealed reduced fractional anisotropy in temporal lobe epilepsy [22,23] and other structural network alterations in epilepsy [24–26]. However, static brain networks have limited ability to explain emergent functional and pathological spatiotemporal dynamics, such as seizures.

Dynamical systems models, when combined with patient-specific structural connectomes, enable the construction of personalized models that can simulate possible spatiotemporal dynamics arising from each network structure. Importantly, they can also simulate spatiotemporal dynamics arising from *changes* to patient-specific connectomes (e.g., due to surgery or disease progression). When validated, these models can then be applied to predict treatment outcome or design treatment strategies.

Some of the early work simulating brain dynamics based on changes to structural connectomes was not in the context of epilepsy. For example, Honey and Sporns illustrated the effect of cortical lesion induced changes in simulated brain dynamics using the macaque structural brain connectivity network as the coupling parameter in two different models [27]. Lesioning was performed by removing connections to/from specific nodes, and model outputs compared pre- and post-lesioning. The authors showed that the effect on cortico-cortical interactions due to lesioning the high degree nodes was most widespread. Community architecture was highlighted as a significant predictor in determining whether the dynamical consequences of lesions should remain confined to a cluster. This work illustrated a framework for how model simulations, combined with structural connectomes, could be used to study the behavior arising from a static structural network.

In the context of epilepsy, some publications used the framework above to study the effect of epilepsy surgery. For example, in an exploratory study, Hutchings *et al.* (2015) [13] used a bistable phenomenological model for each node (brain region) that could transition between non-seizure and seizure-like states. The coupling parameters were derived from the dMRI from patients with temporal lobe epilepsy. Node excitability parameters were set higher in more atrophied areas in a data-driven manner using healthy control volumetrics as a reference, i.e., the excitability was proportional to the abnormality of the brain region. Upon simulation, the model exhibited transitions to seizure-like states more often using the patient parameters than those of the healthy controls. Notably, the amygdala, hippocampus, and parahippocamphal gyrus – which are routinely removed clinically – were also predicted among the most seizure prone by the model. Surgical outcomes were also predicted by simulating the changes in transition time due to given (planned) clinical resections compared with the resection performed in random areas. A limitation of that study was that the simulated surgeries did not account for individual variations in surgery [21], nor was the model validated with personalized patient outcomes. However, it did demonstrate the group level finding of wide variations in post-operative surgical changes in seizure likelihood between patients, similar to those observed clinically [28].

A more recent study by Jirsa et al. [29] used the "Epileptor," a phenomenological model comprising two oscillators coupled by a slow variable. In the model, transitions were simulated though saddle node and homoclinic bifurcations at seizure onset and offset, respectively. These two types of bifurcations had previously been shown to replicate features of seizure onset and offset well [30]. The brain network model was designed by placing the Epileptor at each network node and coupled to each other using the patient's diffusion MRI-inferred connectome. Excitability parameters of local nodes were set according to whether the node was deemed an epileptogenic zone or a propagation zone based on clinical assessment. The parameter space was then explored for simulating network seizure dynamics. Extending the modeling framework in [29], seizure propagation was modeled by Proix et al. [31]. Specifically, the hypothesized epileptogenic zone was quantified from neuroimaging data (MRI and intracranial EEG) collected during the presurgical evaluation of intractable epilepsy patients. Setting the parameter of nodes in the hypothesized epileptogenic zone to be more excitable, linear stability analysis was applied to identify nodes in the propagation zone. The model was validated by computing the accuracy of the predicted propagation zone with its clinical estimates. Further, the authors showed a correspondence between the surgical outcomes and the proportion of propagation zones outside the coverage of invasively placed intracranial EEG electrodes, i.e., the number of unexplored regions in the propagation zone was significantly higher in the poor surgical outcome group. This suggests that in those patients who were not-seizure-free, the epileptogenic and/or propagation zone was not fully captured by iEEG. Obvious clinical applications would be to use this approach to guide electrode placement, as well as to predict post-operative seizure freedom.

Proix et al. [32] then used the Epileptor in a multi-scale approach to model spatiotemporal patterns of seizure spread and termination. The Epileptor model was extended to a neural field model in which the short-range connectivity was incorporated by homogeneous coupling and long-range connectivity with heterogeneous coupling. The interplay between spatial and temporal scales in the model explained two observations of spike-wave discharge (SWD) type focal seizures: (i) propagation of slow ictal wavefront and fast SWDs, and (ii) asynchronous termination of seizures in clusters. This study suggested that these dynamics, together with variations in short- and long-range connectivity strength, play a central role in seizure spread, maintenance and termination.

In contrast to the studies above, which simulate focal onset seizures, other studies have performed personalized brain network modeling of patients with generalized seizures. Yan and Li investigated the role of structural connectivity in

inducing abnormal hypersynchrony during seizure [33]. There, the anatomical connectivity and conduction delay between different cortical areas were inferred from healthy subjects' dMRI. By modeling different cortical areas using a coupled system of four Kuramuto oscillators at each area, the authors investigated the role of connectivity and delays on large-scale synchronization. Importantly, the model quantified the degree of synchronization of each cortical area locally as well as the whole cortex globally. It was apparent that some cortical areas ("hot spots") have a higher propensity of inducing global synchronization than others; this is not otherwise observable on the recordings of an SWD electroencephalogram. To our knowledge this was the first study to simulate dynamics on a human dMRI structural network in the context of epilepsy. Even though the networks used were derived from healthy subjects, the same approach could be applied using patient data.

In another early study of generalized epilepsy modeling, Taylor et al. also used a multi-scale approach to simulate between-subject variations in generalized spike-and-wave seizure dynamics [34]. There, four neural population models were coupled locally to represent the dynamics within an individual node/brain region. Whole-brain scale long-range connections between regions were then inferred from healthy subjects' dMRI. In other words, different "patients" were simulated, although the connectome underlying each patient's simulation was derived from healthy subjects. Using this multi-scale approach, the authors demonstrated that the model can reproduce the prototypic waveform of SWDs. Simulated electrographic data closely resembled the clinical recordings of absence seizures. The simulated SWD seizure dynamics showed higher within-"patient" similarity than between "patients," thus hypothesizing that variations in SWD dynamics between patents may be due to their personal connectome. This modeling approach facilitated development of an optimal stimulation algorithm for abating seizures in silico where the stimulation was tailored to the individual [16], suggesting a potential therapeutic method toward seizure control in generalized epilepsy. A limitation of both the early studies [33,34] is that they used connectivity derived from healthy control imaging; however, the same approach could be used to simulate emergent dynamics on patient-specific structural networks. This short-coming was partly addressed in the study by [16], which used dMRI acquired from a patient with idiopathic generalized epilepsy.

Two other studies have applied dMRI-informed models to conceptually different questions in the context of epilepsy. In the first study, Lu et al. used connectivity from healthy subjects' dMRI, combined with a neural mass model to simulate EEG and functional MRI [35]. The authors used the model to generate music from a simulated seizure. They suggest that the "level of arousal" while participants listen to the music could be used as a potential tool to discriminate patient populations. In a second study, Abdelnour et al. modeled the atrophy pattern in mesial temporal lobe epilepsy using two network-based models: (i) propagation of epileptogenic activity (i.e., extra-hippocampal spread of seizure activity), and (ii) progressive neurodegenerative process whereby loss in hippocampal neurons leads to loss in other connected regions [36]. Both network models simulate a diffusion process on the whole-brain structural connectivity network. The latter model of atrophy spread reproduced the empirically observed atrophy significantly better than the former. Although the structural connectivity was acquired from healthy controls, atrophy measurements were derived from patients. These models might be helpful in predicting future spread of atrophy which may pave the way for a tailored surgical therapy to prevent progressive degeneration.

5.3 Functional Connectivity-Based Modeling

While determining structural connectivity helps reveal alterations in brain structure in epilepsy, it is also important to understand the changes in neural dynamics that occur in this disorder. In particular, the high temporal resolution of electroencephalographic (EEG) recordings allows clinicians to identify abnormal patterns of activity during both interictal and ictal periods. The easiest recording to obtain is scalp EEG, where electrodes placed on the scalp record neural activity generated by the underlying cortex. However, in order to finely localize the origin of seizures in candidates for resective surgery, a more localized recording is required. Some patients therefore undergo intracranial EEG (iEEG) monitoring, in which contacts are surgically placed either directly on the surface of the brain (typically in grid or strip arrangements), or into deeper structures using depth electrodes [3,37,38]. Due to the invasive nature, iEEG provides a finer spatial resolution and less noisy recording than scalp EEG; and can also be used to observe the dynamics of deep brain regions such as the hippocampus. The overall spatial coverage provided by iEEG, though, is more limited; in each patient, only certain regions are recorded from based on the hypothesized epileptogenic zone.

Section 5.2 described computational models in which brain regions were coupled based on patient-specific structural connectivity. Likewise, the coupling parameters of such network models can be defined by functional connectivity, derived from scalp or intracranial EEG [17,39–42]. In this case, each node represents the brain region recorded by a single electrode, while edges correspond to the statistical relationship (e.g., correlation or coherence) between each pair of EEG signals. While structural connections provide opportunities for neural interactions, functional connectivity describes the actual changes in measured interactions during different brain states, such as seizures. Many studies have used functional connectivity to elucidate how spatiotemporal brain dynamics change before, during, and after seizures [43–45], and the epileptogenic zone also appears to have unique functional network properties [44]. As such, computational models incorporating patient-specific functional networks can explore how functional interactions may contribute to epileptic mechanisms in each patient.

Studies have used scalp EEG recordings to infer functional connectivity and applied them in the context of modeling generalized seizures. For example, the pioneering study by Benjamin et al. [46], used a bistable model to investigate the impact of noise and network structure on seizure-like transitions in a model constrained by scalp EEG. There, the authors showed that the model produced significant differences between patients and controls in terms of the model output. Further work from the same group suggested the potential for EEG-based modeling to discriminate between patients and controls [47]. Finally, the study by Taylor et al. used correlations between EEG channels to constrain a network model of the thalamocortical loop, generating generalized spike-and-wave seizures [48]. The authors further examined the effect of stimulation in this model, and found a spatial heterogeneity in terms of the stimulation response duration. This heterogeneity was suggested to account for spatial variability observed after stimulation in experimental models of spike-and-wave seizures [49].

Meanwhile, models based on iEEG data from patients with focal epilepsy have focused on understanding and predicting the effects of surgical resection. Sinha et al. created patient-specific computational models based on interictal iEEG functional connectivity in a cohort of six patients with focal epilepsy [39], an approach that was later extended to a study of 16 patients [17]. In their study, each node of the network is a bistable model at the cusp of a subcritical Hopf bifurcation, and the nodes are coupled by the patient's interictal functional connectivity. Noise and external inputs have the potential to push each node into an oscillatory state, reminiscent of epileptic discharges. To quantify each model's seizure likelihood, the authors measure the "escape time" of each node – the amount of time it takes for the node to switch from a resting state to the oscillatory dynamics. In good outcome patients, removing the resected nodes from the model increases escape time (i.e., decreases seizure likelihood) more than a random resection. Meanwhile, alternative resection for bad-outcome patients are proposed based on which nodes have the highest seizure likelihood. The authors suggest the modeling approach for predicting the outcome of surgery based on interictal data and suggesting alternative resection strategies.

Using ictal iEEG data, Goodfellow et al. simulated dynamics on functional networks using a separate cohort of sixteen patients with focal epilepsy who underwent iEEG monitoring and surgical resection [40]. They modeled the dynamics at each node using a neural mass model set close to a saddle node on invariant circle bifurcation [50]. Coupling between nodes was proportional to patient-specific functional networks, which were derived from the first half of seizure activity. Because the node dynamics are close to a bifurcation, noisy inputs produce simulated discharges. They define "brain network ictogenicity" (BNI) as the proportion of time the model spends in discharges, thus allowing them to quantify the effects of perturbations on the model dynamics. First,

they observed that if the resected nodes are removed from the network, BNI is reduced more for patients that had good surgical outcomes; in other words, successful interventions had a greater impact on model dynamics than unsuccessful surgeries. They then proposed alternative resections based on which nodes produced the greatest reduction in discharges upon removal, and found their proposed resections were consistent with the actual resections of good, but not bad, outcome patients. In a later study, Lopes et al. used the same concept of BNI to explore how patient-specific network dynamics change close to and during seizures [41]. They demonstrated that surgical outcome predictions are more reliable for patients that consistently have an increase in BNI during seizures, compared to pre- and post-ictal periods. They propose that in these patients, the ictogenic network is well-represented by the patient-specific functional connectivity, which can therefore be used to devise an optimal resection strategy.

Despite some differences in their approaches, these studies all suggest that modeling dynamics on patient-specific functional networks can identify the drivers of abnormal neural activity, predict the outcome of a proposed resection, and suggest both more effective and less extensive surgical targets [17,40]. While early work focused on static network representations of ictal [40] or interictal [17] activity, there has been recent interest in exploring how changing functional interactions influence model behavior [41,42]. Interestingly, in all of these models, the intrinsic dynamics of each node are assumed to be the same – it is solely the model network structure that produces differences in the nodes' dynamics. This observation is consistent with theoretical studies demonstrating that network structure, rather than node properties, can be the primary source of abnormal dynamics [51]. However, this is in contrast to some previously mentioned approaches using structural connectivity, where both intrinsic node dynamics and network structure give rise to the model behavior [13,31]. A recent review further highlights this question of node vs. network cause of focal seizures [52]. Personalized network modeling approaches using structural and functional connectivity may prove crucial in future to answer this question.

5.4 Opportunities and Future Applications

The studies highlighted above suggest the potential benefits of a personalized modeling approach in the context of epilepsy; however, there are still some challenges to overcome in order for the approach to be useful for real-world clinical applications. Here, we highlight some areas which we consider to be unsolved challenges or underdeveloped research areas thus far. We suggest they may serve as fruitful avenues of future investigation.

5.4.1 Multimodal Data Integration

Currently, personalized models are usually created with one patient-specific component (e.g., the patient's structural brain network) and validated against a variable, such as surgical outcome. However, in the era of multimodal data, it is unclear how to best include all the available information into one personalized model. One excellent example of how this challenge may be tackled is given by Proix et al. [31]. On top of the patients' structural connectivity this model additionally used EEG-derived information to further parametrize the model (in terms of local excitability of each node), and predict the propagation of ictal activity beyond the recording sites. The validation of those predictions with another data modality – the actual patient outcomes – serves as an example of how the field can progress.

Another possibility is to consider multiple modalities for the validation of a model. For example, the study by Proix *et al.* predicted the existence and location of possible epileptogenic tissue in areas not recorded by iEEG. Their validation was essentially patient outcomes. However, additional validation from e.g., source localized MEG, high density scalp EEG, or fMRI, could also be used to investigate the presence of abnormalities on other modalities (e.g., interictal spikes). Some recent multimodal imaging analyses show that, for example, congruency/discrepancy between two modalities can in itself be a predictor of the epileptogenic zone, or good surgical outcome (e.g., [4,53]).

Model inversion techniques also offer an alternative way to integrate multimodal data. Model inversion can be used to estimate model parameters given an empirical time series and a computational model capable of reproducing features of the signal. In the context of epilepsy, several studies have used model inversion to explore possible physiological bases of epileptic activity [54–60]. However, these studies usually only model the activity of a localized area (or independently model the activity of each brain region), as model inversion of large, spatially coupled systems is typically computationally intractable. Although methods of model inversion for coupled systems are under development [60], data from another modality (e.g., a dMRI derived network) may provide a way to constrain the coupling between brain regions [61]. Such models could potentially reveal the neural mechanisms underlying both local and global brain dynamics in epilepsy.

However, fully understanding how different modalities can inform personalized models will most likely require a more principled understanding of the relationship between modalities in the context of epilepsy. This will most likely entail mapping what the modalities really capture onto a biological basis, and relating them to each other, in the context of epilepsy. A related and similar argument also applies to different measures within the same modality. For example, structural connectivity strength can be defined in various ways (e.g., fractional anisotropy, streamline density), and a number of different measures have also been used to define functional connectivity. Different measures can lead to different predictions or validation outcomes. Again, a more principled understanding of different measures and their relationship to clinical variables is required.

5.4.2 Long-Term Longitudinal Properties in Epilepsy

Epilepsy symptoms change over timescales of years. For example, around 75% of patients are seizure-free after surgery for the first year. However, of those seizure-free patients, around a third will relapse to seizures again within five years [28]. The long-term changes in seizure relapse/relief – and corresponding brain structure, dynamics, and treatment impact – has barely been explored by the modeling community. The fact that patient retention is reasonably high means that longitudinal studies are possible. Models are ideal for studying dynamics regardless of the timescale; however, there are very few examples of disease progression modeling in epilepsy that are constrained by EEG or MRI [36]. Future studies should investigate long-timescale brain network changes and their relation to patient symptom changes, and could take inspiration from previous work in Alzheimer's research [62,63].

Other than investigating long-term surgery outcome, the impact of medication can also be modeled by longitudinal personalized network models. To our knowledge, there are currently no such studies, which is surprising since antiepileptic drugs (AEDs) are known to cause changes in the EEG [64] and MRI properties [65]. The lack of studies may be due to the lack of longitudinal data acquisition, and the fact that seizure frequency changes over time; therefore, it is difficult to confirm if medication is responsible for any observed differences in dynamics. The ability to predict AED efficacy in new onset patients would be highly clinically valuable, and network-based modeling offers opportunities to complement clinical decision making.

A related avenue of research that is currently not tackled in epilepsy is that of drug side-effect modeling, although outside of epilepsy, some general attempts in this direction are being made [66]. Drug side effects have a huge impact on the quality of life in epilepsy patients, and are often linked to non-adherence and poor seizure management. It is conceivable to build personalized models to predict such side effects, although some systematic steps have to be made to quantify (ideally in an objective way) such side effects. Objective behavioral quantification methods (such as body sensor technologies) may open the door to this avenue in future.

5.4.3 Within-Subject Variability

While this chapter is concerned with building patient-specific models for prediction, one key aspect that has not been touched on is that of within-subject variability. For example, it is known that some patients may have different populations of seizures [67], some of which may be linked to specific brain states (e.g., awake vs. asleep [68]). Some populations may also be resistant to treatment. Even within a population, no two seizures ever look exactly alike. It has also been documented that seizures of shorter durations may preferentially appear together, as opposed to longer seizures in the same patient [69]. Similarly, short seizures appear to have a different underlying parameter evolution as compared to long seizures in the same patient [57]. This within-patient heterogeneity has serious consequences for treatment strategies. For example, surgical resection has to consider different epileptogenic zones for different seizure populations. Brain stimulation devices to prevent seizures, again, have to account for heterogeneous seizures within the same patient [70].

Thus, it is also important to consider how personalized models can account for the within-subject variability across different brain states, times of day/week/months, and other modulatory processes. Essentially, we need to avoid overfitting our personalized models to particular (one-off) measurements, and be able to generalize them to "the patient," not just "the patient at one point in time." One way to begin to overcome this challenge is to understand the seizures in a patient as arising against a background of ongoing activity. The ongoing activity will modulate and influence how a seizure is going to occur and evolve [43]. Hence understanding the interplay of the interictal state with the seizure mechanism through personalized models would be the next step forward.

In this chapter we have reviewed how dynamical systems models can be constrained by personalized patient data at the macroscopic scale with network interactions. We suggest that the development of models at multiple timescales (e.g., short-term seizure prediction and long-term disease progression) to predict and compare multiple treatment strategies is something the field of personalized modeling should strive toward.

References

1. Truccolo, W., Donoghue, J.A., Hochberg, L.R., et al. Single-neuron dynamics in human focal epilepsy. *Nat. neurosci.*, 14(5), 635 (2011).

2. Merricks, E.M., Smith, E.H., McKhann, G.M., et al. Single unit action potentials in humans and the effect of seizure activity. *Brain*, 138(10), 2891–2906 (2015).

3. Cook, M. J., O'Brien, T. J., Berkovic, S. F., et al. Prediction of seizure likelihood with a long-term, implanted seizure advisory system in patients with drug-resistant epilepsy: a first-in-man

study. *Lancet Neurol.*, 12(6), 563–571 (2013).

4. Coan AC, Chaudhary UJ, Grouiller F., et al. EEG-fMRI in the presurgical evaluation of temporal lobe epilepsy. *J. Neurol. Neurosurg. Psychiatry*, 87(6), 642–9, (2016).

5. Moeller, F., Siebner, H. R., Wolff, S., et al. Simultaneous EEG-fMRI in drug-naive children with newly diagnosed absence epilepsy. *Epilepsia*, 49 (9), 1510–9 (2008).

6. Duncan, John S., Winston, Gavin P., Koepp, Matthias J., and Ourselin, Sebastien. Brain imaging in the assessment for epilepsy surgery. *Lancet Neurol.*, 15(4), 420–33 (2016).

7. Lossius, M. I., Hessen, E., Mowinckel, P., et al. Consequences of antiepileptic drug withdrawal: a randomized, double-blind study (Akershus Study). *Epilepsia*, 49(3), 455–63 (2008).

8. Wilson, H. R., and Cowan, J. D. Excitatory and inhibitory interactions in localized populations of model neurons. *Biophys. J.*, 12(1), 1–24 (1972).

9. Jansen, B. H., and Rit, V. G. Electroencephalogram and visual evoked potential generation in a mathematical model of coupled cortical columns. *Biol. Cybern.*, 73(4), 357–66 (1995).

10. da Silva, F. L., Blanes, W., Kalitzin, S.N., et al. Epilepsies as dynamical diseases of brain systems: basic models of the transition between normal and epileptic activity. *Epilepsia*, 44, 72–83 (2003).

11. Baier, G., Goodfellow, M., Taylor, P. N., Wang, Y., and Garry, D. J. The importance of modeling epileptic seizure dynamics as spatio-temporal patterns. *Front. Physiol.*, 3, 281 (2012).

12. Wang, Y., Goodfellow, M., Taylor, P. N., and Baier, G. Phase space approach for modeling of epileptic dynamics. *Phys. Rev. E Stat. Nonlin. Soft Matter Phys.*, 85(6 Pt 1), 061918 (2012).

13. Hutchings, F., Han, C. E., Keller, S. S., et al. Predicting Surgery Targets in Temporal Lobe Epilepsy through Structural Connectome Based Simulations. *PLoS Comput. Biol.*, 11(12), 1–24 (2015).

14. Taylor, P. N., Kaiser, M., and Dauwels, J. Structural connectivity based whole brain modelling in epilepsy. *J. Neurosci. Methods*, 236, 51–7 (2014).

15. Richardson, M. P. Large scale brain models of epilepsy: dynamics meets connectomics. *J. Neurol. Neurosurg. Psychiatry*, 83, 1238–48 (2012).

16. Taylor, P. N., Thomas, J., Sinha, N., et al. Optimal control based seizure abatement using patient derived connectivity. *Front. Neurosci.*, 9, 1–10 (2015).

17. Sinha, N., Dauwels, J., Kaiser, M., et al. Predicting neurosurgical outcomes in focal epilepsy patients using computational modelling. *Brain*, 140(2), 319–32 (2017).

18. Hagmann, P., Cammoun, L., Gigandet, X., et al. Mapping the structural core of human cerebral cortex. *PLoS biol.*, 6(7), e159 (2008).

19. Winston, G. P., Yogarajah, M., Symms, M. R., et al. Diffusion tensor imaging tractography to visualize the relationship of the optic radiation to epileptogenic lesions prior to neurosurgery. *Epilepsia*, 52(8), 1430-8 (2011).

20. Winston, G. P., Daga, P., Stretton, J., et al. Optic radiation tractography and vision in anterior temporal lobe resection. *Ann. Neurol.*, 71 (3), 334–41 (2012).

21. Taylor, P. N., Sinha, N., Wang, Y., et al. The impact of epilepsy surgery on the structural connectome and its relation to outcome. *Neuroimage Clin.*, 18, 202–14 (2018).

22. Ahmadi, M. E., Hagler, D.J., McDonald, C. R., et al. Side matters: diffusion tensor imaging tractography in left and right temporal lobe epilepsy. *Am. J. Neuroradiol.*, 30(9), 1740–7 (2009).

23. Concha, L., Beaulieu, C., and Gross, D. W. Bilateral limbic diffusion abnormalities in unilateral temporal lobe epilepsy. *Ann. Neurol.*, 57(2), 188–96 (2005).

24. Bonilha, L., Nesland, T., Martz, G. U., et al. Medial temporal lobe epilepsy is associated with neuronal fibre loss and paradoxical increase in structural connectivity of limbic structures. *J. Neurol. Neurosurg. Psychiatry*, 83(9), 903–9 (2012).

25. Besson, P., Dinkelacker, V., Valabregue, R., et al. Structural connectivity differences in left and right temporal lobe epilepsy. *Neuroimage*, 100, 135–44 (2014).

26. DeSalvo, M. N., Douw, L., Tanaka, N., Reinsberger, C., and Stufflebeam, S. M. Altered structural connectome in temporal lobe epilepsy. *Radiology*, 270(3), 842–8 (2014).

27. Honey, C. J., and Sporns, O. Dynamical consequences of lesions in cortical networks. *Hum. Brain Mapp.*, 29(7), 802–9 (2008).

28. de Tisi, J., Bell, G. S., Peacock, J. L., et al. The long-term outcome of adult epilepsy surgery, patterns of seizure remission, and relapse: A cohort study. *Lancet*, 378 (9800), 1388–95 (2011).

29. Jirsa, V. K., Proix, T., Perdikis, D., et al. The virtual epileptic patient: individualized whole-brain models of epilepsy

spread. *Neuroimage*, 145, 377–88 (2017).

30. Jirsa, V. K., Stacey, W. C., Quilichini, P. P., Ivanov, A. I., and Bernard, C. On the nature of seizure dynamics. *Brain*, 137 (8), 2210–30 (2014).

31. Proix, T., Bartolomei, F., Guye, M., and Jirsa, V. K. Individual brain structure and modelling predict seizure propagation. *Brain*, 140(3), 641–54 (2017).

32. Proix, T., Jirsa, V. K., Bartolomei, F., Guye, M., and Truccolo, W. Predicting the spatiotemporal diversity of seizure propagation and termination in human focal epilepsy. *Nat. Commun.*, 9(1), 1088 (2018).

33. Yan, B., and Li, P. The emergence of abnormal hypersynchronization in the anatomical structural network of human brain. *Neuroimage*, 65, 34–51 (2013).

34. Taylor, P. N., Goodfellow, M., Wang, Y., and Baier, G. Towards a large-scale model of patient- specific epileptic spike-wave discharges. *Biol. Cybern.*, 107, 83–94 (2013).

35. Lu, J., Guo, S., Chen, M., Wang, W., Yang, H., Guo, D., & Yao, D. (2018). Generate the scale-free brain music from BOLD signals. *Medicine*, 97(2).

36. Abdelnour, F., Mueller, S., and Raj, A. Relating cortical atrophy in temporal lobe epilepsy with graph diffusion-based network models. *PLoS Comput. Biol.*, 11(10), e1004564 (2015).

37. Javidan, Manouchehr. Electroencephalography in mesial temporal lobe epilepsy: A review. *Epilepsy Res. Treat.*, 2012, 637430 (2012).

38. Taussig, D., Montavont, A., and Isnard, J. Invasive EEG explorations. *Neurophysiologie Clinique/Clinical*

Neurophysiology, 45(1), 113–9 (2015).

39. Sinha, N., Dauwels, J., Wang, Y., Cash, S. S., and Taylor, P. An in silico approach for pre-surgical evaluation of an epileptic cortex. *Annu. Int. Conf. IEEE Eng. Med. Biol. Soc.*, 2014, 4884–7 (2014).

40. Goodfellow, M., Rummel, C., Abela, E., et al. Estimation of brain network ictogenicity predicts outcome from epilepsy surgery. *Scientific reports*, 6, 29215 (2016).

41. Lopes, M. A., Richardson, M. P., Abela, E. An optimal strategy for epilepsy surgery: Disruption of the rich-club? *PLoS Comput. Biol.*, 13 (8), e1005637 (2017).

42. Yang, C., Luan, G., Wang, Q., et al. localization of epileptogenic zone with the correction of pathological networks. *Front. Neurol.*, 9, 143 (2018).

43. Khambhati, A. N., Davis, K. A., Lucas, T. H., Litt, B., and Bassett, D. S. Virtual cortical resection reveals push-pull network control preceding seizure evolution. *Neuron*, 91 (5), 1170–82 (2016).

44. Burns, S.P., Santaniello, S., Yaffe, R.B., et al. Network dynamics of the brain and influence of the epileptic seizure onset zone. *Proc. Nat. Acad. Sci.*, 111(49), E5321–30 (2014).

45. Kramer, M. A., Eden, U.T., Kolaczyk, E.D., et al. Coalescence and fragmentation of cortical networks during focal seizures. *J. Neurosci.*, 30 (30), 10076–85 (2010).

46. Benjamin, O., Fitzgerald, T. H., Ashwin, P., et al. A phenomenological model of seizure initiation suggests network structure may explain seizure frequency in idiopathic

generalised epilepsy. *J. Math. Neurosci.*, 2(1), 1 (2012).

47. Schmidt, H., Petkov, G., Richardson, M. P., and Terry, J. R. Dynamics on networks: The role of local dynamics and global networks on the emergence of hypersynchronous neural activity. *PLoS Comput. Biol.*, 10 (11), e1003947 (2014).

48. Taylor, P., Baier, G., Cash, S., et al. A model of stimulus induced epileptic spike-wave discharges. *2013 IEEE Symposium Computational Intelligence, Cognitive Algorithms, Mind and Brain.* 53–59 (2013). doi:10.1109/ccmb.2013.6609165.

49. Zheng, T. W., O'Brien, T. J., Morris, M. J., et al. Rhythmic neuronal activity in S2 somatosensory and insular cortices contribute to the initiation of absence-related spike-and-wave discharges. *Epilepsia*, 53(11), 1–11 (2012).

50. Wendling, F., Bartolomei, F., Bellanger, J. J., and Chauvel, P. Epileptic fast activity can be explained by a model of impaired GABAergic dendritic inhibition. *Eur. J. Neurosci.*, 15, 1499–1508 (2002).

51. Hebbink, J., Meijer, H., Huiskamp, G., van Gils, S., and Leijten, F. Phenomenological network models: Lessons for epilepsy surgery. *Epilepsia*, 58, e147–51 (2017).

52. Smith, E. H., and Schevon, C. A. Toward a mechanistic understanding of epileptic networks. *Curr. Neurol. Neurosci. Rep.*, 16(11), 97 (2016).

53. Ridley, B., Wirsich, J., Bettus, G., et al. Simultaneous intracranial EEG-fMRI shows inter-modality correlation in time-resolved connectivity within normal areas but not

within epileptic regions. *Brain Topogr.*, 30(5), 639–55 (2017).

54. Papadopoulou, M., Leite, M., van Mierlo, P., et al. Tracking slow modulations in synaptic gain using dynamic causal modelling: Validation in epilepsy. *Neuroimage*, 107, 117–26 (2015).

55. Papadopoulou, M., Cooray, G., Rosch, R., et al. Dynamic causal modelling of seizure activity in a rat model. *Neuroimage*, 146, 518–32 (2017).

56. Rosch, R. E., Wright, S., Cooray, G., et al. NMDA-receptor antibodies alter cortical microcircuit dynamics. *Proc. Nat. Acad. Sci.*, 115(42), E9916–25 (2018).

57. Karoly, P.J., Kuhlmann, L., Soudry, D., et al. Seizure pathways: A model-based investigation. *PLoS Comput. Biol.*, 14(10), e1006403. (2018).

58. Aarabi, A., and He, B. Seizure prediction in hippocampal and neocortical epilepsy using a model-based approach. *Clin. Neurophysiol.*, 125(5), 930–40 (2014).

59. Wendling, F., Hernandez, A., Bellanger, J. J., Chauvel, P., and Bartolomei, F. Interictal to ictal transition in human temporal lobe epilepsy: insights from a computational model of intracerebral EEG. *J. Clin. Neurophysiol.*, 22(5), 343–56 (2005).

60. Freestone, D. R., Karoly, P. J., Nešić, D., et al. Estimation of effective connectivity via data-driven neural modeling. *Front. Neurosci.*, 8, 383 (2014).

61. Stephan, K. E., Tittgemeyer, M., Knösche, T. R., Moran, R. J., and Friston, K. J. Tractography-based priors for dynamic causal models. *Neuroimage*, 47(4), 1628–38 (2009).

62. Raj, A., Kuceyeski, A., and Weiner, M. A network diffusion model of disease progression in dementia. *Neuron*, 73(6), 1204–15 (2012).

63. Young, A.L., Oxtoby, N.P., Daga, P., et al. A data-driven model of biomarker changes in sporadic Alzheimer's disease. *Brain*, 137(9), 2564–77 (2014).

64. Wu, X., and Ma, J. J. Sodium valproate: Quantitative EEG and serum levels in volunteers and epileptics. *Clin. Electroencephalogr.*, 24(2), 93–9 (1993).

65. Pardoe, Heath R., Berg, Anne T., and Jackson, Graeme D. Sodium valproate use is associated with reduced parietal lobe thickness and brain volume. *Neurology*, 80 (20), 1895–1900 (2013).

66. Alberti, P., and Cavaletti, G. Management of side effects in the personalized medicine era: chemotherapy-induced peripheral neuropathy. In *Pharmacogenomics in Drug Discovery and Development*. New York, NY: Humana Press. 2014. pp. 301–22.

67. Cook, M. J., Karoly, P. J., Freestone, D. R., et al. Human focal seizures are characterized by populations of fixed duration and interval. *Epilepsia*, 57(3), 359–68 (2016).

68. Bazil, C. W., and Walczak, T.S. Effects of sleep and sleep stage on epileptic and nonepileptic seizures. *Epilepsia*, 38(1), 56–62 (1997).

69. Karoly, Philippa J., Nurse, Ewan S., Freestone, Dean R., et al. Bursts of seizures in long-term recordings of human focal epilepsy. *Epilepsia* 58(3), 363–72 (2017).

70. Ewell, L.A., Liang, L., Armstrong, C., et al. Brain state is a major factor in preseizure hippocampal network activity and influences success of seizure intervention. *J. Neurosci.*, 35(47), 15635–48 (2015).

The Baseline and Epileptiform EEG
A Complex Systems Approach

Giridhar P. Kalamangalam and Mircea I. Chelaru

6.1 Introduction

Many will trace the earliest articulation of what we may today call the science of complexity to Weaver's [1] classic essay. In this work, Weaver distinguished between (i) the science of "simplicity" with phenomena that could be understood when reduced to a few variables, such as classical mechanics in two dimensions, (ii) the science of "disorganized complexity" concerning systems with large numbers of variables analyzed by a process of averaging, such as statistical thermodynamics, and (iii) an emerging field of "organized complex" systems, also with large numbers of variables, that was not amenable to either approach. This third middle region, Weaver wrote, would form the next significant challenge for science, needing both the power of machines (computers) and large interdisciplinary scientific teams for progress. Today, the field of complex systems, though lacking a universally accepted definition, studies entities – physical, biological, or social – united by the presence of large numbers of nonlinearly interacting agents that yield collective behavior not directly predictable from the laws governing interactions of the individual agents [2]. The thesis of complexity is therefore in direct opposition to the philosophy of reductionism and the source of an important debate regarding the foundations of science itself [3]. Examples of collective behavior in complex systems include, for instance, the "emergent" phenomena of macroscopic patterns [4] and phase transitions [5]. These coherent structures occur at scales far removed from those governing the interaction of the individual entities of the system and are due to bifurcation and symmetry breaking [6] involving macroscopic "collective" variables. On the other hand, the large size and nonlinearity of complex systems endow them with a measure of unpredictability – arising from deterministic chaos as well as inherent "fluctuations" – that naturally invokes a probabilistic

description. Complex systems are thus said to have an "open" future that generates information and "surprise" as they evolve [7].

In neuroscience, the notions of complexity were arguably implicit in Sherrington's evocative "enchanted loom" metaphor [8]; recent decades have seen more explicit application of the field's central ideas [9]. The metaphor of complexity may resonate particularly with epileptologists: the cellular components of the brain and its pathways are nothing if not nonlinear (from the all-or-none character of the action potential in individual neurons to the thresholding, adaptive, and saturating characteristics of neuronal populations), multi-component (millions of neurons and orders of magnitude more synapses in even a cubic centimeter of cortical tissue), energy-consuming ("far-from-equilibrium") and pattern-forming at a macroscopic level (e.g., the rhythms of the EEG). In this article we introduce the EEG as a complex system, and follow this with two example applications to real scalp and intracranial data. We end with a brief general discussion.

6.2 Pattern Formation in EEG

Figure 6.1A shows a single 10-second epoch of resting scalp EEG in an adult subject whose eyes are closed. This depiction – often the first visual image presented to the new student of EEG – shows the alpha rhythm in the posterior head regions (the channel P4-O2, for example) as an undulating sinusoidal oscillation. The alpha rhythm was the first-discovered of such "resting" rhythms of the brain – two others are beta over the frontocentral regions and mu over the Rolandic area [10]. The alpha can be recorded from all over the back of the head with scalp electrodes, though it is best defined in the posterior-most channels. It appears in the first six months of life, persists through the healthy lifespan and is stable on short time scales: eye

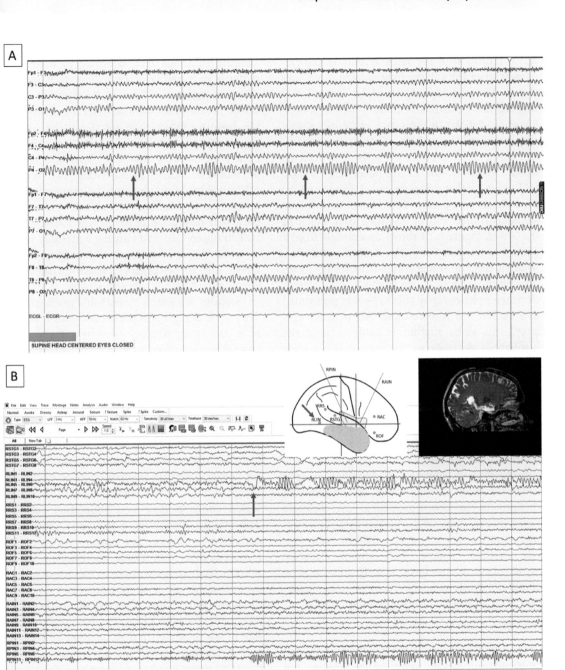

Figure 6.1 Behavior of the alpha rhythm at different spatial scales. A) 10-s scalp EEG page (longitudinal bipolar montage, gain 7μV/ mm) in a normal subject resting with eyes closed. The alpha is seen as a near-perfect modulated sinusoid in the posterior derivations. B) The alpha rhythm in the intracranial EEG, seen in an SEEG implant undertaken to investigate seizure recurrence in a patient with previous right anterior temporal lobe resection. The implant scheme (inset left) shows the region of previous resection (shaded gray) with orange dots and straight lines indicating planned electrode trajectories. Sagittal view of the medial right hemisphere of the pre-operative MRI volume with the reconstructed electrodes in situ (inset right) shows the position of the entry of the electrodes including the medial contacts of the lingular electrode (red arrow) that is situated in the posterior cortex. These are also shown on the implant scheme. The EEG page shows the right-sided SEEG channels in bipolar montage (gain 30 μV/mm; passband 3–70 Hz; gridlines are spaced apart by 1s). Mid-page, the patient is asked to close the eyes and stop moving: the visual alpha rhythm immediately appears (red arrow) as ~10 Hz sinusoidal oscillation maximum in the RLIN5-RLIN6 derivation. That the alpha rhythm exists in bipolar montages in both scalp and intracranial EEG suggests the alpha rhythm is not a unitary entity, but as a hierarchy spanning a spatial scale of at least an order of magnitude (see text).

opening and the transition to sleep abolishes it, and it returns with the same amplitude and frequency when the subject fully awakens with eyes closed. The stability of the alpha immediately suggests it is an attractive limit cycle (i.e., a nonlinear oscillation) in the phase space of suitably chosen collective variables. What dynamic elements cooperate to produce the scalp-EEG detected alpha? Studies by the EEG pioneer Grey Walter [11] revealed that when recorded intracranially, the alpha is not a unitary rhythm, but that various alpha "rhythms" can be recorded over much of the cortex. Figure 6.1B shows an example from a patient in our practice with an intracranial electrode in their posterior cortex (this study – with indwelling depth electrodes – stereo-electroencephalography (SEEG) – was performed as a clinical test to investigate this patient's epilepsy). An alpha rhythm is easily seen at the highlighted electrode as the patient closes their eyes. Yet the receptive field of an intracranial electrode contact is under a cubic centimeter, an order of magnitude smaller than that of a scalp electrode [12,13]. Thus, the alpha must be hierarchical – a macroscopic scalp-EEG alpha comprises the "superposition" of alpha rhythms at smaller spatial scales across the cortex. This superposition is evidently a combination of a neurophysiological interaction of neighboring rhythms in the brain, as well as the algebraic superposition imposed by a single recording electrode contact whose receptive field includes several rhythms. Figure 6.1A shows algebraic superposition at the level of scalp EEG: a slow amplitude modulation of the sinusoidal oscillation. That is, if we consider the sum

$$A \sin kt + A \sin (k + 2\delta)t$$

of two neighboring alpha sub-oscillations of equal amplitude but slightly different frequencies, the resultant oscillation

$$2A \sin (k + \delta)t \cos \delta t$$

is a slowly-modulated sinusoid of an intermediate frequency for small δ. The waxing and waning characteristic of the alpha rhythm constitutes its essential clinical description: the consideration of alpha rhythm families suggests how such amplitude modulation naturally arises. If the sub-alpha rhythms were instead coherent over a larger surface area of the cortex, the scalp electrode would record an unmodulated rhythm. How might such

spatial coherence arise? Here, we are not considering sinusoids that summate to modulated patterns in a particular recording electrode, but rather an interaction between the rhythms themselves in the brain, so that interacting rhythms synchronize, rather than interfere. The idea of the emergence of alpha as the collective oscillation of a population of sub-oscillations is originally attributed to Wiener in the 1950s [14]. Winfree [15] developed the "phase-model" approximation to analyze populations of coupled oscillators, a particular realization of which was solved exactly by Kuramoto [16]. We visit the Kuramoto model in some detail below, not with respect to the alpha, but an "emergent" behavior that is the epileptologist's daily concern: seizure.

Seizures are a truly remarkable phenomenon. They arise abruptly from the background activity of a generating network of neural tissue as an ensemble oscillation, evolving in frequency and spatial extent before subsiding (typically also abruptly). The wide variety of brain pathologies associated with seizures (e.g., tumor, stroke, cortical dysplasia), and the occurrence of seizures without brain pathology at all but as a consequence of systemic illness (e.g., seizures in the neonate from hypoglycemia), indicate that the tendency for seizure is perhaps implicit in the normal operating mechanisms of the brain. That is, the physiological cortex is close to a bifurcation point to pathological behavior along an inhibition-excitation continuum. For clinicians dealing with human epilepsy there is little opportunity to methodically study transitions across this hypothesized bifurcation point, with the exception of after-discharge (AD). First observed by Adrian [17], ADs are paroxysms of local epileptiform activity that follow focal electrical stimulation of the cerebral cortex that typically last a few seconds before reverting to the baseline. ADs are visually striking on the EEG directly recorded from the brain surface (the electrocorticogram; ECoG) as large-amplitude, well-organized rhythms that stand out from the baseline. Early simultaneous microelectrode and surface EEG recordings [18] established that ADs are rhythmic large-scale fluctuations of the local field potential that, at onset, are independent of individual neuronal action potentials but later synchronously entrain single units. ADs in human subjects are commonly observed during cortical stimulation mapping (CSM) carried out for localization of eloquent function prior to resective surgery for refractory focal epilepsy or brain tumors [19]. Stimulation parameter prerequisites for ADs are, in general, sufficient current intensity (amperage) and stimulus duration [20]. In patients with partial epilepsy, as in animal experiments, ADs are readily elicited over normal brain areas, but are seen at lower stimulation thresholds in proximity to epileptic foci [21]. In addition, seizure-like symptoms may be seen with ADs occurring over eloquent cortex [22], and indeed ADs may evolve to full-blown seizures. For these reasons, cortical stimulation mapping seeks to minimize the occurrence of ADs, though it is not uncommon for a few ADs to occur in a typical mapping session. Despite their immediacy to processes underlying localization-related epilepsy, and a wealth of observation since Adrian's original report, ADs historically remained poorly understood. Their phenomenology at a more abstract level however is clear: the baseline EEG is a mix of rhythms, and the electrical stimulation somehow disrupts this tendency for a mixture to create a synchronous ensemble that persists for a few seconds before returning to the baseline mix. We therefore suggested that ADs might be a collective oscillation [23], arising similarly to the process studied by Wiener, Winfree, and Kuramoto [14–16]. Viewing the time domain baseline ECoG as a distribution of modes in the frequency domain, we proposed ADs as arising by "condensation" of distribution into a tighter grouping to yield a rhythm more narrowly centered around an average mode. In the extreme case, the distribution would collapse into a single frequency, yielding a pure sine wave in the time domain. Conversely, when the effect of the stimulation wore off, the condensed cluster of frequencies would spread out again and the mixed-frequency baseline ECoG would reassert itself in the time domain. A key prediction of such a theory was that the dominant frequency of the condensed cluster (the AD) would arise from within the original mix and this was verified to be the case. Fuller details are provided in [23], but in brief we performed a systematic review of ECoG AD data acquired in 15 epilepsy patients undergoing extra-operative cortical stimulation mapping with subdural grid electrodes. Single-channel power spectra of length-matched AD epochs, baseline epochs, and epochs following sub-threshold stimulation were computed. We found that the major power peak in the baseline epoch was indeed more pronounced

in the AD spectrum, with less of a distribution around the mean, minor variable shift of the mean itself, and relatively reduced power in frequencies away from the mean. Figure 6.2A illustrates an example. Other details outside the scheme developed above, such the presence of harmonic frequencies of the main power AD peak, the presence of multiple AD morphologies, and the spontaneous "switching" of one morphology to another within the same AD, are discussed in [23].

As a model of spectral condensation underlying AD, we consider the Kuramoto formalism describing the phases of a system of N oscillators

$$\dot{\theta}_n = \omega_n, \quad n = 1, 2, 3, \ldots N,$$

where the dot represents the time derivative, with each oscillator's intrinsic frequency assumed to be drawn from a distribution with a certain mean and variance. For the human alpha rhythm in a single individual this might be a distribution in the range 9–11 Hz, for example. The oscillators are assumed to interact with each other in an equal "all-to-all" fashion, and with the interaction term being a sinusoidal function of the phase differences, such that we have the system

$$\dot{\theta}_n = \omega_n + \frac{k}{N} \sum_{m=1}^{N} \sin(\theta_n - \theta_m), \, m = 1, 2, 3, \ldots N.$$

Here, the coupling parameter k determines the degree of "binding" of an oscillator to the rest of the population. For $k = 0$ the system is globally decoupled; each oscillator runs free and the ensemble rhythm is their algebraic sum. As k increases from zero, the oscillators begin to increasingly influence each other until a critical value of k is crossed and the system synchronizes into a unitary rhythm. Figure 6.3A–C shows computer simulations of the Kuramoto model for $N = 20$ oscillators for linearly increasing, and then decreasing, k. Synchronization is readily appreciated as the sharply defined sinusoidal rhythm in the middle of the time segment (Fig. 6.3A); Fig. 6.3C shows the growth of the "order parameter" φ defined by

$$\varphi = \left| \sum_{n=1}^{N} e^{i\theta_n} \right|$$

to its asymptotic value of 20 as k increases beyond ≈ 15. The spectral peak at synchronization is seen near the middle of the original frequency mix (Fig. 6.3B).

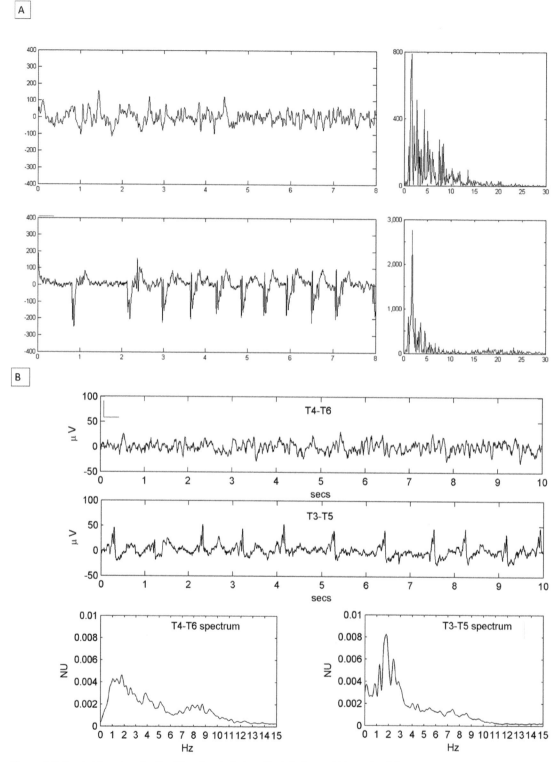

Figure 6.2 Spectral "condensation" in AD and periodic lateralized discharge. A) Example of the "condensation" relationship between the baseline electrocorticogram and the ensuing AD following supra-threshold stimulation. (Top left) An 8-second epoch from a single channel of a lateral temporal subdural grid electrode contact, prior to any stimulation. *x*-axis: time (seconds); *y*-axis:

Is there evidence of a Kuramoto-like process occurring in the cortex to create AD? Single pulses of stimulating current applied to the cerebral cortex, if sufficiently strong, cause depolarization of single units; high frequency currents cause repetitive depolarization that is rate-limited only by the neurons' absolute refractory period [24]. If carried out for a sufficient length of time, high frequency (> 15 Hz) stimulation leads to a state of synaptic depression that suppresses further action potentials; it is from this state of local cortical neural "exhaustion" that AD emerges [20]. Between the two main single unit types in the cortex (principal cells and interneurons) action potential thresholds are lower in interneurons [25]. It is plausible that prolonged repetitive stimulation exhausts interneurons more than other neuronal populations, and following sustained stimulation, interneurons lag behind principal units in recovery, and the cortex for a brief period of time is inhibition-deficient. That is, high frequency (≈50 Hz) electrical stimulation may "homogenize" the cortical volume around the stimulating contact by weakening inhibitory interactions more than excitatory ones to create a uniform excitatory "mean field." Adjacent local field potentials, no longer walled off from one other by inhibitory influence, readily phase-lock into a common rhythm. The constructive effect of phase-locking causes neighboring amplitudes to add up on average, producing a large-amplitude ensemble rhythm that stands out from the background ECoG. The later recovery of interneurons re-establishes the inhibitory interactions between adjacent cortical domains; inter-LFP coupling weakens and the AD desynchronizes to the baseline ECoG. In the Kuramoto metaphor, k, the coupling constant that favors synchronization increases due to the lack of mutual inhibition in the post-stimulation period and synchronization occurs. k decreases as inhibition returns and the system subsequently desynchronizes (Fig. 6.3A–B).

The spatial scale at which ADs occur are those determined by the dimensions of typical intracranial electrode implants. Intracranial electrode contacts (through which CSM is performed) are commonly a few millimeters apart within a single electrode, and adjacent electrodes may be separated by distances of the order of a centimeter. When CSM is applied between contacts of adjacent electrodes, ADs are typically seen at those contacts, though they may also be seen at distant electrode sites that are connected (through white matter pathways) to the primary site of stimulation. Regardless, one may approximate the scale of the electrodes to the scale of the AD phenomenon. Given the discussion about alpha rhythm above, and the presence of various alpha "rhythms" across the brain at multiple spatial hierarchies, one may ask whether AD-like phenomena occur at other scales in the brain. Remarkably, the answer seems to be yes. Originally called periodic lateralized epileptiform discharges (PLEDs) when they were described over 50 years ago [26], whole-brain AD-like events are large (100–300 μV or higher), sharp, and repetitive (usually close to 1 Hz) potential on scalp EEG, usually seen in patients with serial seizures and acute structural brain lesions, and may be present for hours or days. A significant descriptive literature exists on lateralized periodic discharges (LPDs) as the EEG signature of an unstable brain state related to the combination of one or more of seizures, structural injury, and metabolic derangement [27]. Yet – like ADs – it was unclear why they occur at all, let alone what factors determine their periodicity, large amplitude and sharp contour, and association with seizures. We do not know of a neurophysiological

---

Figure 6.2 (cont.) waveform amplitudes referenced to a common average (μvolts). (Top right) The power spectrum of the baseline epoch is an irregular mix of components that is biased toward the lower frequencies. x-axis: frequency (Hz); y-axis: power spectral density (μvolts2/Hz). (Bottom left) An 8-second AD elicited by a 6 mA stimulus at the same electrode. (Bottom right) The AD's power spectrum is a "condensed" version of the baseline spectrum: less spread out, more sharply peaked, and of much greater amplitude at the maximum, as if the spectral modes comprising the baseline had coalesced toward a common average. B) LPD (PLED) in a patient with an acute left posterior quadrant lobar hemorrhage. (Top) A10-s EEG epoch from the normal right hemispheric mid-temporal derivation, showing a mix of polymorphic fast and slow rhythms and irregular larger amplitude transients. (Middle) A typical epoch of the homologous left mid-temporal chain showing LPDs at frequency ~1 Hz. (Bottom left) Power spectrum of the entire T4-T6 EEG epoch. The spectrum is wide-band with broad maxima in the δ and α Berger bands, the latter indicating a preserved posterior dominant rhythm. (Bottom right) Power spectrum of the entire T3-T5 EEG epoch. Comparison of the spectra illustrates spectral condensation, with the broad δ band of the normal side appearing to coalesce into sharply defined peaks in the LPD spectrum. Indeed, the small local maximum on the normal side (at ~2 Hz) "grows" in the same location into the dominant frequency component of the LPD.

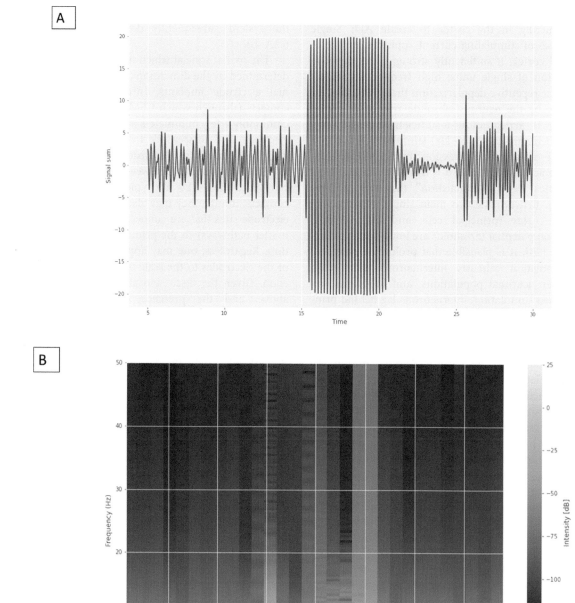

Figure 6.3 Numerical simulation of N=20 Kuramoto oscillators. The initial frequencies of the oscillators are chosen from a uniform distribution spanning the range 3–7 Hz, with k=0 initially and rapidly increasing linearly beyond t=15, and reducing to zero starting at t=20. A) The ensemble signal is a mixed frequency sum of the initial oscillator distribution until t=15. The ensemble synchronizes rapidly thereafter to yield a monomorphic high amplitude rhythm at ≈5 Hz, thereafter desynchronizing rapidly at t>20 as k is reduced to zero. B) Spectrogram to follow the changes described in A) above. The yellow band of frequencies at t<15 coalesces into a single narrow band at ≈5 Hz; the frequencies disperse at t >20 as k is reduced. C) Behavior of the order parameter φ for increasing k. It grows rapidly beyond k≈15 to its asymptotic maximum of φ=20.

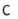

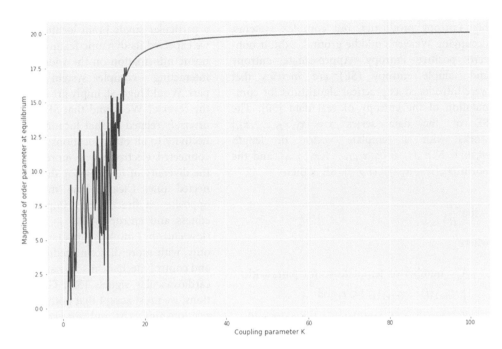

Figure 6.3 *(cont.)*

continuum that traces a path from AD to LPD in terms of cell populations and network architecture, but to us there was an unambiguous phenomenological similarity between ADs and LPDs. We sought therefore to explore the prediction of a Kuramoto-like mechanism to LPDs by evaluating the position of the maxima of the spectra of scalp EEG tracings between channels of the EEG showing LPDs in relation to those that were LPD-free. We refer to [28] for details, but the data-processing approach was similar to [23]. Scalp EEG data from 22 patients with EEG LPDs were analyzed. All patients were hospitalized with the usual range of conditions associated with LPDs – acute brain lesions (commonly hemorrhage or tumor) or chronic brain lesions with seizures. Comparison of power spectra of regular LPDs with those derived from length-matched non-LPD EEG epochs from the homologous channel again revealed the "condensation" of the spectrum: the major power peak in the contralateral spectrum was represented more prominently in the LPD spectrum, with less of a distribution around the mean, variable but modest shift of the mean itself, and relatively reduced power in frequencies away from the mean (Fig. 6.2B).

The emergence of macroscopic coherence in complex systems is one of the chief fascinations of the discipline. In fact, the field of clinical EEG may be thought of as the classification of coherent waveforms corresponding to physiological and pathological brain states. The examples of AD and LPD demonstrate the capacity for even basic complex-systems inspired analytic methods to yield insight not obtainable by purely descriptive accounts of the biology.

6.3 Statistical Complexity in EEG

A complementary approach to complex systems seeks to diagnose or characterize these systems by observables. Here, one is less concerned with modeling the components of the system to explain behavior. The focus instead is to obtain a signature, or metric, of complexity. For dynamical systems, one such metric is the Kolmogorov–Sinai (KS) entropy, a measure of the uncertainty or information content associated with successive values of the dynamical variables [29]. Fully deterministic noise-free dynamical systems have zero KS entropy. Heuristically, their future is already known from the equations of motion and initial

79

conditions and they do not "produce" new information as they evolve. Stochastic systems are high-entropy producing, but complex systems, occupying Weaver's middle ground, exhibit non-zero positive entropy. Approximate entropy and sample entropy (SE) are metrics that were introduced as practical algorithms for computation of the entropy of real data [30]. The SE of the data series $x = [x_1, x_2, \ldots, x_N]$ works with a template vector of length $m, m \ll N, x_m(i) = [x_i, x_{i+1}, \ldots, x_{i+m-1}]$, and the norm $|x_m(i) - x_m(j)|$ $(i \neq j)$. SE is then

$$-\log \frac{A}{B},$$

where

A = number of template vector pairs with $| x_{m+1}(i) - x_{m+1}(j) | < r$, and

B = number of template vector pairs with $| x_m(i) - x_m(j) | < r$.

The embedding dimension, m, is an estimate of the length of feature being diagnosed, and r, the tolerance, is the allowable error between similar features. Conventional choices are $m = 2$ and $r = 0.2$. SE was originally introduced as a metric to quantify irregularity in physiological time series [31], for example to serve as a diagnostic to distinguish healthy from diseased states. Small (close to zero) values of SE imply more frequent instances of patterns, recognizable features or regularity in the data, and large positive values imply greater randomness, information content, or irregularity.

With respect to EEG, one might expect SE to follow the conventionally-described differences in EEG between brain states, and within brain regions during the same state. An example of the former would be the difference between the wake and sleep EEG at a particular location; an example of the latter would be the abundance of alpha over the posterior cortex in contrast to the frontal lobe. Our motive in what follows was not simply to document the variation in SE in different brain regions, but to relate the computed SE to an aspect of the EEG that underlay its complexity – the connectivity of that particular recorded brain region. The assumption was that the EEG at a brain location would be influenced by its wider network of connections and aspects of the network would be reflected, or diagnosable, from activity at just a single location. Thus, considering a particular single brain location as a "variable," we expected its dynamic features to provide diagnostic information on the wider – multivariable, interacting – complex system of which it was a part. Would high SE imply greater connectivity or the reverse? We found that SE at a location was *inversely* related to that location's averaged connectivity to all other locations, implying a highly connected electrode was more "constrained" in the diversity of its behavior than a sparsely connected one. Clearly, one might imagine the opposite – a direct relationship between connectedness and entropy. That is, greater regularity (low entropy) implying greater subsystem autonomy, with more disconnectedness from coupling and control mechanisms, as has been described in cardiovascular signals [32]. Given our observations, we must accept that both direct and inverse relationships exist and are eventually dependent on the nature of the system: the particular dynamics of the variable involved and the pattern of coupling. For instance, a self-oscillating system, say the signal from a small cortical region generating an intrinsic rhythm, when connected to sources of neural noise, might indeed exhibit more entropy when coupled than when in a free-running mode. On the other hand, a cortical region with highly complex intrinsic dynamics and exhibiting wide-band signals might decrease its entropy when networked to a regularly oscillating external influence. This issue of connectivity and entropy abuts an important theme in the field that we do not address but return to briefly in Section 6.4. This is the issue of topology and individual detail – the internal architecture of a complex system with its specific pattern of interactions – in determining system dynamics.

We [33] studied SE and connectivity of resting state intracranial EEG data from the lateral frontal lobe from seven patients denoted S1–S7 undergoing subdural grid evaluation. The latter are a type of intracranial EEG recording – different to the SEEG technique alluded to earlier – where arrays of recording electrodes are placed directly over the cortex through an opening in the skull (craniotomy). Figure 6.4 illustrates the reconstructed positions and size of the lateral frontal grid for all seven patients, projected on their individual reconstructed brain surfaces. The yellow line marks the position of the central (Rolandic)

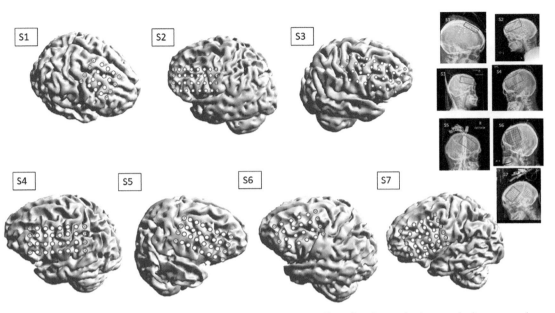

Figure 6.4 Representations of cortical surfaces of the subject group S1–S7. The yellow line marks the central sulcus over each cortical surface. Each subject's post-implant skull x-ray is shown in the group to the right, with the entire subdural implant scheme seen as patterned high-attenuation artifact in each image. The blue rectangles in these images denoted the lateral frontal electrode group (grid), whose recordings provided the data presented here.

sulcus in each case, with the gyri immediately in front and behind it representing the primary motor and sensory areas, respectively. The SE of an electrode (electrode SE (ESE)) was computed from the Hilbert amplitude of the EEG time series of that electrode. The Hilbert amplitude of a function $x(t)$ is the magnitude $| Z |$ of the associated analytic function

$$Z(t) = x(t) - i\mathcal{H}(x(t)),$$

where $\mathcal{H}$ denotes the Hilbert transformation, and is the envelope of that function. Functional connectivity between a pair of electrodes for a data epoch was measured with amplitude cross-correlation (ACC), the Pearson correlation of their respective Hilbert amplitudes. At time point n we defined the *electrode connectivity* (EC) of a certain electrode as the average of its functional connectivity with all the other electrodes of the grid over a 5-s epoch starting at n. The time dependence of EC was computed in moving windows of 5s that overlapped by 4s that yielded a value of EC every second. Figure 6.5A–D are heat maps of the EC-ESE results for subject S2, one for each of the wake and sleep states. The disposition of the frontal grid electrodes is redrawn from this subject's reconstructed lateral brain surface (Fig. 6.4), with the central sulcus

marked in yellow. The cortical connectivity pattern in the wake and sleep states (5A–B) are highly congruent. A reciprocal relationship between mEC and mSE is clearly seen in the sleep state (compare 5B–D), where areas of heat and cold literally "exchange places" on the brain surface. This reciprocal relationship is present, but somewhat less precise, in the wake state (5A–C). The eight electrode contacts at the posterior portion of the grid have the lowest (highest) ECs (ESEs) of all, and these are seen to be overlying lower peri-Rolandic sensorimotor cortex. Figure 6.6 shows all values of EC and ESE for all seven subjects S1–S7. Each separate figure consists of two scatter plots, one each for the wake (red) and sleep (blue) conditions. Each dot represents the ordered pair (ESE, EC) values for a single 5-s epoch. Given that ESE and EC were computed every second for every electrode, the number of data points in each scatter plot is the number of seconds in the concatenated (awake or asleep) data multiplied by the number of electrodes. The inverse relationship between ESE and EC is clear in every case, with a trend for the effect to be larger in the sleep state.

We believe these results are interesting for two reasons. First, a *local* measure of signal complexity – SE of the EEG from a particular brain

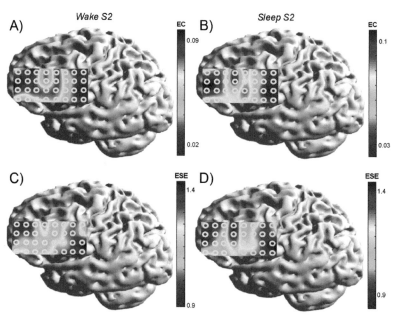

Figure 6.5 Heat maps showing the spatial variation of mean EC and mean SE over the lateral frontal cortex of subject S2. Wake states are to the left, sleep states to the right. Top-down comparisons (A–C and B–D) reveal a reciprocal relation between EC and SE with areas of heat and cold showing a complementary relationship. This reciprocal relationship is particularly vivid in the sleep state, but also clearly appreciated in wakefulness. In addition, electrodes overlying or in closest proximity to the Rolandic area (the posterior two columns of electrodes) have the lowest (highest) ECs (ESEs) values.

location – reflected an aspect of that cortical location's *nonlocal* neurobiological properties (EC), i.e., its averaged network connectivity. Put differently, the novelty or "surprise" metric of an electrode location's dynamics was related to a biologically meaningful "collective variable," its averaged connectivity to the rest of the grid. Second, and from a purely biological standpoint, there was an anterior-posterior (rostro-caudal) gradient in the magnitude of the electrode sample entropy, with lower entropies anteriorly, over the anterior frontal regions, and higher entropies posteriorly, with highest entropies of all being over primary sensorimotor (peri-Rolandic) cortex. This finding of such a gradient is in fact concordant with a number of other studies that document a "rostro-caudal axis" to the organization in the human frontal lobe [34,35], thought to relate to development and myelination of the neocortex and its functional specialization in the adult.

6.4 Conclusions

We have alluded to the spatiotemporal patterns constituting the clinical study of EEG – the cataloging of myriad waveform types that relate to age, brain state, and disease. We have also briefly considered the probabilistic (entropic) aspects of the EEG. The complex systems approach now asks why and how these features arise from the population of underlying elements. These questions adopt a certain universality of perspective that is independent of specific details in favor of generative mechanisms. It is this "universality" that allowed us to think of ADs, for instance, as the emergence of a collective oscillation. Yet, it is clear that the details do matter and that abstractions have limitations that can quickly become evident. The Kuramoto model for AD, for instance, has no capacity to evolve to seizure, nor indeed exhibit the varieties of AD morphologies that are clinically observed [19,23]. Thus, there is the need for the approach of universality to be tempered and informed by relevant details of the biology of the brain. As emphasized by several authors [3,4,7], it is this interplay of abstraction and experimental observation that is the true spirit of the complex systems approach.

What of applications? For a line of inquiry that has yet to mature in epileptology, the greatest "application" of a complex system perspective is perhaps just that: a perspective. A different issue is whether given the very wide scale of neural operations (from single neurons to cortical columns to the entirety of the cerebral hemisphere) the perspective may differ from scale to scale, or whether the brain exhibits Simon's [36] hierarchical organization of "near-decomposability." The latter is the notion that complex systems are fundamentally defined by a hierarchy of scales, and that interactions within a scale are stronger than interaction across scales. We have the hint of a hierarchy in the

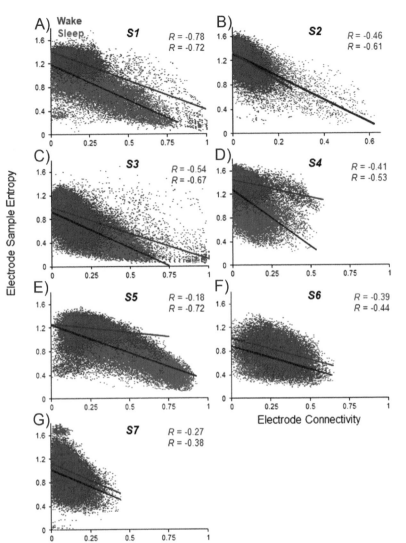

Figure 6.6 A)–G). Scatter plots of all the pairs (EC, ESE) computed from the wake (red) and sleep (blue) states for all the subjects S1–S7, together with regression lines and Pearson correlations R between EC and ESE for the wake (red) and sleep (blue) states.

AD-LPD story above: similar behavior of the spectra with periodicity at widely different spatial scales and fundamentally similar dynamic mechanisms. The emergence of the scalp-EEG alpha as an ensemble of smaller-scale alphas is another instance of hierarchy. Yet another – not discussed here – is the periodicity of spontaneous epileptiform discharge at the AD length scale in foci of cortical dysplasia [37], and at even smaller length and time scales within epileptic foci [38]. Thus, is near-decomposability relevant to brain operations? This is clearly a profound question at the foundations of neuroscience. To turn to a question of clinical applicability, the idea of epilepsy being a "network" disorder is now mainstream, such that even surgical approaches to epilepsy are conditioned by the network hypothesis [39]. Thus, the surgical excision of a diseased epileptic brain area is conceptualized as the removal or disabling of a node in a network, rather than the more conventional view of the excision of a disease focus (as would be, for example, when a brain tumor is removed). If the epileptic network had any more than a few nodes, it would be considered a complex system that evolved on a network. What perspectives of dynamics on complex networks [40] may we bring to focal epilepsy? Can these perspectives reach beyond simple clinical heuristics to advance surgical or neuromodulatory treatments for epilepsy? How can we incorporate knowledge of system topology – the connectomics of brain structure [41–43] – into our understanding of brain dynamics? On the other hand, theory demonstrates that that in Kuramoto-like systems, dynamics may secondarily predict topology [44]; can we use such methods to ascertain self-consistency between the EEG signals we obtain from epileptic foci and their supposed network architecture?

Ending his 1932 Nobel lecture [45], Edgar Adrian – champion of Hans Berger's work on the EEG and discoverer of afterdischarge – remarked "…within the central nervous system the events in each unit are not so important. We are more concerned with the interactions of large numbers, and our problem is to find the way in which such interactions can take place." Adrian's words may be taken as the mission of complex systems research in neuroscience. With their rich store of fundamental problems, the clinical disciplines of EEG and epileptology are an ideal testbed.

Acknowledgement

GPK thanks Mark Ettinger, PhD, for producing Figure 6.3 and for helpful comments on the manuscript.

References

1. Weaver, W. Science and complexity. *Am. Sci.*, 36, 536–44 (1948).

2. Anderson, P. W. More is different. *Science*, 177(4047), 393–6 (1972).

3. Laughlin, R. B., and Pines, D. The theory of everything. *Proc. Natl. Acad. Sci.*, 97(1), 28–31 (2000).

4. Ball, P. *The Self-Made Tapestry: Pattern Formation in Nature*, Oxford: Oxford University Press. 1999.

5. Sole, R. *Phase Transitions*, Princeton, NJ: Princeton University Press. 2011.

6. Nicolis, C., and Prigogine, I. *Exploring Complexity*, New York: WH Freeman. 1984.

7. Nicolis, G., and Nicolis, C. *Foundations of Complex Systems: Emergence, Information and Prediction*. NJ: World Scientific. 2012.

8. Sherrington, C. S. *Man on His Nature*, Cambridge: Cambridge University Press. 1942.

9. Kelso, J. A. S. *Dynamic Patterns: The Self-Organization of Brain and Behavior*, Cambridge, MA: MIT Press. 1995.

10. Chang, B. S. et al. (2011) Normal EEG in wakefulness and sleep. In *Niedermeyer's Electroencephalography* (Schomer, D.L. and Lopes da Silva, F.H. eds), pp. 202–29, New York: Oxford University Press.

11. Grey Walter, W. (1950) Normal rhythms: Their development, distribution and significance. In *Electroencephalography: A Symposium on Its Various Aspects*. (Hill, D. and Parr, G. eds) p. 83, New York: MacMillan.

12. Kahane, P., and Dubeau, F. Intracerebral depth electrode electroencephalography. In *Current Practice of Clinical Electroencephalography* (Ebersole, J. S. ed), pp. 393–441, Philadelphia: Wolters Kluwer. 2014.

13. Tao, J. X., Ray, A., Hawes-Ebersole, S., and Ebersole, J. S. Intracranial EEG substrates of scalp EEG interictal spikes. *Epilepsia*, 46(5), 669–76 (2005).

14. Strogatz, S. H. Norbert Wiener's brain waves. In *Frontiers in Mathematical Biology* (Levin, S. A. ed), pp. 122–38, Berlin: Springer-Verlag. 1994.

15. Winfree, A. T. Biological rhythms and the behavior of populations of coupled oscillators. *J. Theor. Biol.*, 16 (1), 15–42 (1967).

16. Kuramoto, Y. *Chemical Oscillations, Waves, and Turbulence*, Berlin: Springer-Verlag. 1984.

17. Adrian, E. D. The spread of activity in the cerebral cortex. *J. Physiol.* 88, 127–61 (1936).

18. Gerin, P. Microelectrode investigations on the mechanisms of the electrically induced epileptiform seizure ("afterdischarge"). *Arc. It. Biol.*, 98, 21–40 (1960).

19. Blume, W. T., Jones, D. C., and Pathak, P. Properties of after-discharges from cortical electrical stimulation in focal epilepsies. *Clin. Neurophysiol.*, 115(4), 982–9 (2004).

20. Pinsky, C., and Delisle Burns, B. Production of epileptiform after-discharge in cat's cerebral cortex. *J. Neurophysiol*, 25, 359–79 (1962).

21. Wyler, A. R. and Ward, A. A., Jr. Neuronal firing patterns from epileptogenic foci of monkey and human. *Adv. Neurol.*, 44, 967–89 (1986).

22. Carreño, M., and Luders, H. O. General principles of presurgical evaluation. In *Textbook of Epilepsy Surgery* (Luders, H. O. ed), pp. 410, Boca Raton, FL: CRC Press. 2008.

23. Kalamangalam, G. P., Tandon, N., and Slater, J. D. Dynamic mechanisms underlying afterdischarge: A human subdural recording study. *Clin.*

Neurophysiol., 125(7), 1324–38 (2014).

24. Koester, J. and Seigelbaum, S. A. Propagated signaling: The action potential. In *Principles of Neural Science* (5th edn) (Kandel, E., et al. eds) p. 148, New York, NY: McGraw-Hill. (2013).

25. Csicsvari, J., Hirase, H., Czurko, A., and Buzsáki, G. Reliability and state dependence of pyramidal cell-interneuron synapses in the hippocampus: An ensemble approach in the behaving rat. *Neuron*, 21(1), 179–89 (1998).

26. Chatrian, G. E., Shaw, C. M., and Leffman, H. The significance of periodic lateralized epileptiform discharges in EEG: An electrographic, clinical and pathological study. *Electroencephalogr. Clin. Neurophysiol.*, 17, 177–93 (1964).

27. Pohlmann-Eden, B, Hoch, D. B., Cochius, J. I., and Chiappa, K. H. Periodic lateralized epileptiform discharges – a critical review. *J. Clin. Neurophysiol.*, 13(6), 519–30 (1996).

28. Kalamangalam, G. P., and Slater, J. D. Periodic lateralized epileptiform discharges and afterdischarges: Common dynamic mechanisms. *J. Clin. Neurophysiol.*, 32(4), 331–40 (2015).

29. Grassberger, P., and Procaccia, I. Estimation of the Kolmogorov entropy from a chaotic signal. *Phys. Rev. A.* 28 (4), 2591–3 (1983).

30. Delgado-Bonal, A., and Marshak, A. Approximate entropy and sample entropy: A comprehensive tutorial. *Entropy*, 21(6), 541 (2019).

31. Richman, J. S., and Moorman, J. R. Physiological time-series analysis using approximate entropy and sample entropy. *Am. J. Physiol. Heart Circ. Physiol.*, 278(6), H2039–49 (2000).

32. Costa, M., Goldberger, A. L., and Peng. C. K. Multiscale entropy analysis of biological signals. *Phys. Rev. E Stat. Nonlin. Soft Matter Phys.*, 71(2 Pt 1), 021906 (2005).

33. Kalamangalam, G. P., and Chelaru, I. M. Functional connectivity in dorsolateral frontal cortex: An intracranial electroencephalogram study. *Brain Connect*, 11(10), 850–64 (2021).

34. Thiebaut de Schotten, M., Urbanski, M., Batrancourt, B., et al. Rostro-caudal architecture of the frontal lobes in humans. *Cereb. Cortex*, 27 (8), 4033–47 (2017).

35. Amiez, C., and Petrides, M. Functional rostro-caudal gradient in the human posterior lateral frontal cortex. *Brain Struct. Funct.*, 223(3), 1487–99 (2018).

36. Simon, H. A. The architecture of complexity. *Proc. Am. Phil. Soc.*, 106 (6), 467–82 (1962).

37. Dubeau, F., Palmini, A., Fish, D., et al. The significance of electrocorticographic findings in focal cortical dysplasia: A review of their clinical, electrophysiological and neurochemical characteristics. *Electroencephalogr. Clin. Neurophysiol. Suppl.*, 48, 77–96 (1998).

38. Stead, M., Bower, M., Brinkmann, B. H., et al. Microseizures and the spatiotemporal scales of human partial epilepsy. *Brain*, 133(9), 2789–97 (2010).

39. Kokkinos, V., and Richardson, M. *Epilepsy Surgery: The Network Approach*, New York: Elsevier. 2020.

40. Barrat, A., Barthelélemy, M., and Vespignani, A. *Dynamical Processes on Complex Networks*, New York: Cambridge University Press. 2008.

41. Glasser, M. F., Smith, S. M., Marcus, D. S., et al. The Human Connectome Project's neuroimaging approach. *Nat. Neurosci.*, 19(9), 1175–87 (2016).

42. Thompson, P. M., Stein, J. L., Medland, S. E., et al. The ENIGMA Consortium: Large-scale collaborative analyses of neuroimaging and genetic data. *Brain Imaging Behav.*, 8(2), 153–82 (2014).

43. Engel, J., Jr., Thompson, P. M., Stern, J. M., et al. Connectomics and epilepsy. *Curr. Opin. Neurol.*, 26(2), 186–94 (2013).

44. Panaggio, M. J., Ciocanel, M.-V., Lazarus, L., Topaz, C. M., and Xu, B. Model reconstruction from temporal data for coupled oscillator networks. *Chaos* 29(10), 103116 (2019).

45. Adrian, E. D. The Activity of the Nerve Fibres. Nobel Lecture. www.nobelprize.org/ prizes/medicine/1932/adrian/ lecture/. 1932.

Neuronal Approaches to Epilepsy

Aswin Chari, Rod C. Scott, and J. Matthew Mahoney

The previous chapters have dealt with the complex adaptive nature of the genome. Similar concepts in terms of interacting elements, self-organization and adaptation can be applied at other hierarchical scales. In this chapter we will show how complex adaptive systems (CAS) concepts can be usefully applied at the level of action potential firing patterns of single neurons in terms of seizure generation and of associated morbidities.

7.1 Introduction

The epilepsies are associated with reductions in quality of life that are a function of seizure frequency as well as the presence of associated cognitive, behavioral, and psychiatric morbidities. Despite the introduction of multiple new antiepileptic medications since the beginning of the 21st century, the number of patients with medically intractable seizures has remained stable, and there has been virtually no impact on associated morbidities. Therefore, it is critical that new approaches to treatment for epilepsy are identified. Most therapies target mechanisms at the level of receptors and neurotransmitters. However, in a CAS framework (Fig. 7.1), mechanisms can be conceptualized at other scales including at the level of neural dynamics, raising the possibility that therapies can be targeted at neural dynamics directly. The hierarchical scales displayed in Fig. 7.1 are usually studied in isolation although a growing wave of multiscale integration studies are shedding new light on how activity integrates across scales to result in the emergence of structure and function both in health and disease (Fig. 7.1) [1–3]. In this chapter we describe the neuronal scale (single unit and multi-unit activity). We introduce the concept of single and multi-unit recordings and their computational analysis. We then summarize the literature on the unit level mechanisms underlying seizures, epilepsy, and associated conditions and

end by postulating how progress in this domain may improve our treatment of epilepsy.

7.2 What Are Single and Multi-Unit Recordings?

> it is the spatiotemporal variation of neuronal activity that causes behavioral variability
>
> *(Gyorgy Buzsaki, originally written in 2001, published in 2020)[4]*

The description of the spatiotemporal variation of neuronal activity, and its relationship to behavior, requires recording of neuronal activity in awake and behaving animals. Single and multi-unit activity during behavior can be recorded from the intracellular (e.g., in vivo patch clamp) and extracellular (from microelectrodes) compartments. High frequency (30–40kHz) amplifiers are required to capture the very fast timescale of action potentials. Almost all studies to date have used extracellular electrodes as in vivo patch clamp recordings can only be done in one neuron at a time. Traditionally, the number of neurons that could be recorded simultaneously from the extracellular compartment was relatively small (~10s) but recent advances in technology and processing power have opened up the possibility of recording 100–1,000s of neurons simultaneously, with the potential to record 1–2 magnitudes of scale more in the near future [5–7]. Thus, technical advances hold much promise in terms of improving our understanding of brain dynamics in health and disease.

Any single extracellular electrode may record action potentials from more than one neuron simultaneously. Thus, to get single unit activity, spike sorting applications that isolate similarly shaped action potentials from different neurons are required. At times when this is not possible, the recordings can be taken as a whole and considered as a multi-unit activity. While the

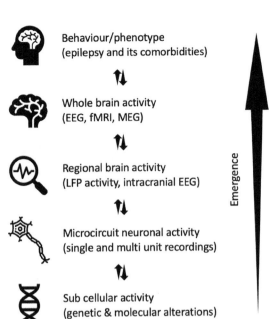

Behaviour/phenotype
(epilepsy and its comorbidities)

Whole brain activity
(EEG, fMRI, MEG)

Regional brain activity
(LFP activity, intracranial EEG)

Microcircuit neuronal activity
(single and multi unit recordings)

Sub cellular activity
(genetic & molecular alterations)

Emergence

Figure 7.1 Multiscale approaches to understanding the neurobiological mechanisms behind epilepsy. This takes a complex system approach, establishing levels in a biological hierarchy that interact in nonlinear ways and influence each other, ultimately resulting in the emergence of function.

technicalities of spike sorting are beyond the scope of this chapter and are comprehensively considered in other reviews [8–10], it is worth mentioning that the fidelity of spike sorting is improved by the use of multiple microelectrode contacts in close proximity (e.g., tetrodes). Spiking properties can subsequently be used to identify putative cell types for each of those neurons [11,12]. There are an increasing number of sorting algorithms that are semiautomatic, of increased fidelity and often increase the yield over manual sorting approaches [10]. These sorts of approaches mean that the techniques for single unit recording are becoming more mainstream, making it more likely that this level of the complex adaptive brain system will be studied.

It is recognized that the coordinated activity of the roughly 10^{11} neurons in the human brain underlies function, including generating motor output, processing sensory input, cognition, and emotion. It is striking that an essay suggesting this was rejected in 2001 but accepted for publication in its original form in 2020 [4], highlighting the fact that studies of these phenomena remain in their infancy, particularly with respect to brain disease. Observed behaviors emerge from specific firing patterns of action potentials in neurons

embedded into, and modulated within, neuronal networks. These networks can be robustly interrogated by evaluating the specific spatiotemporal patterning of action potential firing over time in awake behaving animals. Although we are describing a particular level of the brain CAS (Fig. 7.1), it is important to recognize that this level is deeply integrated with all the other hierarchical levels. For example, neuronal firing can affect subcellular activity by inducing alterations in gene expression and ion channel behavior and vice versa. Similarly, the local field potential (LFP) generated from synaptic currents can influence firing of neurons and vice versa.

Observed patterns of action potential firing can be considered as system level mechanisms of brain function during physiological behavior. In epilepsy, neuronal networks, by definition, are dysfunctional and, in this case, it could be expected that the outputs of the systems will manifest abnormal patterns of action potential firing. This generates the view that strategies to directly modify action potential patterning are likely to alter emergent phenotypes.

There are many ways in which a neuronal network can be perturbed such that action potentials fail to self-organize in a way that can sustain normal functioning. Although the nature of the primary perturbation may be diverse, such as genetic alterations or larger structural changes within the brain (e.g., malformations of cortical development, trauma, and brain tumor), there may be some convergence to common abnormal patterns at the level of neuronal dynamics. An understanding of the neuronal dynamics (see below) beyond the scope of the traditional excitatory-inhibitory imbalance paradigm can be subsequently interpreted at the other levels (e.g., molecular or whole brain) to understand mechanisms of current treatments (e.g., drugs or neurostimulation) and explore novel treatment paradigms [13].

The two key questions that arise from this framework that will be addressed in this chapter are:

1) What patterns of neuronal dynamics initiate, propagate, and terminate a seizure (in the context of an underlying "epileptic brain")?
2) What patterns of neuronal dynamics in the underlying "epileptic brain" predispose to seizures and the associated cognitive, psychological, and behavioral sequelae?

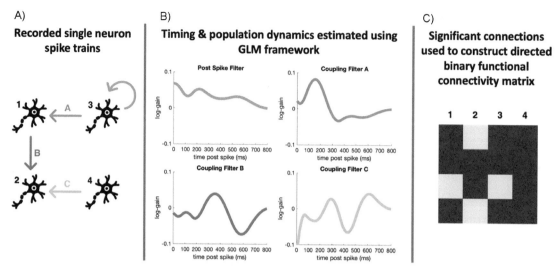

Figure 7.2 Examples of contemporary neuronal computation results that can be used to construct functional connectivity networks. A) Recording of four neurons at steady state. B) Significant post-spike (top left) and coupling filters were found for four connections in these neurons. They provide independent measures of timing and population dynamics of single neurons using the GLM framework as outline. C) These post-spike and coupling filters may be utilized to construct functional connectivity networks (in this case, a binary, directed network), providing an opportunity to study changes in these network dynamics in health and disease.

Action potential firing can be interrogated in a number of ways. *Rate dynamics* refers to changes in the firing rate of action potentials as a function of sensory input. For example, neurons that change firing rate as a function of position in space are called place cells; in this circumstance the increase in firing rate is coding position in space. However, it has become clear that a simplistic view of merely "counting spikes," while undoubtedly useful, is insufficient to fully explain behavior. Other important dynamics include *population dynamics*, which refers to the dynamical interaction between neurons, and *timing dynamics*, which refers to the short timescale modulation of action potential firing (Fig. 7.2). Together, these dynamics are critical for the coding and transfer of information within the brain. The ultimate aim is to explain or predict behavior from these dynamics, but the brain has a number of special features that mean that the "code" is not fixed (the representation of a particular stimulus may change over time), there is considerable "noise" or background activity in the "code", and it has only been possible to record from a small number of neurons thereby getting only a snapshot of part of the "code." [14,15]. When combined with the "many-to-many" problem of the same neuronal network activity leading to different behavioral phenotypes and different neuronal network activity leading to the same behavioral

phenotypes, it becomes clear that developing a thorough understanding of this code in a context-independent manner may be extremely difficult; however, evidence from animal work suggests that artificial networks may be able to simulate the behavior of biological neuronal networks in simpler organisms and technological advances could see this translated into humans [16,17].

A key question is whether unit level recordings add to understanding over and above other electrophysiological recordings. It has been thought that high gamma band (80–150Hz) LFP and functional MRI BOLD signal are correlates of multi-unit activity [18–21], both of which are technically much easier to record. However, more recent data disputes this, arguing that much of the cortically recorded high gamma band LFP signal arises from the superficial layers of the cortex, which has a poor correlation with the deeper unit activity [22]. In addition, LFP and, specifically, the high gamma band, can be contaminated by transient increases in spectral power associated interictal epileptiform discharges, which may be detrimental to studies seeking to analyze cognitive mechanisms at the LFP level [23]. We can therefore conclude that neuronal scale activity contains information that cannot be obtained at other scales and is therefore worthy of independent study.

7.3 An Introduction to Contemporary Neuronal Computation

Traditionally, neuronal dynamics have been evaluated using tools such as peri-event time histograms (PETH) to assess rate dynamics as a function of sensory input, autocorrelograms to identify timing dynamics and crosscorrelograms to assess population dynamics with respect to other neurons. Unfortunately, there are several technical issues that impact inferences that can be drawn from these techniques and therefore newer approaches to spiking data are becoming more popular. In this section, we briefly outline the mathematical theory behind contemporary neuronal computation.

7.3.1 Neuronal Firing May Be Modeled as Point Processes

An action potential, or *spike*, from a single neuron is an "all or nothing" event that is highly localized in time. It is therefore natural to mathematically model a sequence of action potentials, i.e., a *spike train*, as a discrete set of points in time. At a high level of theoretical abstraction, such data are described probabilistically as *point processes*, which are mathematical models that assign probabilities to every possible discrete set of times [24]. The theory of point processes is well developed and has been extensively applied to spike train analysis, which has adopted much of the nomenclature of point process theory (25). However, for the practical modeling of spike trains from neural recordings, the full generality of point process theory is not required and can obfuscate the core intuitive ideas. In this section, we will outline the point process modeling of spike trains using an intuitive approach that is widely used in the neurophysiology literature.

Let $\{t_i\}$ be a spike train, where t_i is the time of the ith spike. Because a physiological spike has a short duration compared to behavioral timescales, we can *bin* the spike train into a vector of counts, r_t, where $r_t = k$ if there are k spikes in the interval $[t, t + dt]$.

The bin size, dt, is an analytical choice, but a typical value is 1ms, as this is small enough to ensure that only zero or one spikes will occur within any given bin. The goal of spike train analysis is to model r_t as a function of experimental or electrophysiological covariates. To begin to do this, we assume that in any given time bin there is a time-dependent *intensity function,* λ_t, that encodes the *firing rate* of the neuron at time t. Over a short time interval, $[t, t + dt]$, the expected number of spikes in the interval is $\lambda_t * dt$, which is much smaller than one. The condition that $\lambda_t * dt \ll 1$ allows us to write the probability of r_t spikes in the interval $[t, t + dt]$ using a Poisson distribution:

$$P(r_t = k) = (\lambda_t \, dt)^k \, \frac{e^{-\lambda_t * dt}}{k} . \tag{1}$$

This is a standard "law of rare events" argument and it applies in this case because the probability of observing a spike in any given 1ms bin is low [26]. Note that, although the Poisson distribution technically allows $r_t \geq 2$, the probability of more than one spike is negligible. The probability, p_t, of observing a spike in the interval $[t, t + dt]$ is therefore

$$p_t = \lambda_t dt e^{-\lambda_t * dt} \approx 1 - e^{-\lambda_t dt}. \tag{2}$$

7.3.2 Neuronal Firing May Be Modeled Using a Generalized Linear Model (GLM) Approach

In order to model the spike train, r_t, we need to estimate the time-varying firing rate λ_t, but at present this only defines notation. A particular analysis for a particular experiment requires specifying how we estimate λ_t as a function of time-varying covariates.

The simplest nontrivial case is when the firing rate of the neuron covaries with some externally measurable factor. For example, the firing rate of a neuron might depend simply on one of a set of experimentally provided cues, in which case, λ_t is a piecewise constant function of which cue is present at a given time [27]. Beyond piecewise constant functions, a neuron's firing rate may have a stereotyped dynamical response to a discrete cue, e.g., a change in context or pressing lever in a behavioral apparatus. In this case, λ_t is modeled as a time-varying function of the discrete event and the strategies for modeling this are discussed below. A neuron's firing rate can also have complex nonlinear tuning, as is the case for example in place, grid, and head-direction cells in the hippocampus and entorhinal cortex [28]. In these cases, λ_t is a complex function of time that depends on both the spatial tuning of the neuron to position and the behavioral trajectory of the animal. In all these cases, the firing rate is modeled as tuned to some external factor that has some semantic meaning to the experimenter – cues, lever presses, physical position.

It is also possible to model a neuron's firing rate as a function of other neural signals. In the hippocampus, for example, there are well-established phenomenological properties of neural firing, including *theta phase preference*, in which a neuron preferentially fires at particular phases within the local theta cycle, and *theta phase precession*, in which a neuron's preferred firing phase changes as a function position within a place field [29–31]. In these cases, λ_t is modeled as a function of the instantaneous theta phase and physical position of the animal [30]. Finally, a neuron's firing rate can be a function of the past firing of itself and other neurons. These models account for the auto- and cross-correlation of single unit firing within an ensemble and provide measures of functional connectivity within and between neural ensembles [25,32].

To estimate a neuron's firing rate as an explicit mathematical model, the standard approach is to use a *generalized linear model (GLM) with exponential link function*. We explain this phrase with the aid of a few examples: a theta phase preference model for a hippocampal neuron, peri-event rate modulation in a behavioral experiment, and auto- and cross-correlation of neurons.

First, consider a hippocampal pyramidal cell. Let r_t be its binned spike train, as above, and suppose φ_t is the instantaneous phase of the local hippocampal theta rhythm (compare with [33]). Phase preference means that the firing rate λ_t oscillates as function of φ_t. Naively, it makes sense to consider λ_t as a sinusoidal function of φ_t, but probabilities must be positive. Thus, it makes sense to consider instead the functional form

$$\lambda_t = e^{(a_0 + a\cos(\varphi_t) + b\sin(\varphi_t))}. \tag{3}$$

Alternative models have been proposed, e.g., [34], but the above serves as a minimal model to develop intuition. In this model, the coefficient a_0 encodes the background firing rate with no phase modulation, and the coefficients a and b together determine the strength of the modulation and the preferred phase. Note that $\cos(\varphi_t)$ and $\sin(\varphi_t)$ are two "external" functions that are supplied as covariates to predict firing rate. The model combines these covariates linearly and then exponentiates them to predict the Poisson firing rate of the cell at an instant in time. In the general terminology of GLMs, the exponential function in this case is termed the *link function* as it links the linear combination of predictors to the mean firing rate. The values of a_0, a, and b must be estimated from a given spike train. Typically, this is done through maximum likelihood estimation, which searches for the parameter values that maximize the log-likelihood function. This optimization cannot be performed in closed form and requires nonlinear optimization software. It is worth noting that a GLM with exponential link function yields a particularly tractable optimization problem, namely that the log-likelihood is *convex*, which mean there are no spurious *local optima* in the parameter space. Other link functions are possible and have been considered in the systems neuroscience literature, although some do not have convex log-likelihood functions [35]. However, beyond technical issues of model fitting, a major conceptual advantage to the exponential link function is that, because an exponential of a sum is a product of exponentials, each time-varying term of an exponential link GLM can be directly interpreted as a dynamical *gain* on the baseline firing rate. In the above example, the theta phase cyclically "turns the firing rate up and down" about the baseline firing rate given by e^{a_0}.

As a second type of GLM, consider the modulation of a neuron as a function of a set of discrete events, for example, a lever press or an interictal discharge. Let r_t be the binned spike train and e_t a binned set of event times. Descriptively, it is common to compute a PETH for the spike train around the event, which captures the rate modulation of firing around an event and corresponds to the cross-correlogram between the event train and the spike train. To convert the PETH into a GLM model, we start with a finite set of *basis functions*, $\{f^{i_t}\}$, that we expect to capture the structure of the PETH. We then convolve the basis functions with the event train to generate a set of putative predictor functions, $g^{i_t} = e_t * f^{i_t}$, that we linearly combine to predict firing rate:

$$\lambda_t = e^{(b_0 + b_1 g^{1_t} + \dots + b_k g^{k_t})}. \tag{4}$$

As in the previous example, the coefficient b_0 encodes the background firing rate, independent of any event-based rate modulation. The remaining coefficients capture the amount of gain modulation that matches each of the basis functions. Because the convolution operation is linear, we can interpret time-varying terms in the exponent as:

$$b_1 g_1(t) + \ldots + b_k g_k(t)$$
$$= e_t * (b_1 f_1(t) + \ldots + b_k f_k(t)) = e_t * f(t). \qquad (5)$$

This shows that that these terms define an *event filter*, which is a linear combination of the basis functions and that, when convolved with the event train, encodes the event-related gain modulation of the firing rate. One advantage of the GLM approach over a purely descriptive approach, is that all neurons can be modeled using the same set of basis functions, and therefore directly compared to each other. Furthermore, the basis functions can be chosen so that the predicted PETHs are smooth, which can help alleviate challenging analytical issues such as choosing a bin size for a PETH for every neuron.

As a final example, we note that the above example can be readily adapted to model the auto-correlation of a single neuron and the cross-correlation of pairs of neurons. If we replace e_t in the above example with r_t, then the above model yields a *post-spike filter* that encodes the rate modulation of the neuron's firing as a function of its past firing (Fig. 7.2) [25]. Similarly, if we replace e_t with the spike train for a second neuron, then the above model yields a *coupling filter* that encodes the rate modulation of the target neuron as a function of a source neuron (Fig. 7.2). While operationally the same as event filters, post-spike and coupling filters encode the functional connectivity within the neuronal network. Note that these are estimated jointly in the GLM, so that modeled connections are "corrected" for the effects of all other covariates, enabling system level inferences.

The use of GLMs per se to model neuronal point processes is convenient, intuitive, and well understood statistically, including goodness of fit metrics [36] and statistical hypothesis testing for the significance of model terms [32]. However, there is an active research field working on broadening the class of point process models using emerging techniques from statistics and machine learning, including stochastic process theory and deep learning. This research parallels the advancing hardware innovations for measuring neural spiking at much larger scales [37]. Thus, GLMs will likely remain a workhorse model for many neuroscience applications.

7.4 Unit Level Mechanisms Underlying Seizures

The cardinal feature of epilepsy is seizures. Single unit dynamics surrounding seizures have been studied both in animal models and in humans undergoing neurosurgical procedures for the treatment of epilepsy. The recordings use cortical microelectrode arrays that allow the high resolution study of spatiotemporal dynamics within a small area (Fig. 7.3) [38]. This body of work has elucidated a number of important mechanisms and features at different stages of a seizure.

Primarily, rate dynamics have been studied during seizures. There is debate on the nature of the patterns of activity during a seizure based on whether recordings are from the actual seizure focus or a surrounding area [39–41]. There are studies that have identified heterogeneous changes in neuronal firing at seizure onset, with some neurons increasing their firing, some decreasing firing, and others not changing at all, suggesting a state change that is not as simple as the excitatory-inhibitory imbalance theories would suggest [41]. However, others have argued that this is not reflective of the true "core" of the seizure (see below), where hypersynchronous activity has been observed [40,42,43]. In slice and animal model experiments, irrespective of the location (neocortex vs. mesial temporal structures) and type of seizure onset pattern seen in LFP (low voltage fast vs. hypersynchronous), seizure onset is thought to be caused by hypersynchronous recruitment of pyramidal cells initiated by a loss of inhibition from interneurons [39,44–47]. This loss of inhibition has been postulated to occur due to both excess or inadequate GABA and may be preceded by a period of increased interneuron activity [39,48,49]. If shown to be true in humans, this may have implications for seizure detection (e.g., closed loop neurostimulation devices) that may be able to take advantage of the earlier interneuron activity to terminate seizures before they manifest in the LFP or clinical domains [50,51].

Seizure propagation has been shown to occur via a traveling wavefront, resulting in intense recruitment of almost all pyramidal neurons in the **core** of the seizure (Fig. 7.3) [40,52,53].

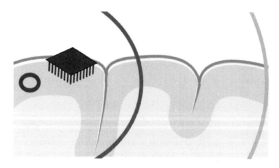

Figure 7.3 Schematic of microelectrode array on the cortical surface, illustrating the concepts of the microelectrode defined ictal onset zone, core, and penumbra. All these zones may show similar LFP activity but the core can be distinguished from the penumbra at microelectrode level due to the intense recruitment and firing of almost all pyramidal neurons.

Ictal Onset Zone
- LFP: Ictal activity
- Microelectrode: Unknown

Core
- LFP: Ictal activity
- Microelectrode: Intense recruitment and firing of almost all pyramidal cells

Penumbra
- LFP: Ictal activity
- Microelectrode: Variable unit activity with some neurons, increasing, some decreasing, and others not changing firing rates

Interestingly, the **penumbra** outside of this traveling wavefront may show similar LFP activity to the "core" but does not have this concurrent pyramidal cell recruitment (Fig. 7.3). Mechanistically, this traveling wave phenomenon may be a feature of self-organizing network dynamics with pyramidal cells in the core recruiting fast-spiking interneurons in the penumbra that delay or prevent further pyramidal cell recruitment [39,54,55]. It would follow that these dynamics have a key role in the extent of propagation (is there a similar phenomenon in the thalamus that prevents/facilitates generalization) and termination (at some point, the self-organizing behavior succeeds) although these have not been formally tested. The concept of the core and penumbra could also explain the finding from other studies that show heterogeneous unit level activity at LFP seizure onset, suggesting that they were recording from the penumbra [41,56,57].

From a therapeutic perspective, phase locked high gamma (80–150Hz activity phase locked to lower frequency 4–30Hz activity) has been shown to be a marker for the ictal core and the resection of a larger proportion of areas with this activity has been shown to correlate with post-resection outcomes in patients, suggesting a refinement of the traditional LFP-defined seizure onset zone is needed [52,58,59]. It is possible that single unit studies will allow such a refinement and thus improve surgical approaches to epilepsy. The key role of interneurons in seizure propagation also underpins the concept of interneuron transplantation as a therapy for epilepsy, although there remain multiple challenges to overcome prior to consideration of clinical translation [60,61]. Selective optogenetic neurostimulation of interneurons has also been used to terminate seizures, although, in the interictal phase, this same stimulation was ictogenic [62]. Patterns of interneuron firing characteristics, and their relationships with pyramidal cell firing, have not yet been formally defined. Clarity on these patterns is likely to influence the design of stimulation approaches in order to recapitulate normal microcircuit dynamic neuronal activity, thereby terminating seizures.

Increased unit firing is observed toward the end of a seizure, followed by a period of almost silence that may last many seconds before a slow recovery to baseline levels [41,56,63]. Patterns of cessation have been shown to be inconsistent with depolarizing block caused by changes in neurotransmitter or electrolyte concentrations following rapid firing, suggesting that the hypersynchronous activity and sudden cessation could be emergent properties of large-scale networks themselves. Elucidation of these mechanisms may allow us to replicate or induce such changes to trigger earlier termination of seizures or even provide a therapeutic strategy for the treatment of severe status epilepticus being treated in intensive care units.

A limitation of this approach in humans is that recordings are limited to those undergoing neurosurgical procedures (presurgical evaluation or surgical resection for presumed focal epilepsy). Other seizure types, such as absence seizures, may have different dynamic perturbations and involve distinct brain regions for initiation and termination, although there is a widening scope for capturing these dynamics through closed loop neuromodulatory treatments [64]. Animal models will remain an important part of the armamentarium and facilitate translation of such therapies.

7.5 Unit Level Mechanisms Underlying Epilepsy

Given that epilepsy is defined as an "enduring predisposition to generate epileptic seizures," it follows that there may be microcircuit level changes that are detectable outside the context of seizures [65].

Studies in animals and humans have shown that the cortex displays specific properties during normal function such as a delicate excitatory-inhibitory balance (at neuronal level) or self-organized criticality (at neuronal and LFP levels). Perturbations of these dynamics can manifest as the emergent phenomenon of seizures [66–70]. These intrinsic properties may be abnormal even in the interictal state, making certain brains (or particular areas of brain) more susceptible to seizure generation/propagation and others more resistant [71]. Indeed, treatment with antiepileptic drugs have been shown to induce subcritical network dynamics at the LFP level, a novel mechanistic insight into drugs that are usually understood at the molecular level [72]. Animal models (using similar recordings from animals with and without epilepsy) and human microelectrode recordings will facilitate advancement of this understanding. The therapeutic potential of such approaches includes better localization of focal epilepsy and the tailoring of therapies (resection, stimulation, and pharmacological treatments) to target these specific areas or mechanisms.

Microcircuit networks are likely to be affected by more than just the cause of epilepsy. The dynamic nature of the brain means that unit level dynamics may also be altered by other factors such as ongoing seizures and antiepileptic medication; as alluded to above, the "code" is not fixed [72]. Indeed, induced status epilepticus in animal models has been shown to result in both disproportionate loss and increased firing of certain interneuron populations and these may have subsequent effects on the population and timing dynamics of the remaining cells in the microcircuits that may manifest as ongoing propensity to seizures and cognitive deficits [73,74].

Unit dynamics can also be used to explore mechanisms behind interictal phenomena such as interictal epileptiform discharges. The

characteristic interictal spikes have been shown to probably be generated from sparse neuronal networks, distinct to both ictal onset and physiological "spikes" of spontaneous population activity [48,75] and the spread depends upon important GABAergic input [76]. Pathological high frequency oscillations (HFOs) have also emerged as important interictal phenomena since they were described in around 2010. Indeed, resection of areas with increased HFO activity have been shown to correlated with better clinical outcome and we stand to gain from exploring the mechanisms behind such phenomena at the neuronal level [77,78]. Slice electrophysiology work has again highlighted the importance of inhibitory barrages from interneurons as crucial to the generation of HFOs [79]. Exactly how these inhibitory barrages link to the inhibitory restraints during seizure initiation and propagation remain to be elucidated and could shed light on why resection of these areas may be important in the context of the surgical treatment of focal epilepsy.

7.6 Unit Level Mechanisms Underlying Cognitive Dysfunction in Epilepsy

Cognition is characterized by constantly changing dynamics, as the brain acquires and processes information, and updates attention, goals, and behavior. In mathematical terms, it is a high-complexity state.

Work since the beginning of the 21st century on the mathematical modeling of seizures has made clear that low-dimensional dynamical systems suffice to explain the core features of their dynamics [80,81]. Physiological neuronal dynamics, on the other hand, do not appear to have any such reduction in the degrees of freedom beyond that required for robust computation. For example, in the V1 area of the visual cortex of primates, the number of bits of visual information transmitted per action potential is near the theoretical maximum, and this information capacity appears to require complex, correlated timing dynamics among neurons [82]. From first principles, one would expect evolution to optimize cognitive circuitry to be highly efficient, squeezing out any useless redundancies. Therefore, we expect that these visual system results to generalize to higher cognitive functions, which many studies are beginning to show.

In the context of epilepsy research, this presents a tantalizing opportunity. Given that behavior is a function of underlying microcircuit dynamics, which are abnormal in patients and in animal models of epilepsy, then it follows that we can probe the dynamical abnormalities of the brain in the high-complexity state with more degrees of freedom.

Some of the first work on the unit level dynamics of cognition in the context of epilepsy concerned the so-called place field system in the rodent hippocampus [83,84]. This pathbreaking work showed that the rate-based encoding of animal position by the hippocampus was significantly impaired in a rat model of temporal lobe epilepsy, which correlated with behavioral deficits in tasks of spatial memory [84]. Taking this further, we have shown that these rate level dynamics in other disease models are strongly associated with abnormalities in oscillatory dynamics at the theta timescale (6–12 Hz), where oscillatory features of neural firing directly predict the quality of place fields on a per neuron basis [85]. Going beyond spatial cognition, we recently showed that rate-based cognitive encodings in a working memory task were also associated with these same timing features, suggesting that timing properties that encode neural circuit dynamics indeed ramify to the cognitive encodings in the hippocampus [86]. From a mechanistic point of view, Bui et al. have used large-scale simulations of the hippocampal formation to argue that dentate gyrus granule cells control seizure activity and spatial memory [87]. This study underscores the value of systems neuroscience in connecting "neurology" on one hand with "psychology" on the other.

Going forward, the pressing clinical question for physicians is to develop therapies that can ameliorate seizures and cognitive deficits. Here too, the complex systems framework and the cognitive approach are potentially powerful. Given that cognition activates many more dynamical brain regimes than seizures, it stands to reason that, beyond purely targeting seizures, we could directly target interictal dynamical abnormalities, particularly those that correlate with cognitive encodings. Recent work has shown that electrical stimulation can restore memory in humans, with corresponding changes in LFP-level neurophysiological encoding states [88–90]. This proof-of-concept work shows that it is possible to acutely perturb the brain to alter neurophysiological dynamics although the current studies have only explored this at the LFP level. The next frontier is to design personalized stimulation paradigms that induce the brain to durably reorganize in a "pro-cognitive" way that also suppresses the ability of the neural circuit to generate seizures.

7.7 Conclusions

Emergent behavioral phenotypes, in health and disease, are functions of the patterns of firing of action potentials in the brain. While significant progress has been made from studying epilepsy at larger (structural, electrophysiological) and smaller (genetic, epigenetic, molecular) scales, units provide an attractive level at which there may be common underlying abnormalities that explain both the seizures and the associated cognitive, psychiatric, and behavioral comorbidities.

Despite being available for over 50 years, increases in the number of potential neurons that can be recoded simultaneously and data processing power are only now bringing large-scale unit level recordings in behaving human subjects into their prime [38,91]. While the first stage involves using such data to understand the neuronal network abnormalities in epilepsy, there is also potential to alter these dynamics through established (medication, surgical resection/ablation) and novel (neuromodulation, stimulation, cell transplantation) treatments in a more holistic way that addresses both the seizures and associated comorbidities.

References

1. Driscoll, N., Rosch, R. E., Murphy, B. B., et al. Multimodal in vivo recording using transparent graphene microelectrodes illuminates spatiotemporal seizure dynamics at the microscale. *Commun. Biol.*, 4, 136 (2020).

2. Paquola, C., Seidlitz, J., Benkarim, O., et al. The cortical wiring scheme of hierarchical information processing. 2020. bioRxiv. 2020.01.08.899583.

3. Scott, R. C., Menendez de la Prida, L., Mahoney, J. M., et al. WONOEP APPRAISAL: The

many facets of epilepsy networks. *Epilepsia.*, 59(8), 1475–83 (2018).

4. Buzsáki, G. The brain–cognitive behavior problem: A retrospective. *eNeuro.* 7(4) (2020). doi:10.1523/ENEURO.0069-20.2020

5. Jun, J. J., Steinmetz, N. A., Siegle, J. H., et al. Fully integrated silicon probes for high-density recording of neural activity. *Nature*, 551 (7679), 232–6 (2017).

6. Sahasrabuddhe, K., Khan, A. A., Singh, A. P., et al. The Argo: A high channel count recording system for neural recording in vivo. *J. Neural Eng.*, 18(1), 015002 (2020).

7. Obaid, A., Hanna, M.-E., Wu, Y.-W., et al. Massively parallel microwire arrays integrated with CMOS chips for neural recording. *Sci Adv.*, 6(12), eaay2789 (2020).

8. Carlson, D., and Carin, L. Continuing progress of spike sorting in the era of big data. *Curr. Opin. Neurobiol.*, 55, 90–6, (2019).

9. Rey, H. G., Pedreira, and C., Quian Quiroga. R. Past, present and future of spike sorting techniques. *Brain Res. Bull.*, 119, 106–17 (2015).

10. Magland, J., Jun, J. J., and Lovero, E., et al. SpikeForest, reproducible web-facing ground-truth validation of automated neural spike sorters. *eLife*, 9, e55167 (2020).

11. Buccino, A. P., Ness, T. V., Einevoll, G. T., Cauwenberghs, G., and Hafliger, P. D. A deep learning approach for the classification of neuronal cell types. *Annu. Int. Conf. IEEE Eng. Med. Biol. Soc.*, 2018, 999–1002 (2018).

12. Trainito, C., von Nicolai, C., Miller, E. K., and Siegel, M. Extracellular spike waveform dissociates four functionally distinct cell classes in primate cortex. *Curr. Biol.*, 29(18), (2019).

13. O'Donnell, C., Gonçalves, J. T., Portera-Cailliau, C., and Sejnowski, T. J. Beyond excitation/inhibition imbalance in multidimensional models of neural circuit changes in brain disorders. *Elife*, 6, e26724 (2017).

14. Kreiman, G. Neural coding: Computational and biophysical perspectives. *Phys. Life Rev.*, 1 (2), 71–102 (2004).

15. Reinartz, S. Long-term activity dynamics of single neurons and networks. *Adv. Neurobiol.*, 22, 331–50 (2019).

16. Ahrens, M. B. Zebrafish neuroscience: Using artificial neural networks to help understand brains. *Curr. Biol.* 29(21), R1138–40, (2019).

17. Haesemeyer, M., Schier, A.F., and Engert, F. Convergent Temperature Representations in Artificial and Biological Neural Networks. *Neuron*, 103 (6), 1123–34.e6 (2019).

18. Nir, Y., Fisch, L., Mukamel, R., et al. Coupling between neuronal firing rate, gamma LFP, and BOLD fMRI is related to interneuronal correlations. *Curr. Biol.* , 17(15), 1275–85 (2007).

19. Rich, E. L., and Wallis, J. D. Spatiotemporal dynamics of information encoding revealed in orbitofrontal high-gamma. *Nat. Commun.*, 8(1), 1139 (2017).

20. Ray, S., Crone, N. E., Niebur, E., Franaszczuk, P. J., and Hsiao, S. S. Neural correlates of high-gamma oscillations (60–200 Hz) in macaque local field potentials and their potential implications in electrocorticography. *J. Neurosci.*, 28(45), 11526–36 (2008).

21. Mukamel, R., Gelbard, H., Arieli, A., et al. Coupling between neuronal firing, field potentials, and FMRI in human auditory cortex. *Science*, 309 (5736), 951–4 (2005).

22. Leszczyński, M., Barczak, A., Kajikawa, Y., et al. Dissociation of broadband high-frequency activity and neuronal firing in the neocortex. *Sci. Advances.*, 6 (33), eabb0977 (2020).

23. Ammanuel, S. G., Kleen, J. K., Leonard, M. K., and Chang, E. F. Interictal epileptiform discharges and the quality of human intracranial neurophysiology data. *Front. Hum. Neurosci.*, 14, 44 (2020).

24. Jacobsen, M. *Point Process Theory and Applications: Marked Point and Piecewise Deterministic Processes*. Basel: Birkhäuser. 2006.

25. Truccolo, W., Eden, U. T., Fellows, M. R., Donoghue, J. P., and Brown, E. N. A point process framework for relating neural spiking activity to spiking history, neural ensemble, and extrinsic covariate effects. *J. Neurophysiol.*, 93(2), 1074–89 (2005).

26. Grinstead, C. M., and Snell, J. L. *Introduction to Probability*. 2nd edition. Providence, RI: American Mathematical Society. 2012. p. 510.

27. Binev, P., Cohen, A., Dahmen, W., DeVore, R., Temlyakov, V. Universal algorithms for learning theory part I: Piecewise constant functions. *J. Mach. Learn. Res.*, 6(2), 1297–321 (2005).

28. Barbieri, R., Wilson, M. A., Frank, L. M., and Brown, E. N. An analysis of hippocampal spatio-temporal representations using a Bayesian algorithm for neural spike train decoding. *IEEE Trans. Neural. Syst. Rehabil. Eng.*, 13(2), 131–6 (2005).

29. Newman, E. L., and Hasselmo, M. E. Grid cell firing properties vary as a function of theta

phase locking preferences in the rat medial entorhinal cortex. *Front. Syst. Neurosci.*, 8, 193 (2014)

30. Bose, A., and Recce, M. Phase precession and phase-locking of hippocampal pyramidal cells. *Hippocampus*, 11(3), 204–15 (2001).

31. Buzsáki, G., Moser, E. I. Memory, navigation and theta rhythm in the hippocampal-entorhinal system. *Nat. Neurosci.*, 16(2), 130–8 (2013).

32. Kim, S., Putrino, D., Ghosh, S., and Brown, E. N. A Granger causality measure for point process models of ensemble neural spiking activity. *PLoS Comput. Biol.*, 7(3), e1001110 (2011).

33. Hasselmo, M. E. What is the function of hippocampal theta rhythm? – Linking behavioral data to phasic properties of field potential and unit recording data. *Hippocampus*, 15(7), 936–49 (2005).

34. Johnson, T. D., Coleman, T. P., and Rangel, L. M. A flexible likelihood approach for predicting neural spiking activity from oscillatory phase. *J. Neurosci. Methods.*, 311, 307–17 (2019).

35. Paninski, L. Maximum likelihood estimation of cascade point-process neural encoding models. *Network*, 15(4), 243–62 (2004).

36. Brown, E. N., Barbieri, R., Ventura, V., Kass, R. E., and Frank, L. M. The time-rescaling theorem and its application to neural spike train data analysis. *Neural Comput.*, 14(2), 325–46 (2002).

37. Zoltowski, D. M., and Pillow, J. W. Scaling the Poisson GLM to massive neural datasets through polynomial approximations. *Adv. Neural Inf. Process Syst.*, 31, 3517–27 (2018).

38. Chari, A., Thornton, R. C., Tisdall, M. M., and Scott, R. C.

Microelectrode recordings in human epilepsy: A case for clinical translation. *Brain Commun.*, 2(2), fcaa082 (2020).

39. Trevelyan, A. J., Muldoon, S. F., Merricks, E. M., Racca, C., and Staley, K. J. The role of inhibition in epileptic networks. *J. Clin. Neurophysiol.*, 32(3), 227–34 (2015).

40. Schevon, C.A., Weiss, S.A., McKhann, G., et al. Evidence of an inhibitory restraint of seizure activity in humans. *Nat. Commun.*, 3(1), 1060 (2012).

41. Truccolo, W., Donoghue, J. A., Hochberg, L. R., et al. Single-neuron dynamics in human focal epilepsy. *Nat. Neurosci.*, 14(5), 635–41 (2011).

42. Merricks, E. M., Smith, E. H., McKhann, G. M., et al. Single unit action potentials in humans and the effect of seizure activity. *Brain*, 138(Pt 10), 2891–906 (2015).

43. Merricks, E. M., Smith, E. H., Emerson, R. G., et al. Neuronal firing and waveform alterations through ictal recruitment in humans. *J. Neurosci.*, 41(4), 766–79 (2021).

44. McCormick, D. A., and Contreras, D. On the cellular and network bases of epileptic seizures. *Annu. Rev. Physiol.*, 63, 815–46 (2001).

45. Köhling, R., D'Antuono, M., Benini, R., de, Guzman, P., and Avoli, M. Hypersynchronous ictal onset in the perirhinal cortex results from dynamic weakening in inhibition. *Neurobiol. Dis.*, 87, 1–10 (2016).

46. Trevelyan, A. J., Sussillo, D., Watson, B. O., and Yuste, R. Modular Propagation of Epileptiform Activity: Evidence for an Inhibitory Veto in Neocortex. *J. Neurosci.*, 26(48), 12447–55 (2006).

47. Weiss, S. A., Staba, R., Bragin, A., et al. Interneurons and principal cell firing in human

limbic areas at focal seizure onset. *Neurobiol. Dis.*, 124, 183–8 (2019).

48. Kandrács, Á., Hofer, K. T., Tóth, K., et al. Presence of synchrony-generating hubs in the human epileptic neocortex. *J. Physiol.*, 597(23), 5639–70 (2019).

49. Köhling, R. Translational perspectives: Interneurones start seizures. *J. Physiol.*, 597(23), 5525–6 (2019).

50. Avoli, M., and de Curtis, M. GABAergic synchronization in the limbic system and its role in the generation of epileptiform activity. *Prog. Neurobiol.*, 95(2), 104–32 (2011).

51. Elahian, B., Lado, N.E., Mankin, E., et al. Low-voltage fast seizures in humans begin with increased interneuron firing. *Ann. Neurol.*, 84(4), 588–600 (2018).

52. Weiss, S. A., Banks, G. P., McKhann, G. M., et al. Ictal high frequency oscillations distinguish two types of seizure territories in humans. *Brain*, 136(Pt 12), 3796–808 (2013).

53. Timofeev, I., and Steriade, M. Neocortical seizures: Initiation, development and cessation. *Neurosci.*, 123(2), 299–336 (2004).

54. Cammarota, M., Losi, G., Chiavegato, A., Zonta, M., and Carmignoto, G. Fast spiking interneuron control of seizure propagation in a cortical slice model of focal epilepsy. *J. Physiol.*, 591(4), 807–22 (2013).

55. Parrish, R. R., Codadu, N. K., Scott, C. M.-G., and Trevelyan, A. J. Feedforward inhibition ahead of ictal wavefronts is provided by both parvalbumin- and somatostatin-expressing interneurons. *J. Physiol.*, 597(8), 2297–314 (2019).

56. Lambrecq, V., Lehongre, K., Adam, C., et al. Single-unit activities during the transition to seizures in deep mesial

structures. *Ann. Neurol.*, 82(6), 1022–8 (2017).

57. Bower, M. R., Stead, M., Meyer, F. B., Marsh, W. R., and Worrell, G. A. Spatiotemporal neuronal correlates of seizure generation in focal epilepsy. *Epilepsia*, 53(5), 807–16 (2012).

58. Weiss, S. A., Lemesiou, A., Connors, R., et al. Seizure localization using ictal phase-locked high gamma: A retrospective surgical outcome study. *Neurology*, 84 (23), 2320–8 (2015).

59. Eissa, T. L., Tryba, A. K., Marcuccilli, C. J., et al. Multiscale aspects of generation of high-gamma activity during seizures in human neocortex. *eNeuro*, 3 (2), ENEURO.0141–15.2016 (2016).

60. Hunt, R. F., and Baraban, S. C. Interneuron transplantation as a treatment for epilepsy. *Cold Spring Harb. Perspect. Med.*, 5 (12), a022376 (2015).

61. Harward, S. C., and Southwell, D. G. Interneuron transplantation: A prospective surgical therapy for medically refractory epilepsy. *Neurosurg. Focus*, 48(4):E18 (2020).

62. Assaf, F., and Schiller, Y. The antiepileptic and ictogenic effects of optogenetic neurostimulation of PV-expressing interneurons. *J. Neurophysiol.*, 116(4), 1694–704 (2016).

63. Weiss, S. A., Alvarado-Rojas, C., Bragin, A., et al. Ictal onset patterns of local field potentials, high frequency oscillations, and unit activity in human mesial temporal lobe epilepsy. *Epilepsia*, 57(1), 111–21 (2016).

64. Young, J. C., Nasser, H. M., Casillas-Espinosa, P. M., et al. Multiunit cluster firing patterns of piriform cortex and mediodorsal thalamus in absence epilepsy. *Epilepsy Behav.*, 97, 229–43 (2019).

65. Fisher, R. S., Acevedo, C., Arzimanoglou, A., et al. ILAE official report: A practical clinical definition of epilepsy. *Epilepsia*, 55(4), 475–82 (2014).

66. Dehghani, N., Peyrache, A., Telenczuk, B., et al. Dynamic balance of excitation and inhibition in human and monkey neocortex. *Sci. Rep.*, 6 (1), 23176 (2016).

67. Meisel, C., Storch, A., Hallmeyer-Elgner, S., Bullmore, E., and Gross, T. Failure of adaptive self-organized criticality during epileptic seizure attacks. *PLoS Comput. Biol.*, 8(1), e1002312 (2012).

68. Hahn, G., Ponce-Alvarez, A., Monier, C., et al. Spontaneous cortical activity is transiently poised close to criticality. *PLoS Comput. Biol.*, 13(5), e1005543 (2017).

69. Beggs, J. M., and Plenz, D. Neuronal avalanches in neocortical circuits. *J. Neurosci.*, 23(35), 11167–77 (2003).

70. Bravo-Martínez, J., Rivera, A. L., Toledo-Roy, J. C., et al. Dynamical phase transition in spike neuronal firing patterns of hippocampal cells. *Biochem. Biophys. Res. Commun.*, 516(4), 1216–21 (2019).

71. Suzuki, J., Ozawa, N., Murashima, Y. L., Shinba, T., and Yoshii, M. Neuronal activity in the parietal cortex of EL and DDY mice. *Brain Res.*, 1460, 63–72 (2012).

72. Meisel, C. Antiepileptic drugs induce subcritical dynamics in human cortical networks. (2019) arXiv:190413026 [q-bio]

73. Wang, L., Liu, Y.-H., Huang, Y.-G., and Chen, L.-W. Time-course of neuronal death in the mouse pilocarpine model of chronic epilepsy using Fluoro-Jade C staining. *Brain Res.*, 1241, 157–67 (2008).

74. Stief, F., Zuschratter, W., Hartmann, K., Schmitz, D., and Draguhn, A. Enhanced synaptic excitation-inhibition ratio in hippocampal interneurons of rats with temporal lobe epilepsy. *Eur. J. Neurosci.*, 25(2), 519–28 (2007).

75. Alvarado-Rojas, C., Lehongre, K., Bagdasaryan, J., et al. Single-unit activities during epileptic discharges in the human hippocampal formation. *Front. Comput. Neurosci.*, 7, 140 (2013).

76. Sabolek, H. R., Swiercz, W. B., Lillis, K. P., et al. A candidate mechanism underlying the variance of interictal spike propagation. *J. Neurosci.*, 32(9), 3009–21 (2012).

77. Jacobs, J., Staba, R., Asano, E., et al. High-frequency oscillations (HFOs) in clinical epilepsy. *Prog. Neurobiol.*, 98 (3), 302–15 (2012).

78. Frauscher, B., Bartolomei, F., Kobayashi, K., et al. High-frequency oscillations: The state of clinical research. *Epilepsia*, 58 (8), 1316–29 (2017).

79. Trevelyan, A. J. The Direct Relationship between Inhibitory Currents and Local Field Potentials. *J. Neurosci.*, 29 (48), 15299–307 (2009).

80. Jirsa, V. K., Stacey, W.C ., Quilichini, P. P., Ivanov, A. I., and Bernard, C. On the nature of seizure dynamics. *Brain*, 137 (8), 2210–30 (2014).

81. Houssaini, K. E., Bernard, C., and Jirsa, V. K. The Epileptor model: A systematic mathematical analysis linked to the dynamics of seizures, refractory status epilepticus, and depolarization block. *eNeuro*, 7 (2), ENEURO.0485–18.2019 (2020).

82. Pillow, J. W., Schlens, J., Paninski, L. et al. Spatio-temporal correlations and visual signalling in a complete neuronal population. *Nature*, 454 (7207), 995–9 (2008).

83. Zhou, Jun-Li, Shatskikh, T. N., Liu, X., and Holmes, G. L. Impaired single cell firing and long-term potentiation parallels memory impairment following recurrent seizures. *Euro. J. Neurosci.*, 25(12), 3667–77 (2007).

84. Lenck-Santini, P.-P., and Holmes, G.L. Altered phase precession and compression of temporal sequences by place cells in epileptic rats. *J. Neurosci.*, 28(19), 5053–62 (2008).

85. Hernan, A. E., Mahoney, J. M., Curry, W., et al. Environmental enrichment normalizes hippocampal timing coding in a malformed hippocampus. *PLoS One*, 13(2), e0191488 (2018).

86. Hernan, A. E., Mahoney, J. M., Curry, W., Mawe, S., and Scott, R. C. Fine spike timing in hippocampal-prefrontal ensembles predicts poor encoding and underlies behavioral performance in healthy and malformed brains. *Cereb. Cortex*, 31(1), 147–58 (2020).

87. Bui, A. D., Nguyen, T. M., Limouse, C., et al. Dentate gyrus mossy cells control spontaneous convulsive seizures and spatial memory. *Science*, 359(6377), 787–90 (2018).

88. Goyal, A., Miller, J., Watrous, A. J., et al. Electrical stimulation in hippocampus and entorhinal cortex impairs spatial and temporal memory.

J. Neurosci., 38(19), 4471–81 (2018).

89. Ezzyat, Y., Kragel, J. E., Burke, J. F., et al. Direct brain stimulation modulates encoding states and memory performance in humans. *Curr. Biol.*, 27(9), 1251–8 (2017).

90. Ezzyat, Y., Wanda, P. A., Levy, D. F., et al. Closed-loop stimulation of temporal cortex rescues functional networks and improves memory. *Nat. Commun.*, 9(1), 365 (2018).

91. Topalovic, U., Aghajan, Z. M., Villaroman, D., et al. Wireless programmable recording and stimulation of deep brain activity in freely moving humans. *Neuron.*, 108(2), 322–334.e9 (2020).

Mapping Epileptic Networks with Scalp and Invasive EEG

Applications to Epileptogenic Zone Localization and Seizure Prediction

Manel Vila-Vidal and Adrià Tauste Campo

8.1 Introduction

Since the early 2000s, the growing field of computational neuroscience has shown remarkable applicability in the study of epilepsy. A number of different and complementary approaches have been applied to brain signals obtained with scalp and invasive electroencephalography (EEG) to address a variety of fundamental and clinical problems. Historically, researchers have focused on overt changes in brain electrical signals, which can be detected using signal processing techniques. More recent advances have also shown that connectivity and network-level effects can provide critical information that complements the classical brain regional perspective. Thus, the modern toolkit for epilepsy electrophysiology now includes complex systems approaches such as network science (e.g., graph theory), nonlinear signal processing, information theory, and machine learning techniques. Complex systems approaches have made their contribution to our understanding of epilepsy and to the development of new tools that might improve its diagnosis and treatment.

In this chapter, we provide the reader with an overview of these new approaches, stressing the value that a network-level perspective can bring to address both clinical and research questions. To organize the material and guide the reader, we have structured the chapter around two main problems that have driven research in the field. First, some studies have aimed to extract spatial information about networks that might play a role in the genesis and maintenance of epileptic activity. Complementarily, others have aimed to analyze the dynamics of those networks, either by detecting or predicting changes in brain activity. In Section 8.2 we introduce the main biomarkers

that have been applied to scalp and intracranial EEG to address the first problem. We build up from single-node metrics, through pairwise connectivity measures, to topological features, discussing the advantages and limitations of each of these approaches in mapping epileptic networks. In Section 8.3 we discuss how complex system techniques help us better track the evolution of epileptic network properties across time. In addition, we also show how this perspective can provide insight into the development of seizure prediction algorithms that could open up new possibilities for the treatment of drug-resistant epilepsy.

8.2 Spatial Map of Epileptic Networks: Toward Localization of the Epileptogenic Zone

A diagnosis of epilepsy is based on a combination of different sources of information, including the patient's medical history, seizure semiology, and a number of different tests aimed at detecting brain anatomical or functional abnormalities.[1] Among these, electroencephalography (EEG) is widely used to detect changes in the normal pattern of brain electrical activity. In clinical practice, EEG recordings are visually reviewed by specialized clinicians that target a number of stereotypical patterns of activity associated with epilepsy.

---

[1] Electroencephalography (EEG), long-term video-EEG, computerized tomography scan (CT), magnetic resonance imaging (MRI), functional magnetic resonance imaging (fMRI), positron emission tomography (PET), and ictal single photon emission tomography (SPECT).

In particular, EEG monitoring has become the gold standard diagnostic procedure for MRI lesion negative drug-resistant patients, for which resective surgery might be the only available treatment. The success of resective surgery depends on the correct identification of the epileptogenic zone (EZ), which is defined as the region of the cortex that can generate epileptic seizures and whose removal or complete disconnection is necessary and sufficient to attain seizure freedom. The EZ is a theoretical concept that is related to but different from the seizure onset zone (SOZ), which is the area of the cortex from which clinical seizures are actually generated [1]. Note that the relationship between the two areas is not trivial, as the EZ may include the actual SOZ plus additional areas of the cortex taking the role of

seizure generators after removal of the primary presurgical SOZ.

The EZ cannot be measured directly, and its location must be inferred by defining the SOZ and other affected regions. In combination with structural MRI, scalp EEG is the most important technique to identify the EZ. Scalp EEG is a non-invasive electrophysiological monitoring method that is used to record the electric field generated by neurons with very high temporal resolution (order of ms) by means of electrodes that are placed along the scalp (Fig. 8.1A). However, scalp EEG has a relatively low sensitivity to detect the SOZ and EZ because electrodes are placed relatively far from the cortex and across a number of barriers that significantly alter the recorded signals (meninges, skull, and scalp).

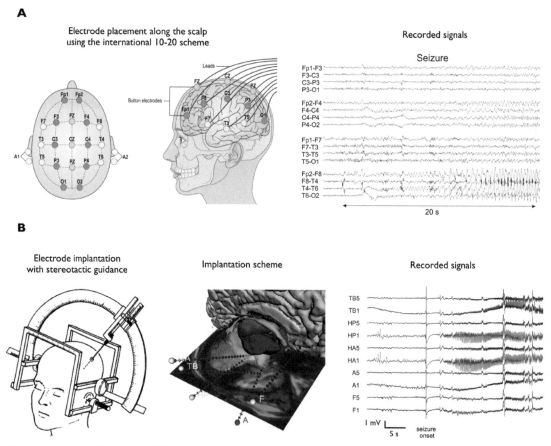

Figure 8.1 Scalp and intracranial EEG recordings. From left to right, examples of electrode implantation, implantation scheme, and recorded signals for each EEG type. A) Scalp EEG. (Left). Reprinted from *Elsevier Fitzgerald's Clinical Neuroanatomy and Neuroscience* (7th ed.), Estomih Mtui, Gregory Gruener, Peter Dockery, "Chapter 30. Electroencephalography," pp. 289–97 [109], Copyright © 2016 Elsevier Ltd., with permission. (Right) Adapted from Hindawi *Epilepsy Research and Treatment*, vol. 2012, article id 637430, Manouchehr Javidan, "Electroencephalography in Mesial Temporal Lobe Epilepsy: A Review" [110], Copyright © 2012 Javidan, under CC BY 3.0. B) Intracranial EEG. (Left) Reprinted from Elsevier *Neurology and Neurosurgery Illustrated* (5th ed.), Kenneth W. Lindsay, Ian Bone, Geraint Fuller, "Section IV. Localized neurological disease and its management: A. Intracranial," pp. 217-388 [111], Copyright © 2011 Elsevier Ltd., with permission.

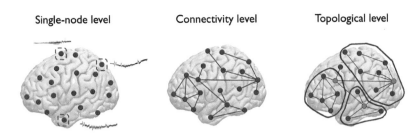

Figure 8.2 **Scheme representing three levels of analysis in network approaches**. (Left) Single-node measures target local properties of brain regions. Three targeted nodes are highlighted in red and their EEG signals are shown. (Middle) Connectivity measures quantify pairwise coactivations of different areas. Connections between pairs of regions are depicted with red edges. (Right) Topological measures quantify global features of the network architecture. In the example, the three red nodes have a high number of connections (hubs). These hubs connect three segregated subnetworks (circled in red). In particular, the subnetwork in the right displays a star-like topology.

When results are contradictory or inconclusive, the patient may undergo invasive EEG (iEEG) monitoring using subdural or depth electrodes that provide direct access to neocortical and deep structures. The most common invasive technique consists of the placement of rigid electrodes into the brain structures that are suspected to be involved in the seizure process. When these electrodes are stereotactically implanted (using three-dimensional systems that allow the precise placement of the electrode in the target sites), the technique is known as stereoelectroencephalography (SEEG). Other invasive recordings might involve the placement of grid or strip electrodes directly on the exposed surface of the brain to record activity from the cortex; this technique is known as electrocorticography (ECoG). In either case, invasive recordings provide continuous monitoring of key regions at a very high temporal resolution for presurgical diagnosis and might be required to precisely determine the cortical areas to be resected (Fig. 8.1B) [2–8].

The current gold standard in epilepsy diagnosis is retrospective visual inspection of EEG recordings, a time-consuming process where highly specialized neurologists target a number of visually observed patterns that might correlate with the EZ. In a subset of patients, estimation of EZ with this procedure might be difficult because of complex, more distributed patterns of activity. In addition, certain features of the signals might remain invisible to the human eye. Overall, the simultaneous and direct recording of different brain structures provided by intracranial EEG has also shown that epilepsy is a complex neurological disease that involves different interconnected cortical structures that are dynamically coactivated over time. This has given rise to the concept of an "epileptogenic network" [9,10], that complements and enriches that of a localized "EZ" [1].

Based on this new conceptual approach, a number of quantitative techniques have been developed to expedite EZ detection and improve our understanding of ictogenesis and the pathophysiology of epileptogenic networks. Biomarkers based on these techniques can be organized in three groups, depending on the network features they target (Fig. 8.2): 1) single-node biomarkers target local properties of brain regions, 2) pairwise connectivity measures assess coactivations of different areas, and 3) topological measures quantify global properties of the network. In the following sections we will introduce and discuss the most common biomarkers used in epilepsy research at the three levels.

8.2.1 Single-Node Epileptogenicity Biomarkers for Intracranial EEG

Epileptic seizures are characterized by an abnormal and excessive amount of neuronal activity in the brain. This activity is often manifested in complex electrophysiological patterns that gradually propagate from the SOZ to a subset of other brain sites. Time-frequency signal analysis provides a framework to quantify temporal variations in brain signals across different frequency bands and has been extensively used to build biomarkers that quantify the degree of involvement of each monitored brain region in the seizure process. Although these biomarkers are built around single-node spectral features, the gradient of values across brain areas is often conceptualized as mapping the participation of each area in the epileptogenic network, i.e., its epileptogenicity [11].

Typical frequency bands considered in the context of brain signals are: delta (1–4 Hz), theta (4–8 Hz), alpha (8–12 Hz), beta (12–30 Hz), gamma (>30 Hz). For oscillatory-like signals, the signal power is defined as the average square amplitude over time and quantifies the magnitude of the oscillation [12]. However, general signals are a combination of activity at multiple frequencies and different mathematical transformations can be used to extract the signal power carried by each frequency. The Fourier transform is a linear transformation that is used to decompose a signal into its constituent frequencies. When signals are empirically observed in a noisy environment, this transformation assumes that the observed signal is stationary, a condition that is rarely met in the analysis of epileptic brain activity, especially during seizure epochs. To overcome this limitation, sliding window approaches can be used to obtain the temporal evolution of the spectrally decomposed signal. An important limitation of this approach, however, is that the length of the time window must be defined beforehand, a procedure that might yield inaccurate results when the temporal scale of quasi-stationary signal periods is not estimated appropriately.

An alternative approach is provided by the Hilbert transform, a nonstationary nonlinear transformation that describes the temporal evolution of the signal power with the same resolution of the sampled signal. The signal is first decomposed into its constituent frequencies by filtering it in a set of frequency bands covering the broadband spectrum or a desired band of interest. For each bandpass filtered signal, the Hilbert transform quantifies the instantaneous power carried by the signal as time varies. Despite being fully adaptive to changes in the temporal domain, this approach still requires the definition of frequency windows in which the signal is primarily decomposed.

The wavelet transform has been also used for time-frequency analysis, offering a framework in which different temporal and frequency scales can be explored at the same time. However, the wavelet transform depends on the a priori definition of bases functions or fundamental time-frequency patterns that the method seeks. It is worth noting that all described techniques are limited by a fundamental uncertainty principle of signal processing, according to which a signal cannot be precisely localized both in time and frequency. Achieving a better temporal resolution in the temporal domain will result in a higher uncertainty of the frequency at which events occur.

8.2.1.1 Frequency-Specific Biomarkers

Fast discharges in the beta (12–30 Hz) and gamma (>30 Hz) bands are known to be good signatures of epileptogenic tissue [13]. Based on this feature and using time-frequency analysis, the first biomarker to assess the "epileptogenicity" of recorded brain structures from the analysis of intracerebral EEG signals in the ictal period was proposed in 2008 [11]. The epileptogenicity index (EI) was designed to mimic the parameters that are typically assessed by clinicians when examining the signals: the propensity of a given brain region to generate rapid discharges (above 12.4 Hz) and the delay of appearance of such oscillations with respect to the seizure onset.

The EI is based on the computation of the energy ratio (ER) of the signals using a sliding window approach. For each brain site and time window, the ER is defined as the ratio between the signal power carried in the high (beta and gamma) and low (theta and alpha) frequency bands. The time-varying measure obtained with this procedure $ER[n]$ is sensitive to frequency shifts in the signal and is expected to increase when beta-gamma discharges raise above background theta-alpha activity. These increases can be detected by means of a change detection algorithm that raises an alarm every time $ER[n]$ crosses a certain threshold and maintains its activity for a certain amount of time. This provides a detection time for each recording site involved in the generation of fast discharges. In order to quantify the delay of involvement of each brain region in the seizure process, the first detection time is arbitrarily set as the reference time n_0 (corresponding to the first region whose ER increases). Then, for each recording site i, the epileptogenicity index EI_i is defined as $ER[n]$ integrated over a certain time window H divided by the delay Δ_i of involvement of site i with respect to time n_0:

$$EI_i = \frac{1}{\Delta_i + 1} \sum_{n=n_0+\Delta_i}^{(n_0+\Delta_i)+H} ER[n]. \tag{1}$$

This index was applied to a cohort of 17 mesial temporal lobe epilepsy (MTLE) patients using a time window H of 5s, finding higher EI values in mesial structures of the temporal lobe than in structures not involved at seizure onset. The gradient observed in the EI values was interpreted by authors as showing that the EZ is not a clearly delimited structure, but rather involves a number of different brain structures with gradual epileptogenicity that, together, form an epileptogenic network with complex interactions. In this vein, the study also showed that the duration of epilepsy in these patients was positively correlated with the number of regions with high epileptogenicity, suggesting an evolution of the disease which consists of the progressive recruitment of regions within the EZ [11]. Further studies confirmed that the EI is higher in regions suspected, from etiology, to be part of the SOZ [14].

A few years later, methodological advances in neuroimaging were incorporated with intracranial EEG analysis to generate statistical parametric maps of the EI that extend beyond the recording sites per se [15]. On one hand, epileptogenicity was redefined as a significant increase of signal power in high-frequency activity (60–100 Hz) during a time window of 4 s after seizure onset, when compared to a baseline recording of at least 20 s, deliberately chosen not to contain strong artifact or epileptic activity. On the other hand, spatial interpolation of SEEG log-power from the electrode coordinates was used to create spatially extended brain maps. In particular, the epileptogenicity map was defined as the t-value of the differences in smoothed log-power between ictal and baseline activity. By applying a threshold on the associated p-value, regions showing significant rapid discharges after seizure onset were delineated. Epileptogenicity maps at seizure onset were found to pinpoint seizure focus regions in a group of 13 patients. Additionally, this neuroimaging approach renders a significant advantage when compared to studies that limit their conclusions to the recording sites per se.

Further studies have systematically made use of fast activity as a natural biomarker for the SOZ. In particular, a number of recent studies have proposed automatic methods for SOZ localization based on the detection of high-frequency oscillations (HFOs) [16–18]. Nonetheless, HFOs are known to be also present in physiological activity [19].

Moreover, both research and clinical practice have shown that there is a huge variety of electrophysiological patterns associated with seizure genesis and propagation (Fig. 8.3A) [20,21]. Singh et al. reviewed at least 15 different ictal onset patterns (IOPs) appearing in the literature: low-voltage fast activity was the most common pattern among neocortical epilepsies, low frequency high amplitude repetitive spiking (LFRS) was associated with mesial TLE, and slow delta waves (0.5–4 Hz)

were infrequently yet occasionally reported. The conclusion of the review was that "no single IOP is associated consistently with a focal onset" [22].

8.2.1.2 Multispectral Biomarkers

The heterogeneity of emergent electrophysiological seizure patterns renders frequency-specific biomarkers such as the EI practically ineffective to universally characterize the SOZ or EZ in all seizure types and patients. For instance, biomarkers based on HFOs are very specific to fast discharges but might overlook pathological patterns of activity dominated by lower frequency oscillations that evolve over longer temporal scales.

Ictal patterns are varied in frequency, amplitude, and duration, and might evolve in the three domains as the seizure progresses and activity propagates across the network. This feature adds a layer of complexity to the study of seizure generation and propagation and lays bare the need to find more flexible measures that can encompass the multispectral properties of seizure dynamics.

A first approach to address this issue can be to tailor the frequency or frequencies of interest (FOIs) in which signal power is computed depending on the electrophysiological pattern observed in each seizure. Around half of the patients included in a 2011 study [23] exhibited seizures with a focal pattern characterized by a peak in activity below 20 Hz, followed by fast or very fast discharges (100–300 Hz). Patient-specific FOIs at seizure onset and during the following phases of seizures were determined by inspecting the spectral power distribution and finding the frequencies displaying the most prominent activations. In each FOI, the variable used to define the epileptogenicity of brain structures was the integral of each contact's power over the relevant time period, i.e., the total energy carried by the signal in the time period.

Although relying on visual inspection of spectrograms, this study constitutes a first attempt to include the heterogeneity of IOPs and inform the method with seizure-specific features. In particular, recording sites that were responsible for each FOI at seizure onset and for the following FOI patterns were identified and accumulated across frequencies and seizures to map a single EZ per patient. The extension of the EZ defined in eight patients with this procedure was found to correlate well with the clinically-marked EZ, confirming the need for more complex multi-frequency approaches in mapping this network.

A)

Seizure onset patterns

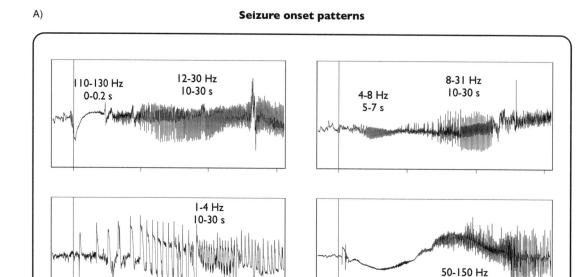

B)

TC-plot

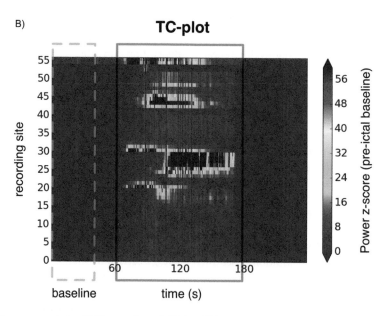

Figure 8.3 Time-frequency analysis of iEEG recordings. A) Distinct EEG patterns associated with seizure onset. Seizure onset is marked with a red vertical line in each EEG trace. Left top: Low-voltage fast activity combined with rhythmic spiking (~10 Hz) initiated from high-frequency oscillations. Left bottom: Very slow spiking activity (~1 Hz) of large amplitude that becomes faster (up to ~4 Hz) as the seizure progresses. Right top: Low-voltage fast activity combined with rhythmic spiking (~10 Hz) initiated from theta activity (4–8 Hz). Right bottom: Spectrally diffuse activity (50–150 Hz) of very low amplitude. B) Time-channel plot quantify seizure initiation and propagation in a given frequency of interest. Time-varying instantaneous activation for 56 channels, obtained by normalization of the frequency-independent instantaneous power with respect to a baseline distribution defined by the power values of all channels during the first 40 s of the preictal period. Reprinted from Elsevier *Clinical Neurophysiology*, vol. 128, no.6, Manel Vila-Vidal, Alessandro Principe, Miguel Ley, et al., "Detection of recurrent activation patterns across focal seizures: Application to seizure onset zone identification" [24], Copyright © 2017 International Federation of Clinical Neurophysiology, with permission. Similarly found in [23].

Ictal onset and propagation patterns can be easily evaluated by means of succinct 2D color intensity maps that display the time evolution of all contacts' power in a given frequency of interest (Fig. 8.3B). As proposed by Vila-Vidal et al. [24], two main variables can be defined to characterize these patterns: the signal power increase (referred to as mean activation (MA)) at a given frequency band, and the delay of this increase with respect to seizure onset (referred to as activation onset (AO)). Specifically, for each targeted brain region, frequency band, and time windows of interest, the former parameter is defined to quantify the average spectral activation with respect to a certain baseline period, while the latter accounts for the onset of this activation defined similarly as in the EI.

In a cohort of seven patients, by Vila-Vidal et al. analyzed the predictive power of both variables for different combinations of frequency of interest (3–8 Hz, 8–20 Hz, 20–70 Hz, 70–165 Hz, and broadband) and time window (5 s after seizure onset and the whole seizure). Interestingly, slow activity (3–8 Hz and 8–20 Hz) achieved the highest discrimination values between SOZ and non-SOZ sites when the whole seizure period was considered, indicating that the choice of frequency and time window of interest in SOZ identification are intimately tied. An open-access Python package with the tools used in that study is publicly available [25].

Both studies, [23] and [24], reported general inter-seizure stability within each patient, with isolated cases of distinct seizure patterns in some patients. In particular, the study by Vila-Vidal et al. was the first to incorporate an automatic step to assess the homogeneity of ictal-driven patterns (MA and AO) across seizures of the same patient.

Following the effort to design a method that can be adapted to seizure specificities, Vila-Vidal et al. developed an algorithm to automatically find the time-frequency windows that characterize the seizure onset pattern in each case [26]. These features are then used to inform a classifier that performs a binary SOZ detection. Central to the proposed analysis is the definition of two novel measures that characterize global coactivations and their spread across the entire network, respectively. These measures are jointly optimized to obtain the time-frequency windows in which the SOZ can be maximally discriminated from the remaining sites. By varying certain parameters,

additional regions of the EZ can be also detected. This methodology was tested in a cohort of 10 temporal lobe epilepsy patients with varied seizure onset patterns, exhibiting remarkable accuracy in identifying both the SOZ and IOPs in each case

Other biomarkers combine a set of parameters that quantify the presence of commonly observed patterns such as fast activity at 80–120 Hz, transient slow potential shift and signal flattening [27] as a way to encompass the described heterogeneity. Alternative approaches coming from dynamical systems and information theory base their predictions on the intrinsic dynamical properties of targeted brain nodes in the whole spectrum, thus avoiding the need of spectral decompositions. In particular, it has been shown that interictal EEG signals from epileptogenic brain areas are less random and more stationary compared to signals recorded from non-epileptogenic brain areas [28]. In addition, EZ signals have stronger mutual nonlinear dependencies on each other than the non-EZ regions. These results led to the definition of the univariate time-varying nonlinear structure index (NLSI) by Andrzejak et al. [29], which quantifies the degree to which present states of the local dynamics allow the prediction of future states of the signal, a way to quantify how random signals are.

Overall, signal analysis can provide a first approximation to classify brain regions according to their electrophysiological patterns and to categorize their participation in the epileptogenic network. In the study done by Andrzejak et al. in 2015 [29], the performance of four single-node biomarkers for EZ characterization [11,15,27,29] was compared in a cohort of four patients. This study concluded that 1) the sensitivity of the four methods to detect the EZ was strongly dependent on the specific seizure pattern and 2) when traditional visual inspection was not successful in detecting EZ on iEEG, the different signal analysis methods produced discordant outputs. From these conclusions, it seems clear that no single univariate parameter can reliably unravel the underpinnings of brain functional interactions that generate and sustain pathological networks. As such, the identification of the epileptogenic network remains elusive, and more sophisticated measures that can explicitly account for node-to-node interactions and network effects might be required in the more complex cases.

8.2.2 Connectivity-Based Methods for Intracranial EEG

The methods in Section 8.2.1 focused on node-level metrics, like stereotyped changes in spectral content as a function of peri-seizure time. However, functional alterations in the brain tissue extend beyond the SOZ proper [11], suggesting distributed, interictal abnormalities in brain dynamics. Following Bartolomei et al., "today, the classical notion of epileptic focus should be replaced by a more complex model that takes into account the potential interactions within the neuronal networks involved in seizures" [30].

This change of perspective has proven fruitful, resulting in a number of studies that have aimed to detect altered interactions and causal relationships between the monitored structures as putative biomarkers for the EZ or related structures. From this point of view, the brain is seen as a network of distributed nodes that interact at different. Graph theory and network analysis techniques can be used to quantify how brain regions are structurally and functionally connected [31]. Three categories of connectivity can be studied in the brain. Structural connectivity quantifies the underlying anatomical connections linking distant neural populations, functional connectivity refers to temporal covariations of the neural activity in different regions that can be statistically tested, and effective connectivity describes the influence or causal effect that one neural population exerts over another, either at a synaptic or a cortical level. More specifically, effective connectivity depends critically on state-space models that try to explain the complex patterns of neural activity covariations observed with measurements [31–33].[2] Connectivity measures can be classified according to a number of additional criteria: they can quantify directed or undirected, linear or nonlinear, associations between either the amplitude or the phase of recorded signals in the time or frequency domains. Additionally, bivariate methods quantify associations between pairs of nodes, while multivariate measures take into account the whole set of signals and can differentiate between direct and mediated relationships. For a comprehensive review and mathematical formulation of connectivity measures and their application in epilepsy research, see [32].

A second level of analysis is provided by graph theory and modern network analysis, which builds upon the estimated connectivity relationships to extract topological features of the brain network. Local indices can be used to characterize the importance of certain nodes within the network, pinpointing hubs where information is integrated and then distributed to other regions. In addition, global indices can be used to assess how the network is organized, whether only neighboring regions exchange information, whether there are generalized long-range interactions or whether information is centralized and then distributed.

In the following list we gather some concepts from network science [34] commonly encountered in epilepsy research. The list is not exhaustive and is intended to serve as a glossary for the reader throughout the rest of the chapter:

- Node degree. The node degree is the number of total connections or edges that link it to other nodes in the network. For directed graphs, two degrees can be defined for each node. The outdegree refers to the total amount of outgoing or efferent connections that emerge from it, while the indegree is the number of incoming or afferent connections.

- Shortest path length. For any given pair of nodes, the shortest path length is the number of connections of the shortest path joining the two nodes, i.e., the smallest number of edges that need to be traversed to go from the first node to the second.

- Centrality. The centrality of a node quantifies its global importance within the network. Different quantifiers can be used to characterize the centrality. For instance, the betweenness centrality of a node is defined as the ratio between the number of shortest paths (between all other node pairs) that cross that node and the total number of shortest paths in the whole network.

- Hub. Hubs are highly interconnected nodes. The hub value of a node can be quantified either with its degree or centrality.

---

[2] The characterization of effective connectivity and its distinction from the functional connectivity at a practical level is not free of controversy. For instance, some of the cited reviews classify Granger-based methods [112] as a measure of effective connectivity between brain regions [33,52], while others define it as a measure of lagged functional connectivity [31,32].

- Clustering coefficient. The clustering coefficient measures the degree to which nodes in a network tend to cluster together. Local and global clustering coefficients can be defined. For a given node, the local clustering coefficient is defined as the ratio between the number of connections that exist between nodes adjacent to it and the maximum number of possible connections. The global clustering coefficient of a network can be defined as the average local coefficient.
- Assortativity. The assortativity is a global index that quantifies the preference of a network's nodes to attach to nodes with similar properties (typically with similar degree or centrality). The assortativity can be computed as a correlation between degrees of connected nodes.

8.2.2.1 Coherence-Based Methods

The first attempts to use connectivity measures to estimate the EZ date back to the 1970s and 1980s [35]. Because effects in brain activity have been found to be strongly dependent on its frequency components, measures in the frequency domain are preferred over their time analogs. To disentangle frequency-specific interactions that might remain invisible in the broadband signal, measures are typically derived from the cross-spectral density function. For each pair of nodes i and j, the cross-spectral density function $S_{ij}(f)$ is the Fourier transform of the cross-correlation and quantifies the strength of the linear coupling between recording sites i and j at each frequency f. Upon normalization by the auto-spectral density functions, the coherency is obtained:

$$C_{ij}(f) = \frac{S_{ij}(f)}{\sqrt{S_{ii}(f)S_{jj}(f)}}. \qquad (2)$$

Note that the coherency is, in general, a complex-valued function. Its module is referred to as coherence and ranges between 0 and 1. Because coherence relies on the use of the Fourier transform of the signal it can only be applied to stationary signals. To meet such a condition, the recordings can be segmented into smaller time periods where stationarity holds.

The coherence is a bivariate measure and can only account for relationships between two signals at a time. Analogously to the partial correlation in the time domain,[3] the partial coherence can be defined to assess conditionally dependent relationships. The partial coherence between two signals is defined as the coherence between their residuals, after the linear effect of the remaining signals has been regressed out. Note that partial coherence captures mutual statistical dependencies between nodes and it cannot, in general, be interpreted as a measure of direct functional interactions. Yet, the phase of the coherency can be used to determine consistent time lags between pairs of signals as proxy for a potential directed interaction of one signal onto the other.

Network-Based Applications

In 1970, Gersch and Godard used these measures to locate the epileptic focus in the brain of a cat with iEEG recordings obtained during a generalized seizure where widespread activations rendered visual detection impossible [36]. For each set of three recording sites, the coherence and partial coherence were compared to infer whether one channel might be driving the other two at a given frequency. The main driver of the seizure was successfully identified using this procedure.

On the other hand, time lags were first used in 1972 by Brazier [37] in patients with stereotactically implanted electrodes to infer the locus whose abnormal discharge precedes other structures in the development of a similar abnormal activity. For each pair of recording sites, the coherence (magnitude of the coherency) was maximized to detect dominant frequencies in wave trains common to both sites and the phase of the coherency was used to determine which site was leading and which was lagging in the course of the abnormal discharge. Interestingly, Brazier tested the general applicability of the method to trace the propagation of wave-like activity in a series of patients with psychiatric disorders that had intracranial electrodes implanted and obtained results that were concordant with well-established anatomical pathways. A similar approach was used in 1983 by Gotman to precisely establish time

---

[3] In a network of multiple nodes, the partial correlation measures the degree of association between the activity of two nodes, after regressing out the effect of the remaining nodes' activity. In general, partial correlation measures are effective in avoiding the confounding effect of observed third-node variables.

differences between the activity of different EEG channels that appeared synchronous on visual inspection [38]. The focus was found to consistently lead other recording sites by 5–30 ms even when the seizure activity was widespread, demonstrating the added value of connectivity measures over visual inspection or single-node measures when describing seizure propagation.

8.2.2.2 MVAR Model and Related Connectivity Measures

A major limitation of coherence analysis is that it merely captures mutual statistical dependencies between brain structures, giving no information about *how* they are functionally linked. In addition, leading and lagging relationships between nodes extracted from the coherence phase can be spuriously generated by uncontrolled variables. To explicitly quantify the direction of information flow over stationary periods of activity over the epileptic brain network, a battery of multivariate measures has been developed on the basis of autoregressive (AR) models. In this framework, signals are represented as linear combinations of their own past plus uncorrelated noise. When multiple signals are jointly considered (as in a network of interconnected nodes) and used as regressors of one another, the model is called multivariate autoregressive model (MVAR). For signals simultaneously recorded from a network of N nodes, the MVAR model can be written as

$$X(t) = \sum_{\tau=1}^{p} A(\tau)X(t - \tau) + E(t), \qquad (3)$$

where $X(t)$ is the state variable at time t (i.e., a vector consisting of the N signals at time t), p is the model order, $A(\tau)$ is the $N \times N$ coefficient matrix for the delay τ that encodes directed connections in the network, and $E(t)$ is the uncorrelated noise. The model order defines the length of the time window that is used to predict the present state of the system, and the coefficient matrix $A(\tau)$ quantifies the influence of the past onto the current network state. More precisely, the matrix entry $A_{ij}(\tau)$ quantifies the linear influence of the past activity at node j on the current values of node i at a time lag τ. For a given problem, the model order can be chosen using model comparison criteria, and the coefficients can be estimated with the ordinary least square procedure or with the method of the moments [39].

As already discussed, in epilepsy-related problems we are typically interested in frequency-dependent relationships. The Fourier transform of the coefficient matrices $A(f)$ quantifies direct interrelations between signals at particular frequencies. Specifically, the coefficient $A_{ij}(f)$ quantifies the effect of node j on node i at frequency f. The normalized version of this measure defines the partial directed coherence (PDC) [40]

$$PDC_{ij}(f) = \frac{A_{ij}(f)}{\sqrt{\sum_{k=1}^{N} |A_{kj}(f)|^2}}, \qquad (4)$$

where $PDC_{ij}(f)$ represents the fraction of information flow from node j to node i at frequency f with respect to the total outgoing flow from node j.

Another connectivity measure commonly used to quantify epileptic network interactions is the directed transfer function (DTF), defined by Kaminski and Blinkowska in 1991 to estimate both direct and indirect information transfer between the signals' nodes at a given frequency of interest [41]. The representation of the MVAR process in the frequency domain can be expressed as

$$X(f) = H(f)E(f), \qquad (5)$$

where $X(f)$ and $E(f)$ are the Fourier transforms of the signals and the random noise, respectively, and $H(f) = A^{-1}(f)$ is the transfer matrix of the system. This equation allows breaking down each node's signal power at a particular frequency as the direct contribution of all other nodes in the network:

$$X_i(f) = \sum_{k=1}^{N} H_{ik}(f)e_k(f), \qquad (6)$$

From this, the DTF is defined as

$$DTF_{ij}(f) = \frac{H_{ij}(f)}{\sqrt{\sum_{k=1}^{N} |H_{ik}(f)|^2}}, \qquad (7)$$

where the numerator represents the information flow from node j to node i and the denominator represents the total incoming flow to node i. Hence, $DTF_{ij}(f)$ quantifies how much oscillations of node i are driven by oscillations at node j at frequency f. The measure can also be integrated over a band of interest to obtain the integrated DTF (iDTF).

The validity of AR-based methods critically depends on the signals being stationary, a condition that is rarely met in the context of epilepsy research. To overcome this limitation, time-varying extensions of the MVAR model and the

DTF measure can be used. Among them, the adaptive DTF (ADTF) [42,43] relies on the use of the Kalman filter algorithm to estimate the autoregressive coefficients of a time-varying multivariate autoregressive model (TVAR).

Network-Based Applications

The PDC was used by Varotto et al. [44] to investigate the synchronization properties of the lesional zone[4] in patients suffering from epilepsy with type II focal cortical dysplasia under inter-ictal, preictal, and ictal conditions. The authors showed that the region inside the dysplasia was characterized by abnormal outgoing connectivity (mainly in the gamma band) in the whole period, pinpointing the leading role of the lesional zone in the generation and spread of seizure events to the rest of the network in this kind of epilepsy. In parallel, the first epilepsy study to use the DTF both with grid and depth electrodes was [45]. Their method was tested in stationary periods of activity obtained from three patients with MTLE. Their method was shown to reveal patterns of seizure onset and propagation, allowing for the localization of the source of seizure activity. The authors suggested that the method could also be used to pinpoint remote areas that might act as secondary generators after seizure onset and that should also be considered for resection. Further studies use DTF-based methods to localize the EZ regions with depth electrodes [45,46] and with grid electrodes in combination with ictal source localization techniques [47,48]. An in-depth overview of these studies can be found in [32].

To deal with nonstationary signals, Van Mierlo et al. tested the ADTF both with simulated data and intracranial recordings from depth and grid electrodes of one patient that remained seizure-free with a follow-up of 3 years [35]. Using a modified version of the ADTF (full-frequency ADTF (ffADTF)) in the range 5–30 Hz, the authors analyzed four seizure onsets and 29 subclinical seizures and studied propagation patterns by thresholding the ffADTF values based on the ffADTF distribution of preictal iEEG epochs. Information flow patterns were similar across all analyzed seizures and highest outflow values were found for nodes within the resected area. In a later study [49], van Mierlo et al. analyzed a total of 27 seizures from 8 patients using another ADTF-based measure (the spectrum-weighted ADTF (swADTF)) in the frequency band 3–40 Hz. The study concluded that in all cases the electrode nodes with the highest outdegree lay within the ictal onset zone defined by the epileptologist and within the resected region that rendered the patient seizure-free.

In a series of studies, Wilke et al. used the iADTF technique to study the connectivity patterns during interictal spikes [43,46]. In 2011, the same group combined the DTF with the network measure of betweenness centrality to find critical nodes during both ictal and interictal states from a cohort of 25 patients [50]. Specifically, using a sliding window approach, they extracted the time-varying DTF betweenness centrality of each node, a measure that is defined as the ratio between the number of shortest paths that cross the node and the total number of shortest paths in a network. Nodes with the highest values of betweenness centrality were found to lie within the resected regions in patients that were seizure-free after surgery, suggesting that critically interconnected nodes play a crucial role in seizure onset and spread. They also found that these network interactions were also present during random non-ictal periods as well as during interictal spike activity, reinforcing the view that pathological functional networks may be also present during seizure-free periods.

8.2.2.3 Phase Synchronization

The main limitation of MVAR modeling is the assumption that the relationships of the underlying process are linear. This is particularly important if we take into account that EEG signals from epileptogenic brain areas may have a strong yet nonlinear coupling [51,52]. To overcome this drawback, nonlinear, mostly bivariate, connectivity measures have also been used in epilepsy research [32,53].

---

[4] The lesional zone or epileptogenic lesion is the portion of the cortex with radiological lesions that might be responsible for the cause of epileptic seizures. Epileptogenic lesions are initially diagnosed with MRI and later confirmed with functional neuroimaging techniques such as EEG [1]. The relationship of the lesional zone and the EZ is not trivial. On one hand, some lesions might not be epileptogenic or might depend on other tissue to elicit seizures. On the other hand, in a number of patients no radiographic lesion is observable.

A first set of measures relies on quantifying the strength of phase couplings between signals. As previously discussed, the coherence can be indirectly used to assess those relationships. However, the most commonly used bivariate measures to assess phase synchronization are the phase locking value (PLV) [54], also called mean phase coherence [55], and the phase lag index (PLI) [56]. The computation of either measure intrinsically assumes that signals are generated from a single oscillatory component (i.e., dominated by a single and clear frequency) and their instantaneous phases can be extracted using the Hilbert or wavelet transforms. This assumption is not true for the case of brain signals, which are typically a combination of activity at multiple frequencies. In this case, spectral decomposition of signals by means of bandpass filtering is a prerequisite to obtain physically meaningful results.

For two given nodes and a particular frequency of interest, the PLV quantifies the spread of the distribution of phase differences across time. Specifically, for two nodes i and j the PLV is defined as:

$$PLV_{i,j} = \frac{1}{T} \left| \sum_{t=1}^{T} e^{-i\left(\phi_i(t) - \phi_j(t)\right)} \right|, \tag{8}$$

where $\phi_i(t)$ and $\phi_j(t)$ are the instantaneous phases of signals i and j, respectively, and T is their total length. When the two nodes display synchronous activity, the phase difference between them is expected to remain constant across time and PLV attains a value of 1. On the contrary, when there is no coupling, the phase differences are randomly distributed and PLV is 0 [54].

The PLI, on the other hand, simply tests whether the phase difference distribution is shifted toward positive or negative values, against the null hypothesis that it is randomly distributed around zero. The PLI is defined as:

$$PLI_{i,j} = \left| \langle sign(\phi_i(t) - \phi_j(t)) \rangle_t \right|, \tag{9}$$

where $\langle \cdot \rangle_t$ stands for the mean across time [54].

Network-Based Applications

In a study performed with interictal recordings from 17 patients with bilateral implantations [55], Mormann et al. found spatial and temporal alterations in PLV that correlated with pathological activity. In the spatial domain, the study revealed increased synchronization even in seizure-free segments on the brain hemisphere containing the EZ in 82% of the patients. Although the authors stressed the difficulty to obtain finer estimates of the EZ due to the non-pathological variations in synchronization across brain structures, this result suggested that the EZ might display altered connectivity in the interictal state with high diagnostic value. This result was complemented with other studies that reported altered network topology in the network state. Using PLI, Van Diessen et al. [57] found that the EZ was associated with a decreased hub value in the theta frequency band. In network science, hubs are highly interconnected brain regions and the hub value of a region refers to the total number of connections that it has with other nodes. Taken together, these results suggest that during interictal periods, the EZ becomes functionally disconnected from other brain structures while exhibiting an increased intra-region connectivity.

8.2.2.4 Nonlinear Correlation Coefficient

Another nonlinear approach was envisaged by Pijn and Lopes da Silva to study propagation in scalp EEG recordings and was then extended to intracranial EEG [58]. These authors introduced the nonlinear correlation coefficient h_{xy}^2, which measures the coupling strength between nodes x and y, based on a nonlinear function estimated from the two nodes' signals. Specifically, the coefficient h_{xy}^2 quantifies the reduction of variance of signal y that can be obtained by predicting its values using the values of signal x with an optimal time lag τ_{xy} and an optimal fitting curve that models their statistical dependence. The asymmetry of this measure led Bartolomei and Wendling to propose the direction index D_{xy} [59], that is based on the sign of $h_{xy}^2 - h_{yx}^2$ (stating which signal best predicts the other) and the sign of $\tau_{xy} - \tau_{yx}$ (stating which signal is leading and which is lagging). The direction index is nonzero only when one signal consistently across time samples depends on and is delayed with respect to the other.

Network-Based Applications

Using a sliding window approach, Wendling and Bartolomei used this method to investigate the coupling between limbic and neocortical structures in TLE patients, and to infer epileptogenic networks that might be responsible for the triggering of seizures in focal epilepsy [60]. In another study done with 13 patients, the nonlinear correlation method was used to study the coupling between the thalamus and temporal structures. The study reported a positive correlation between the degree of thalamocortical ictal synchrony and the surgical outcome, suggesting that an extended reach of the epileptogenic network to the thalamus might have prognostic value.

A very recent study done with SEEG from 51 patients with focal epilepsy proposed a new measure, the connectivity epileptogenicity index (cEI) [61], that combines a directed connectivity measure derived from the nonlinear correlation coefficient and the original EI previously introduced (see Equation (1)) [11]. In particular, for each pair of nodes directionality of information flow in the beta-gamma range (12–45 Hz) was determined in different time windows as described in the previous paragraph. Then, an outdegree measure was defined for each node by computing the total number of outgoing connections and this value was averaged across time windows to obtain a single outdegree value per node. In seizures displaying slow onset patterns the cEI was found to outperform EI, suggesting high-frequency interactions that might remain invisible to the human eye. However, the use of connectivity did not improve the mapping of the epileptic network over the single-node EI measure in seizures displaying fast onset patters. Overall, this exemplifies that the application and utility of connectivity-based biomarkers is not always straightforward and is strongly dependent on the context and specific clinical or research question.

8.2.2.5 Information Theory

A well-known group of nonlinear bivariate connectivity measures originate from information theory. Information theory was originally proposed by Claude Shannon in 1948 [62] to study quantification, storage, and communication of information and has been widely applied in a variety of different fields. Information-based measures have the advantage of being model-free nonlinear techniques that make no assumption on the kind of coupling between nodes.

One of the central measures in information theory is entropy, which quantifies the amount of uncertainty associated with the value of a random variable. For a generic random variable X associated with the time-varying activity of a network node during a time period, the entropy is defined as

$$H(X) = E_X[-\log P_X], \tag{10}$$

where E_X denotes the expectation over the probability distribution P_X. The entropy is maximized when all possible values of X are equiprobable, the activity of the node being most unpredictable. On the contrary, when the node displays constant activity, there is no uncertainty in its future values and, therefore, its entropy is 0.

To quantify undirected associations between nodes in a network, the mutual information (MI) can be used. The MI of two random variables measures the statistical dependence between them by quantifying the amount of information obtained about one random variable that is obtained upon observation of the other, i.e., the reduction of uncertainty over a variable upon observation of the other. Formally, for two nodes, whose activity is described with variables X and Y, respectively, the MI can be expressed as

$$MI(X, Y) = H(X) + H(Y) - H(X, Y), \tag{11}$$

where $H(X, Y)$ is the joint entropy when considering the two nodes together. In the case where the activity of the two nodes is independent, the joint entropy equals the sum of the marginal entropies and the MI is 0. On the other hand, when the two nodes are totally coupled displaying the same behavior, observation of one node is sufficient to predict the other nodes' activity. In this case, the three entropy functions take the same value and the MI coincides with the entropy value of either node.

The MI is a symmetric measure and provides no information about directionality. Another information-theoretic functional that can be used to overcome this limitation is the transfer entropy (TE), a directional biomarker that quantifies the reduction of uncertainty of a variable achieved when incorporating the past values of another variable. More specifically, for two nodes whose activity is represented with two random processes $\{X_t\}$ and $\{Y_t\}$, where t represents time, the TE is formally defined as:

$$TE(\{X_t\} \rightarrow \{Y_t\}) = H(Y_t | Y_{t-1}, \ldots, Y_{t-L})$$
$$- H\left(Y_t | Y_{t-1}, \ldots, Y_{t-L}, X_{t-1}, \ldots, X_{t-L}\right), \tag{12}$$

Where X_t and Y_t are samples of the process, L is the length of the time window used to predict present values, and $H(A|B)$ stands for the conditional entropy, the entropy of variable A when the value of B is known. As previously stated, the TE is an asymmetric measure and can be used to estimate directed causal effects of the first node on the other. Note that the TE from one node to another will be nonzero only when the past activity of the first node is consistently influencing the current value of the second node.

TE considers the influence of $\{X_t\}$ and $\{Y_t\}$ over a limited time window (L steps backward), implicitly assuming that the underlying processes are stationary. An extension of this measure for more general dynamics and interactions is given by the directed information (DI). DI quantifies the total amount of information transferred from one node to another over the whole recording period, imposing no assumptions on the underlying distributions. For two network nodes, the recorded signal of which is represented by two T-length sequences of random variables $X^T = (X_1, \ldots X_T)$ and $Y^T = (Y_1, \ldots Y_T)$, respectively, the DI over the whole recordings is defined as

$$DI(X^T \rightarrow Y^T) = \sum_{t=1}^{T} MI(Y_t; X_1, \ldots X_t | Y_1, \ldots Y_{t-1}).$$

(13)

Although conceptually different from the TE, the general assumptions of DI estimators (stationarity, ergodicity) result in both measures giving equivalent results for practical estimations. In general, results obtained with model-free connectivity measures such as information-theoretic functionals are strongly dependent on the selected estimation method. Our group has also released open-access implementations for DI inference in Matlab and Python [63,64].

Network-Based Applications

In a study performed with strip electrodes implanted in two patients with focal and generalized seizures [65], nodes consistent with seizure onset were found to have increased MI values during the seizure period in patients with focal seizures, while higher MI was generally found for all pairs of sampled network nodes in patients with generalized seizures. However, this method could not identify significant increases in MI between nodes generating seizures and nodes with apparent propagated activity. Based on this result,

the paper concluded that seizure activity in the latter nodes might be independently generated.

Another study done with four patients with TLE [66] used TE to assess causal connectivity patterns. The study showed that this measure can successfully track information flow across the epileptic network even when blindly applied to long EEG segments of interictal activity (around 600 h), potentially helping in the localization of the EZ core when there is no ictal activity available. Finally, the DI has also been used to estimate causal effects on the epileptic network. In particular, Malladi et al. compared two DI estimators [67]. The first estimator assumed an underlying MVAR model, thus quantifying only linear causal interactions in a similar fashion as Granger Causality. In addition, a data-driven estimator based on probability density reconstructions by means of Gaussian kernels was proposed. Both methods were applied to ECoG recordings from five patients with varied epilepsy types to estimate causal connectivity patterns during seizures.

The study showed that SOZ nodes were more isolated from the rest upon seizure onset when quantifying only linear interactions, but they displayed large net outflows when quantifying nonlinear couplings. This result reinforces the idea that seizures are a highly nonlinear phenomenon during which the SOZ paces the rest of the network by means of nonlinear causal influences. Furthermore, this study stressed the strong dependence of the results on the connectivity measure choice.

In summary, nonlinear methods can potentially yield better estimations of node interactions in epilepsy and the results obtained with them can potentially improve our understanding of seizure mechanisms. Nonetheless, the applicability of these measures, most of which are model-free, is not straightforward and each estimation method entails certain assumptions that can have a large influence on the results. The statistical power of estimations can be assessed by performing nonparametric significance tests such as permutation tests. Another limitation of model-free measures derives from the complexity of extending them to encompass multivariate interactions. Estimation of joint or conditional probabilities would require lengthy time series to have enough estimation power, which makes this computationally challenging to date.

8.2.3 Scalp EEG: Source Inversion and Network-Based Applications

Brain activity in patients with epilepsy can also be investigated using the electrophysiological signals recorded from scalp EEG sensors. The main advantage of this technique over iEEG is that it is a cheap noninvasive procedure that requires minimal preparation. In fact, scalp EEG is routinely performed during long-term presurgical investigations, offering a continuous monitoring of neural activity with a high temporal resolution.

The use of this technique supposes a conceptual change with respect to intracranial EEG and has a number of advantages and limitations over its invasive counterpart that are worth discussing. While the former offers direct measurements of targeted brain structures, the latter captures voltage fluctuations at the surface of the scalp resulting from ionic currents originating from sufficiently large neural populations. Thanks to volume conduction, which allows the transmission of electromagnetic fields from primary current sources through biological tissue, these currents can be detected at the level of the scalp as changes in electric potential. The brain activity generating the measured potentials can be inferred by means of certain model-based techniques, as will be discussed later.

From the network point of view, scalp EEG offers larger spatial coverage. However, this is largely restricted to the cortical surface due to the dampening of activity as distance increases. Moreover, standard configurations include around 20 to 40 electrodes, resulting in a poor spatial resolution, an issue that has partially been addressed by increasing the number of sensors (high-density EEG, up to 256 electrodes) and by combining it with other high spatial resolution techniques such as MEG [68,69] or fMRI [70,71].

A number of studies have applied connectivity measures directly to these signals to extract clinically relevant information. Coherence and phase differences of scalp EEG recordings have been related to the surgical outcome and have successfully been used to lateralize seizures in focal epilepsies. The TE has also been used to identify the hemisphere containing the seizure focus, and PDC- and DTF-related measures have provided rough localizations of the focus [32].

However, these approaches suffer methodological limitations such as volume conduction contamination. In general, the most relevant contributions come from combining scalp EEG with a neuroimaging perspective, with the aim of inferring the intracranial activity that might give rise to scalp potentials. This perspective runs into two major challenging issues. On one hand, brain tissues attenuate and modify the potentials before they reach the electrodes. On the other, the activity of all brain regions can be potentially measured by all EEG sensors simultaneously, generating spurious correlations between electrodes. In particular, the visibility of each source to each sensor depends on a number of factors that cannot be fully controlled.

8.2.3.1 EEG Source Inversion

Electrical source imaging (ESI) techniques allow information coming from different sources to be disentangled, thus estimating the neural activity that might have generated the signals recorded by the scalp sensors. From a methodological point of view, this is significantly distinct from the pure signal processing and statistical approaches in the previous sections. ESI requires a generative model based on biophysical mechanisms for the observed signals. This model, more commonly known as forward model, characterizes the electrical field propagation in the subject's head. Individual MRI is used to estimate the size and specific location of each tissue (cerebrospinal fluid, dura, skull, fatty tissue, skin, each with a different conductance) and an individual head model is built to link brain activity to recorded scalp potentials.

The forward model allows the projection of sources of brain activity onto the scalp. Based on the forward model, the inverse problem can be solved assuming a number of constraints. Source inversion refers to the solution of the inverse problem. A number of different techniques are available to perform it. It has been shown that the estimated sources critically depend on the quality of the equipment, the density of electrodes, the forward model, and the source inversion technique being used. An in-depth overview of the technical issues and the available methods to perform ESI can be found in [69].

In general, ESI provides a reconstruction of the EEG time courses in certain brain regions of interest. Upon estimation of the time courses, the same levels of analysis (single-node, connectivity, topological features) that we discussed in Sections

113

8.2.1 and 8.2.2 (intracranial recordings) can be used here to characterize the epileptic network. For instance, at the single-node level, ESI has been mostly used in interictal periods to estimate the irritative zone (IZ),[5] a region that generates inter-ictal spikes. In contrast, ictal recordings are often contaminated by motion artifacts and source reconstruction can be very difficult to perform. Early studies on SOZ estimation from the late 1990s and 2000s showed the feasibility of ictal ESI on artifact-free periods and validated the results in a qualitative way [72]. Ictal source imaging was mainly performed assuming spatially restricted sources, and few studies used distrib-uted source models from which SOZ could be later inferred. An extensive review of these initial works and a proposal for a new strategy for ESI-SOZ estimation based on the largest amplitude changes in specific frequency bands correspond-ing to dominant patterns can be found in [73]. ESI-estimated SOZ regions were concordant with clinical-SOZ in 64% of seizures.

8.2.3.2 Network-Based Applications

Due to the complexity of the techniques required for an accurate source reconstruction during seizures, the first quantitative studies for SOZ localization using ictal scalp EEG did not appear until very recently. In 2007, Ding et al. used the integrated version of the direct transfer function (iDTF) defined above (see Section 8.2.2.2) on 20 seizures from 5 patients (31 electrodes), reporting a localization error for the EZ smaller than 15 mm in 85% of the seizures [74]. In 2012, Lu et al. used DTF analysis to localize the seizure source on 10 patients with focal epilepsy [75], and studied the effect of the number of scalp EEG electrodes (76, 64, 48, 32, and 21). They found a negative correlation between the SOZ localization error and the number of electrodes, suggesting

that high-density EEG might be beneficial for a better mapping of the epileptic network.

In 2017, a very interesting and promising study performed by Staljanssens et al. compared the estimation of the SOZ when using pure single-node measures or connectivity measures [72]. Specifically, they compared the detection accuracy when using the source with maximal power and the source with the strongest swADTF outdegree. As previously defined, swADTF (see Section 8.2.2.2) is the spectrum-weighted adaptive DTF, a measure that averages direct linear connections across dif-ferent frequencies to obtain a time-varying esti-mate of causal interactions in the network. Based on this measure, the node's outdegree is the sum of all swADTF values to every other source, thus quantifying the total amount of efferent functional connections it has. In total, 111 seizures from 27 post-surgical seizure-free patients monitored with a 27-electrode configuration were analyzed. For each patient, the most relevant time epoch and frequency of interest were manually selected by epileptologists. ESI power was reported to localize the SOZ within 10 mm of the border of the resected zone (RZ)[6] in 42.3% of the seizures, while the SOZ detected with the swADTF method laid within 10 mm of the RZ in 93.7% of cases. The authors argued that this superiority can be partly explained because some drivers might be more silent (less power) than the regions they influence, in which case the mapping of connectivity patterns is crucial to SOZ detection. Similar studies should be per-formed with intracranial recordings to assess the extent to which power and connectivity are com-plementary or redundant sources of information for SOZ localization, and whether this is an intrin-sic property of the neural activity or a contingency of the recording modality.

Some studies have also investigated in detail the changes in network topology during the occurrence of a seizure. Of particular interest for the under-standing of the mechanisms that maintain the ictal process after seizure onset is the study performed in 2013 by Elshoff et al. [76]. Using partial directed coherence (PDC; see Equation (4)) on a cohort of 11 patients with focal epilepsy, they showed that

---

[5] The irritative zone (IZ) is defined as the area of the cortex that generates interictal spikes. Interictal spikes can be observed with EEG and MEG, and, in general, do not generate any clinical symptoms regardless of their localization. If they are sufficiently strong in amplitude and generated in eloquent areas, however, they can give rise to transient symptoms, such as myoclonic jerks. The seizure onset zone is usually a portion of the IZ that generates repetitive spikes with sufficient strength to initiate seizures [1].

[6] The resected zone consists of the cortical areas that are excised and removed during surgery. Ideally, the resected zone should coincide with the EZ, but for a number of reasons (blood vessels, eloquent cortex, etc.) this is not always possible.

seizure onset is characterized by a significant information flow from the first dominating source (in all cases fitting the SOZ) to all other sources, demonstrating propagation. The middle part of the seizure was marked by a reorganization of the network in which the topology changes from a star-like map with the SOZ as the main hub, to a closed pattern in which information flow went in circles between all detected sources. It is hypothesized that the circular information flow could be a mechanism of seizure perpetuation. The development of this topological reorganization might also explain why interictal epileptiform discharges are not sufficient to generate seizures. A secondary mechanism by which nodes in the epileptic network resonate with each other must come into play after ictogenesis has occurred for a seizure to fully develop. Elshoff et al. also hypothesized that the sequence of stereotyped symptoms that some patients present might be related not only to the brain structures affected, which would not substantially change over the course of a seizure, but also to the hierarchic functional relationship between them.

Another interesting example of topological alterations was found in interictal idiopathic generalized epilepsy (IGE) by Clemens et al. [77]. Using Pearson correlation, the authors of that study investigated the network patterns in frequency bands of 1 Hz bandwidth from 1 to 25 Hz on a cohort of 19 patients and 19 healthy participants. As pointed out by many other studies, functional connectivity patterns were found to show a strong frequency dependence. Importantly, this study revealed an extraordinary complex organization of the IGE network that spans across multiple frequencies. This observation probably holds true for underlying networks in other epilepsy types and stresses the importance of using frequency-resolved recording modalities (such as EEG) and techniques, while modalities with lower resolution (such as fMRI) and broadband analysis can generate a confounding effect by averaging out anatomically different patterns. In particular, decreased connectivity was consistently found in the 1–6 Hz frequency range, with a certain degree of interhemispheric asymmetry. Because slower rhythms are mostly related to global cofluctuations and are known to be more intimately constrained by the anatomy of the network, the authors hypothesized that this alteration could provide insight into structural disruptions is network pathways, such as white matter pathologies. At higher frequencies,

the connectivity patterns showed a far more complex topological structure, with decreased connectivity in the anterior parts of the cortex, and increased connectivity in its posterior parts, a result that delineated two networks abnormally segregated and regulated according to different still unknown principles. Based on previous pharmacological results, the authors suggested that this pattern might be partially explained by alterations in region-specific neurotransmitters, that may also account for seizure maintenance in IGE.

Overall, the above reviewed studies have found very promising results using source inversions combined with connectivity analysis techniques to characterize epileptogenic networks. Although not fully developed, their potential to identify signatures of seizure typology has also been established. They have also shown the advantage of high-density recordings over lower spatial resolution EEG to get accurate SOZ localization [75,78]. EEG connectivity has also proven useful in increasing the localization accuracy in low density EEG when the analysis is limited to adequate EEG epochs and to the frequency band of interest of the seizure [78], offering a simple pipeline that could be used in clinical settings where hdEEG equipment is not available (see Fig. 8.4 for a summary of the employed methods and reported results). In conclusion, further studies should be performed to validate these techniques with larger cohorts of patients and strongest clinical hypotheses.

8.2.4 Concluding Remarks

Single-node metrics derived from signal analysis, dynamical systems, and ESI are well established and tested both in intracranial and scalp EEG. Their diagnostic power has been shown in a number of studies when compared to the purely visual evaluation of the recordings that remains the gold standard in clinical practice. These studies are likely revealing system level mechanisms of seizure generation and propagation and are therefore potentially targetable therapeutically. Connectivity analysis and network theory can provide further insight into these phenomena, opening up new perspectives on the network component of epilepsy. These provide information about the origin and spread of pathological information, about the topological changes that affect a diseased network both during ictal and interictal periods, and about the

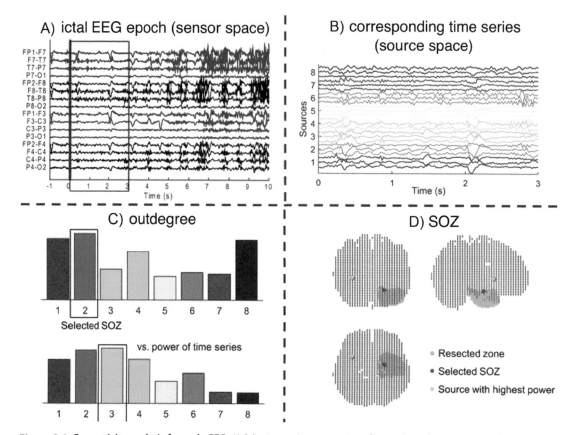

Figure 8.4 Connectivity analysis for scalp EEG. A) Selection and preprocessing of an ictal epoch. B) Time series for x, y, and z direction for extracted sources. C) Summation of the spectrum-weighted adaptive directed transfer function (swADTF) values across sources leading to the outdegree. D) The source with the highest outdegree is selected as seizure onset zone (SOZ). The location of this source is compared with the location of the source with the highest power and with the segmented resected zone. The presented method finds the SOZ in the resected zone (RZ), while the source with the highest power is not located inside the RZ. Adapted from Springer Nature *Brain Topography*, vol. 30, no. 2, Willeke Staljanssens, Gregor Strobbe, Roel Van Holen et al., "Seizure Onset Zone Localization from Ictal High-Density EEG in Refractory Focal Epilepsy" [78], Copyright © 2016 Springer Science Business Media New York, with permission.

mechanisms by which abnormal synchronous activity might be sustained during seizures. However, different studies often provide contradictory results, mostly due to the use of different network metrics or analyses. Currently, there is no gold standard to interpret and combine the information provided by different connectivity-based metrics. Further research is needed to address this issue before these promising perspectives can be integrated into clinical decision making.

8.3 Epileptic Network Dynamics: Toward Seizure Prediction

As pointed out in Section 8.2, epileptic networks are not a static entity with time-invariant properties. Quite the opposite, a core property of these

networks is that their activity and connectivity patterns evolve over time. We have discussed changes in single-node and network metrics upon seizure onset and have introduced some basic principles of topological reorganization that may act as a key mechanism for seizure initiation and perpetuation. In this section, we aim to further develop how complex systems approaches can be used to track epileptic network dynamics. Some metrics used to address this problem have been already introduced, while others are specific to analyze dynamical changes. Likewise, three approaches can be identified in the study of the temporal evolution of these networks. Single-node, connectivity, and topological metrics focus on different but complementary features of the network dynamics.

From a clinical point of view, it is worth noting that gaining insight into the temporal evolution of network patterns could pave the way for a significant breakthrough in the treatment of pharmacoresistant epilepsies. The ability to predict upcoming seizures on the basis of dynamic changes in the EEG recordings would enable the development of new therapeutic approaches that can prevent or mitigate seizure occurrence. Based on these predictions, one could develop closed-loop seizure prevention systems to reset the brain dynamics and abort the development of a seizure. This could be achieved, for instance, with electrical stimulation, or with the release of anticonvulsant medication either locally or intravenously. These systems could then be integrated in small devices that would be implanted subcranially and would function like artificial pacemakers, cardioverters, and defibrillators that are already used to treat life-threatening cardiac disorders.

The possibility of anticipating the occurrence of a seizure depends on how the ictal state is generated. If it is caused by an abrupt and sudden transition in single-node or brain network dynamics, it is very unlikely that one can find EEG biomarkers that anticipate their occurrence. On the contrary, if the ictal state is preceded by a continuous and gradual change in dynamics that eventually leads to seizure onset, the detection of such changes could be used to predict the upcoming seizure [79]. Until the 1970s the common belief among the medical community was that epileptic seizures could not be anticipated. Nonetheless, premonitory symptoms experienced by some patients from minutes to hours before clinical onset and changes observed in vital sign measurements had already been described in the literature and provided evidence that at least some seizures are preceded by a preictal state [80,81]. More recently, several studies have also shown that seizures are indeed preceded by changes in the brain dynamics that can be measured via intracranial recordings [82,83].

8.3.1 Dynamical Traces of the Preictal State in EEG

As described in Iasemidis' historical perspective on the topic [84], it was in the 1970s that the first project to investigate the predictability of grand mal seizures by analysis of scalp EEG recordings was conducted. Using what we would nowadays name machine learning, Viglione and Walsh used pattern recognition techniques to capture preictal features of the intracranial EEG in training sets and then tested them in testing sets [85]. Despite poor results with respect to specificity, this pioneering project paved the way for a number of studies that brought further evidence of the gradual transition between the interictal and ictal states in the 1980s. Other studies investigated the predictive power of spike occurrence rates in the EEG and while most of them found no significant changes before or after seizures, in 1983 Lange et al. reported a consistent change of spike activity prior to the occurrence of a seizure in iEEG [86]. Interestingly, Lange et al. found that it was the spatial pattern of spikes across the whole epileptic network, and not the rate of spikes in single nodes, that carried predictive value for the upcoming seizure. In the 20 minutes before seizure onset, there was an increase in interhemispheric coupling in terms of spike cooccurrence at different sites. This was an early scientific observation of network-level effects predicting seizure onset.

8.3.1.1 Use of Nonlinear Dynamic Measures: Lyapunov Exponent and Correlation Dimension

In the late 1980s, new signal processing methodologies were developed on the basis of the mathematical theory on nonlinear dynamical systems. These methodologies aim to better characterize the complex behaviors that emerge in several biophysical systems. From this perspective, the brain is understood as a system of different components that interact with each other in a nontrivial way. By using EEG recordings, the trajectory of the neural dynamics is described in a multi-dimensional space of "brain states." Iasemidis et al. used the concept of Lyapunov exponent, a measure that characterizes the chaoticity of a complex dynamical system, to monitor the activity of ECoG recordings of epilepsy patients as the upcoming seizure was approaching [87]. Briefly, a dynamical system is said to be chaotic when its dynamics are highly sensitive to initial conditions or perturbations (commonly known as the butterfly effect). These systems are prone to exploring different trajectories at a given moment. A certain degree of chaoticity can be thought of reflecting a healthy brain function, allowing the network to easily switch connectivity patterns to appropriately process and respond to external stimuli and cognitive demands.

The study performed by Iasemidis et al. showed that the system became progressively less chaotic in the minutes before seizure onset. Upon seizure onset, the chaoticity of the SOZ nodes suddenly dropped, followed by the nodes outside the SOZ, until chaotic behavior returned to normal values after seizure offset. The central concept, Iasemidis concludes, "was that seizures represented transitions of the epileptic brain from its 'normal,' less ordered (chaotic) state to an abnormal, more ordered state and back to a 'normal' state along the lines of chaos-to-order-to-chaos transitions" [84]. Further evidence for the orderliness and reduction of chaoticity of the ictal state have been confirmed by the stability of generation and propagation patterns observed inter-seizure by later studies [23,24].

Under similar principles, alternative indices were defined to quantify the complexity of the dynamics of the recorded brain signals (see [79] for a review of these measures), finding consistent evidence for a reduction in the complexity of the brain a few minutes prior to seizures. For instance, Elger and Lehnertz's group used the correlation dimension, a measure used in chaos theory to quantify dimensionality of the space populated by a set of points. In the case of brain signals, this index quantifies the number of independent states that the brain visits when considered holistically, i.e., at the network-level. Elger and Lehnertz reported a transition toward low-dimensional states before the occurrence of epileptic seizures in iEEG [88]. The authors hypothesized that this drop of complexity in the pre-seizure state could be reflecting a gradual increase of synchronicity between pathologically discharging neurons. In this vein, several groups reported increased phase synchronization in the minutes or hours preceding the seizure onset [55,89], inducing a state of higher susceptibility for pathological synchronization and a lowered threshold for seizure activity. Mormann et al. successfully used this feature to detect a pre-seizure state in 12 of 14 analyzed seizures using intracranial recordings [90].

8.3.1.2 Mechanistic Interpretations

From a theoretical perspective, these transitions from functional to abnormal epileptic activity have been modeled as a bifurcation process in which the functional state with distributed integration and segregation becomes unstable and jumps to another pathophysiologic much more synchronous oscillatory state [91,92]. Lopes da Silva et al. proposed that the two states (functional and ictal) coexist in all brains, thus accounting for the fact that all brains are susceptible to having an epileptic seizure under certain circumstances. The difference between healthy brains and those with epilepsy would be the distance between the attractors in the dynamical systems' phase-space, a concept that roughly coincides with the idea of a seizure threshold that needs to be crossed for a seizure to be elicited. In the study, the authors hypothesized that there are two different biologically plausible mechanisms by which this transition might occur. In the first one, the two attractor states (functional and ictal) coexist in close vicinity (low seizure threshold) in a bistable brain network. Small random fluctuations in this bistable network would trigger the jumping from one attractor to the other, resulting in the onset of a seizure. The authors hypothesize that this might be the case of primary generalized epilepsy, a case in which prediction would be unfeasible. In other kinds of epilepsies, on the other hand, the distance between the functional and ictal states is rather large, but networks have abnormal features that are characterized by unstable parameters that may gradually change with time, thus decreasing the seizure threshold until a transition occurs. This explanation would account for the gradual transition that can be measured with EEG in some seizure disorders. This idea is the focus of Chapter 4.

8.3.2 Modern Approaches Based on Network Theory and Machine Learning

From the mid-2000s, modern network science and statistical learning techniques have introduced a myriad of new opportunities to study the brain and its diseases. In particular, since 2010 two different and complementary approaches have been undertaken to study the seizure prediction problem with EEG. A theoretical one, centered on the characterization of the preictal transition at a network/brain state level, and a practical one, relying on the design of seizure prediction algorithms based on either feature-fixed engineering systems or, more recently, advanced machine learning methods.

8.3.2.1 Network Theory Analysis of the Preictal Transition

The first group of studies have aimed to study the topological and dynamic organization of the pre-ictal state, with the aim that a better understanding of the general principles that govern this state would provide insight into seizure prediction and control. These studies adopted network approaches to understand brain dynamics at a global level, identifying graph theoretical properties of preictal functional networks that might later be used as EEG signatures anticipating the advent of a seizure [93]. Preictal, ictal, and postictal network topology have been studied with intracranial EEG recordings to understand the spatiotemporal patterns of activity of epileptogenic networks [57]. Several studies have found that the ictal period is characterized by a shift toward a more regular topology compared to the preictal period in focal seizures using linear and nonlinear connectivity measures [94,95]. Specifically, these studies have found an increased average clustering coefficient and path length, reflecting a fragmented and less integrated configuration of the brain upon seizure onset.

Of particular relevance for seizure prediction is whether these changes can already be measured in the preictal phase. In a study done with intracranial EEG in 2015, Geier et al. studied the long-term evolution of assortativity based on phase synchronization [96], a graph theoretical measure that quantifies the preference of a network's node to attach to nodes with similar properties (in this case with similar degree, i.e., with similar amount of connections). Although a decrease of the assortativity was observed in the preictal state of four patients, this measure presented increased values in one patient. Inconclusive results were also found in another study that concluded that network properties might not be good predictors of seizure onset by themselves, since pre-seizure changes were strongly dependent on the brain states as defined by the degree distribution of the nodes [97]. The authors hypothesized that global trends may be associated with a change of brain states from the interictal to the preictal period, rather than with the network properties per se.

This "brain state" hypothesis has been further elaborated [83,98]. For instance, Khambhati et al. have shown that interictal activity exhibits larger fluctuations than ictal periods over a common set of states suggesting that the preictal state might undergo a change in the sequential occurrence of certain states [98] (See Fig. 8.5 for a scheme of the employed network methodology). On the other hand, Tauste Campo et al. showed that the transition from interictal to ictal periods is characterized by the larger occurrence of high functional connectivity states of short duration during a critical period as compared with time-matched periods from preceding seizure-free days [83] (See Fig. 8.6 for a schematic summary of the reported results). These later results also shed light into the importance of considering circadian rhythms in seizure prediction [99].

8.3.2.2 Machine Learning Algorithms for Seizure Prediction

The second group of studies have adopted a black-box approach by either using predetermined set of features (e.g., [100]) or learned features (e.g., [101]) that anticipate an upcoming seizure without the need for understanding the mechanisms underlying such changes. These EEG features can be linear or nonlinear, univariate or multivariate, and can be based on thresholding of a certain variable, or on the training of machine learning classifiers. In-depth reviews on the topic can be found in [102,103].

Perhaps the first demonstration that seizure prediction may be feasible in a real setting is from Cook et al. [100], who accumulated a data set of continuous intracranial EEG recordings and thousands of seizures from 15 patients with implantable devices undergoing a clinical trial for up to two years. Although the prediction success of the study was, in general, high (sensitivities from 65 to 100% in 11 patients), it was not consistent in all patients. The same authors have later argued that the algorithm suffered from the use of a limited and pre-defined set of features. Instead, they have recently proposed a more sophisticated deep learning algorithm that takes advantage of all data to recognize preictal pattern signatures [104].

Among the machine learning classifiers with best reported results is the work by Park et al. in 2011 [101]. The authors proposed a patient-specific algorithm based on support vector machine (SVM), a classification of features of spectral power extracted in nine bands of interest and a sliding window approach. The algorithm

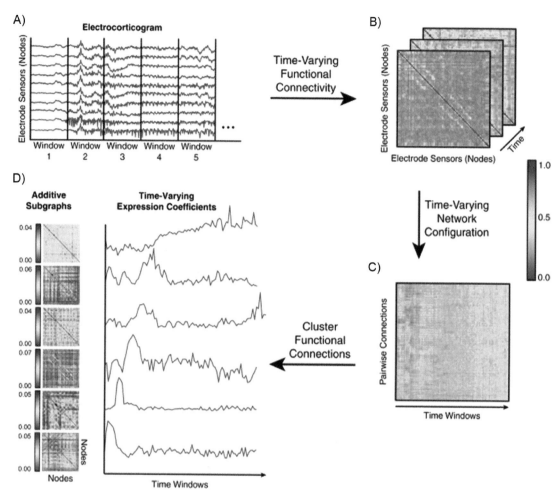

Figure 8.5 Clustering functional connections in epileptic networks. A) Ictal and interictal epochs from ECoG signals collected from patients with drug-resistant neocortical epilepsy implanted with intracranial electrodes. Time-varying functional connectivity networks are estimated in 1-s time windows. Each electrode sensor is a network node, and the weighted functional connectivity between sensors, interpreted as degree of synchrony, is represented as a network connection. B) For each epoch, functional connectivity is estimated by applying a magnitude normalized cross-correlation between each pair of sensor time series in each time window. C) For time-varying functional connectivity, all pairwise connections between nodes are extracted and concatenated over time windows to generate a time-varying network configuration matrix. D) A dimensionality reduction technique named nonnegative matrix factorization is applied to the time-varying configuration matrix from each epoch, resulting in subgraphs that capture frequently repeating patterns of functional connections, and their expression over time. Reprinted from Society for Neuroscience *eNeuro*, vol. 4, no. 1, Ankit N. Khambhati, Danielle S. Basset, Brian S. Oommen, et al., "Recurring Functional Interactions Predict Network Architecture of Interictal and Ictal States in Neocortical Epilepsy" [82], Copyright © 2017 Khambhati et al., under CC BY 4.0.

was designed to raise an alarm for a seizure prediction horizon of 30 minutes. This algorithm was applied to ECoG recordings of 18 patients from the Freiburg EEG database (24 h of preictal recording per patient) achieving high accuracies in detection rates (97.5% of a total of 80 seizure events were detected) with a false alarm rate of 0.27 per hour.

With the appearance of an ever-growing number of seizure prediction algorithms [102],

in 2014 the American Epilepsy Society, the Epilepsy Foundation of America, and National Institutes of Health sponsored an open invitation competition on kaggle.com to stimulate reproducible and competitive research on extended and realistic EEG data sets. These data sets comprised iEEG data from canines (n = 5, total recording time = 28,002 h, total seizures = 101) and humans (n = 2, total recording time = 229.8 h, total seizures = 10) with epilepsy [105]. The contest

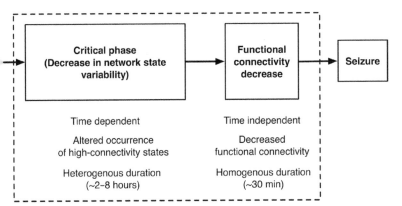

Figure 8.6 Preictal characterization. Scheme representing the preictal characterization with two sequential events of different nature and duration: The critical phase and the global functional connectivity decrease. Reprinted from Public Library of Science *PLOS Biology*, vol. 16, no. 4, Adrià Tauste Campo, Alessandro Principe, Miguel Ley, et al., "Degenerate time-dependent network dynamics anticipate seizures in human epileptic brain" [83], Copyright © 2018 Tauste Campo et al., under CC BY 4.0.

ran from August to November 2014; 654 participants submitted a total of 17,856 classifiers. The overall performance from multiple contestants on unseen data achieved above-chance level performance results, supporting the view that real-time seizure forecasting is indeed feasible. More recent studies have shown that using iEEG and deep learning techniques, seizures can be predicted with a sensitivity of around 80%. An in-depth review of these algorithms and discussion of future perspectives of wearable devices for seizure prediction can be found in [106].

Despite remarkable progress, there is still a long road to understand the principles that guide the dynamics of epileptic network from functional to pathological states. In this vein, we are still far from developing seizure prediction techniques that are sufficiently robust and reliable for their implementation in therapeutic devices [102,103]. Among the most promising lines to accelerate this journey is the use of deep learning in the algorithm implementation and the deployment of such systems on ultra-low power neuromorphic chips that could provide the mobile processing power for a wearable system [104,107].

8.4 Summary and Outlook

Despite many research and clinical efforts, diagnosis and treatment of epilepsy is still far from optimal. Antiepileptic drugs remain ineffective for one-third of all patients for causes that remain largely unknown. In addition, only 60% of patients undergoing resective surgery achieve seizure freedom, while the rest attain moderate to very mild improvement in symptoms and seizure frequency. This can be due to a number of reasons including a wrong identification of the seizure focus, a difficult-to-map complex and

distributed epileptogenic network or surgery technical limitations such as epileptogenic sites overlapping with cortical eloquent areas [108].

Since the beginning of the 21st century, complex network perspectives have been used to study specific properties of what is now understood as a complex network-based disease. Different approaches have been applied to brain EEG signals obtained with scalp and intracranial electrodes to tackle both scientific and clinical questions. Signal processing, dynamical systems, information theory, machine learning, and graph theory, among other techniques, have made their contribution by unveiling some pieces of this complex puzzle. First, single-node biomarkers have been used to classify brain regions based on local properties that might remain invisible to the human eye. Then, connectivity measures have allowed us to track propagation pathways for epileptic activity. Finally, topological features have shown how reorganization in the functional architecture of the brain network might play a central role in sustaining ictal activity. Based on recent results, it is reasonable to envisage a future in which clinicians can simulate the effect of a resection to better tailor surgeries [109] or where drug-resistant patients no longer need to undergo surgery thanks to closed-loop devices that are capable of predicting and aborting seizures [100].

This landscape of promising results contrasts with the fact that clinical procedures have remained mostly unchanged since the 1950s, being the gold standard in diagnosis visual inspection of EEG recordings. Why is it so? On one hand, complex systems approaches are relatively young in the study of epilepsy and evidence is still being gathered. In addition, the myriad of different measures and techniques – sometimes only with slight variations between one another – make it very difficult to establish one line of research along which significant effort can be invested for it to reach a clinical phase. On the other hand, most results still lack a clear explanation in terms of physiological or biochemical mechanisms. As Smith and Stacey comment [108], this arguably turns most biomarkers into a black box for neurologists, that are ultimately responsible for patient management and treatment. However, viewing the current findings as systems level mechanisms that can themselves be targeted therapeutically (e.g., using stimulation approaches) shows that significant progress in

diagnosis and treatment can be made without the need for identifying alternative biological and physiological mechanisms.

In the coming decades, we are facing the challenge of turning the promise offered by complex systems approaches to better diagnose and treat epilepsy into reality. Along the road, this will require further and stronger collaboration between research and clinical practice, conducting more concrete hypothesis-driven research studies and complying with the appropriate protocols to validate the scientific findings in a clinical environment (e.g., epilepsy units) to achieve the desired impact on patients.

References

1. Rosenow, and F., Lüders H. Presurgical evaluation of epilepsy. *Brain*, 124(9), 1683–700, (2001).

2. Talairach, J., Bancaud, J., Szikla, G., et al. Approche nouvelle de la neurochirurgie de l'épilepsie. Méthodologie stéréotaxique et résultats thérapeutiques. 1. Introduction et historique [New approach to the neurosurgery of epilepsy. Stereotaxic methodology and therapeutic results. 1. Introduction and history]. *Neurochirurgie*, 20 Suppl 1, 1–240 (1974).

3. Munari, C., and Bancaud, J. The role of stereo-EEG in the evaluation of partial epileptic seizures. In *The Epilepsies*. London: Butterworths. 1985. p. 267–306.

4. Guenot, M., Isnard, J., Ryvlin, P., et al. Neurophysiological monitoring for epilepsy surgery: The Talairach SEEG method. *Stereotact. Funct. Neurosurg.*, 77(1–4), 29–32 (2001).

5. Kahane, P., Minotti, L., Hoffmann, D., Lachaux, J.-P., Ryvlin, P. Invasive EEG in the definition of the seizure onset zone: depth electrodes. *Handb. Clin. Neurophysiol.*, 1(3), 109–33 (2003).

6. Cossu, M., Cardinale, F., Castana, L., et al. Stereoelectroencephalography in the presurgical evaluation of focal epilepsy: A retrospective analysis of 215 procedures. *Neurosurgery*, 57(4), 706–18 (2005).

7. Engel, A. K., Moll, C. K. E., Fried, I., and Ojemann, G. A. Invasive recordings from the human brain: clinical insights and beyond. *Nat. Rev. Neurosci.*, 6(1), 35–47 (2005).

8. Cardinale, F., Cossu, M., Castana, L., et al. Stereoelectroencephalography: Surgical methodology, safety, and stereotactic application accuracy in 500 procedures. *Neurosurgery.*, 72(3), 353–66 (2013).

9. Chauvel, P., Buser, P., Badier, J., et al. La "zone épileptogène" chez l'homme: représentation des événements intercritiques par cartes spatio-temporelles [The "epileptogenic zone" in humans: Representation of intercritical events by spatio-temporal maps]. *Rev. Neurol.*, 143, 443–50 (1987).

10. Bancaud, J., Angelergues, R., Bernouilli, C., et al. Functional stereotaxic exploration (SEEG) of epilepsy. *Electroencephalogr. Clin. Neurophysiol.*, 28(1), 85–6 (1970).

11. Bartolomei, F., Chauvel, P., and Wendling, F. Epileptogenicity of brain structures in human temporal lobe epilepsy: A quantified study from intracerebral EEG. *Brain*, 131 (7), 1818–30 (2008).

12. Cohen, M. X. *Analyzing Neural Time Series Data: Theory and practice*. Cambridge: MIT press. 2014.

13. Worrell, G. A., Parish, L., Cranstoun, S. D., et al. High-frequency oscillations and seizure generation in neocortical epilepsy. *Brain*, 127 (7), 1496–506 (2004).

14. Aubert, S., Wendling, F., Regis, J., et al. Local and remote epileptogenicity in focal cortical dysplasias and neurodevelopmental tumours. *Brain*, 132(11), 3072–86 (2009).

15. David, O., Blauwblomme, T., Job, A.-S., et al. Imaging the seizure onset zone with stereo-electroencephalography. *Brain*, 134(10), 2898–911 (2011).

16. Geertsema, E. E., Visser, G. H., Velis, D. N., et al. Automated seizure onset zone approximation based on nonharmonic high-frequency oscillations in human interictal intracranial EEGs. *Int. J. Neural. Syst.*, 25(05), 1550015 (2015).

17. Liu, S., Sha, Z., Sencer, A., et al. Exploring the time-frequency content of high frequency oscillations for automated identification of seizure onset zone in epilepsy. *J. Neural. Eng.*, 13(2), 26026 (2016).

18. Murphy, P. M., von Paternos, A. J., and Santaniello, S. A novel HFO-based method for unsupervised localization of the seizure onset zone in drug-resistant epilepsy. *Annu. Int. Conf. IEEE Eng. Med. Biol. Soc.*, 2017, 1054–7. (2017).

19. Jefferys, J. G. R., Menendez de la Prida, L., Wendling, F., et al. Mechanisms of physiological and epileptic HFO generation. *Prog. Neurobiol.*, 98(3), 250–64 (2012).

20. Perucca, P., Dubeau, F., and Gotman, J. Intracranial electroencephalographic seizure-onset patterns: Effect of underlying pathology. *Brain*, 137(1), 183–96 (2014).

21. Lagarde, S., Bonini, F., McGonigal, A., et al. Seizure-onset patterns in focal cortical dysplasia and neurodevelopmental tumors: Relationship with surgical prognosis and neuropathologic subtypes. *Epilepsia*, 57(9), 1426–35 (2016).

22. Singh, S., Sandy, S., and Wiebe, S. Ictal onset on intracranial EEG: Do we know it when we see it? State of the evidence. *Epilepsia*, 56(10), 1629–38 (2015).

23. Gnatkovsky, V., Francione, S., Cardinale, F., et al. Identification of reproducible ictal patterns based on quantified frequency analysis of intracranial EEG signals. *Epilepsia*, 52(3), 477–88 (2011).

24. Vila-Vidal, M., Principe, A., Ley, M., et al. Detection of recurrent activation patterns across focal seizures: Application to seizure onset zone identification. *Clin.*

Neurophysiol., 128(6), 977–85 (2017).

25. Vila-Vidal, M. Epylib v1.0, 2019. github.com/mvilavidal/ Epylib, Zenodo, doi:10.5281/ ZENODO.2630604

26. Vila-Vidal, M., Pérez Enríquez C., Principe, A., et al. Low entropy map of brain oscillatory activity identifies spatially localized events: A new method for automated epilepsy focus prediction. *Neuroimage*, 208, 707497 (2020).

27. Gnatkovsky, V., de, Curtis, M., Pastori, C., et al. Biomarkers of epileptogenic zone defined by quantified stereo-EEG analysis. *Epilepsia*, 55(2), 296–305 (2014).

28. Andrzejak, R. G., Schindler, K., and Rummel, C. Nonrandomness, nonlinear dependence, and nonstationarity of electroencephalographic recordings from epilepsy patients. *Phys. Rev. E Stat. Nonlin. Soft Matter Phys.*, 86(4 Pt 2), 046206 (2012)

29. Andrzejak, R. G., David, O., Gnatkovsky, V., et al. Localization of epileptogenic zone on pre-surgical intracranial EEG recordings: Toward a validation of quantitative signal analysis approaches. *Brain Topogr.*, 28 (6), 832–7 (2015).

30. Bartolomei, F., Wendling, F., and Chauvel, P. The concept of an epileptogenic network in human partial epilepsies. *Neurochirurgie*, 54(3), 174–84 (2008).

31. Sporns, O., Chialvo, D. R., Kaiser, M., and Hilgetag, C. C. Organization, development and function of complex brain networks. *Trends Cogn. Sci.*, 8 (9), 418–25 (2004).

32. van Mierlo, P., Papadopoulou, M., Carrette, E., et al. Functional brain connectivity

from EEG in epilepsy: Seizure prediction and epileptogenic focus localization. *Prog. Neurobiol.*, 121, 19–35 (2014).

33. Friston, K. J. Functional and effective connectivity: A review. *Brain Connect*, 1(1), 13–36 (2011).

34. Bullmore, E., and Sporns, O. Complex brain networks: Graph theoretical analysis of structural and functional systems. *Nat. Rev. Neurosci.*, 10 (3), 186–98 (2009).

35. van Mierlo, P., Carrette, E., Hallez, H., et al. Accurate epileptogenic focus localization through time-variant functional connectivity analysis of intracranial electroencephalographic signals. *Neuroimage*, 56(3), 1122–33 (2011).

36. Gersch, W., and Goddard, G. V. Epileptic focus location: Spectral analysis method. *Science*, 169(3946), 701–2 (1970).

37. Brazier, M. A. B. Spread of seizure discharges in epilepsy: Anatomical and electrophysiological considerations. *Exp. Neurol.*, 36 (2), 263–72 (1972).

38. Gotman, J. Measurement of small time differences between EEG channels: Method and application to epileptic seizure propagation. *Electroencephalogr. Clin. Neurophysiol.*, 56(5), 501–14 (1983).

39. Lütkepohl, H. *New Introduction to Multiple Time Series Analysis*. Berlin: Springer Science & Business Media. 2005.

40. Baccalá, L. A., and Sameshima, K. Partial directed coherence: A new concept in neural structure determination. *Biol. Cybern.*, 84(6), 463–74 (2001).

41. Kaminski, M. J., and Blinowska, K. J. A new method

of the description of the information flow in the brain structures. *Biol. Cybern.*, 65(3), 203–10 (1991).

42. Astolfi, L., Cincotti, F., Mattia, D., et al. Tracking the time-varying cortical connectivity patterns by adaptive multivariate estimators. *IEEE Trans. Biomed. Eng.*, 55(3), 902–13 (2008).

43. Wilke, C., Ding, Lei, and He, Bin. Estimation of time-varying connectivity patterns through the use of an adaptive directed transfer function. *IEEE Trans. Biomed. Eng.*, 55(11), 2557–64 (2008).

44. Varotto, G., Tassi, L., Franceschetti, S., Spreafico, R., and Panzica, F. Epileptogenic networks of type II focal cortical dysplasia: A stereo-EEG study. *Neuroimage.*, 61(3), 591–8 (2012).

45. Franaszczuk, P. J., Bergey, G. K., and Kamiński, M. J. Analysis of mesial temporal seizure onset and propagation using the directed transfer function method. *Electroencephalogr. Clin. Neurophysiol.*, 91(6), 413–27 (1994).

46. Wilke, C., van Drongelen, W., Kohrman, M., and He, B. Identification of epileptogenic foci from causal analysis of ECoG interictal spike activity. *Clin. Neurophysiol.*, 120(8), 1449–56 (2009).

47. Kim, J. S., Im, C. H., Jung, Y. J., et al. Localization and propagation analysis of ictal source rhythm by electrocorticography. *Neuroimage*, 52(4), 1279–88 (2010).

48. Kim, J.-Y., Kang, H.-C., Cho, J.-H., et al. Combined use of multiple computational intracranial EEG analysis techniques for the localization of epileptogenic zones in Lennox–Gastaut syndrome.

Clin. EEG Neurosci., 45(3), 169–78 (2014).

49. van Mierlo, P., Carrette, E., Hallez, H., et al. Ictal-onset localization through connectivity analysis of intracranial EEG signals in patients with refractory epilepsy. *Epilepsia*, 54(8), 1409–18 (2013).

50. Wilke, C., Worrell, G., and He, B. Graph analysis of epileptogenic networks in human partial epilepsy. *Epilepsia*, 52(1), 84–93 (2011).

51. Andrzejak, R. G., Chicharro, D., Lehnertz, K., and Mormann, F. Using bivariate signal analysis to characterize the epileptic focus: The benefit of surrogates. *Phys. Rev. E*, 83(4), 046203 (2011).

52. Sakkalis, V. Review of advanced techniques for the estimation of brain connectivity measured with EEG/MEG. *Comput. Biol. Med.*, 41(12), 1110–7 (2011).

53. Panzica, F., Varotto, G., Rotondi, F., Spreafico, R., and Franceschetti, S. Identification of the epileptogenic zone from stereo-EEG signals: A connectivity-graph theory approach. *Front. Neurol.*, 4, 175 (2013).

54. Lachaux, J. P., Rodriguez, E., Martinerie, J., and Varela, F. J. Measuring phase synchrony in brain signals. *Hum. Brain Mapp.*, 8(4), 194–208 (1999).

55. Mormann, F., Lehnertz, K., David, P. E. and Elger, C. Mean phase coherence as a measure for phase synchronization and its application to the EEG of epilepsy patients. *Phys. D Nonlinear Phenom.* 144 (3–4), 358–69 (2000).

56. Stam, C. J., and Reijneveld, J. C. Graph theoretical analysis of complex networks in the brain. *Nonlinear Biomed. Phys.*, 1(1), 3 (2007).

57. van Diessen, E., Diederen, S. J. H., Braun, K. P. J., Jansen, F. E., and Stam, C. J. Functional and structural brain networks in epilepsy: What have we learned? *Epilepsia*, 54(11), 1855–65 (2013).

58. Pijn, J. P., and Lopes da Silva, F. Propagation of electrical activity: nonlinear associations and time delays between eeg signals. In *Basic Mechanisms of the EEG*. Boston, MA: Birkhäuser Boston. 1993. p. 41–61.

59. Wendling, F., Bartolomei, F., Bellanger, J. J., and Chauvel, P. Identification de réseaux épileptogènes par modélisation et analyse non linéaire des signaux SEEG. *Neurophysiol. Clin. Neurophysiol.*, 31(3), 139–51 (2001).

60. Wendling, F., Chauvel, P., Biraben, A., and Bartolomei, F. From intracerebral EEG signals to brain connectivity: Identification of epileptogenic networks in partial epilepsy. *Front. Syst. Neurosci.*, 25(4), 154 (2010).

61. Balatskaya, A., Roehri, N., Lagarde, S., et al. The "Connectivity Epileptogenicity Index" (cEI), a method for mapping the different seizure onset patterns in StereoElectroEncephalography recorded seizures. *Clin. Neurophysiol.*, 131(8), 1947–55 (2020).

62. Shannon, C. E. A mathematical theory of communication. *Bell Syst. Tech. J.* 27(3), 379–423 (1948).

63. AdTau, and Vila-Vidal, M. DI-Inference-for-Python. 2020. doi:10.5281/zenodo.4067039

64. AdTau. AdTau/DI-Inference v1.0 (v1.0). Zenodo. 2020. https://doi.org/10.5281/zenodo.4059445

65. Mars, N. J. I., Thompson, P. M., and Wilkus, R. J. Spread of

epileptic seizure activity in humans. *Epilepsia*, 26(1), 85–94 (1985).

66. Sabesan, S., Good, L. B., Tsakalis, K. S., et al. Information flow and application to epileptogenic focus localization from intracranial EEG. *IEEE Trans. Neural Syst. Rehabil. Eng.*, 17 (3), 244–53 (2009).

67. Malladi, R., Kalamangalam, G., Tandon, N., and Aazhang, B. Identifying seizure onset zone from the causal connectivity inferred using directed information. *IEEE J. Sel. Top. Signal. Process.*, 10(7), 1267–83 (2016).

68. Plummer, C., Vogrin, S. J., Woods, W. P., et al. Interictal and ictal source localization for epilepsy surgery using high-density EEG with MEG: A prospective long-term study. *Brain*, 142(4), 932–51 (2019).

69. van Mierlo, P., Höller, Y., Focke, N. K., and Vulliemoz, S. Network perspectives on epilepsy using EEG/MEG source connectivity. *Front. Neurol.*, 10, 721 (2019).

70. Centeno, M., and Carmichael, D. W. Network connectivity in epilepsy: Resting state fMRI and EEG–fMRI contributions. *Front,. Neurol.*, 5, 93 (2014).

71. Lei, X., Wu, T., and Valdes-Sosa, P. Incorporating priors for EEG source imaging and connectivity analysis. *Front. Neurosci.*, 9, 284 (2015).

72. Staljanssens, W., Strobbe, G., Van, Holen, R., et al. EEG source connectivity to localize the seizure onset zone in patients with drug resistant epilepsy. *Neuroimage Clin.*, 16, 689–98 (2017).

73. Pellegrino, G., Hedrich, T., Chowdhury, R., et al. Source localization of the seizure onset zone from ictal EEG/MEG data. *Hum. Brain Mapp.*, 37(7), 2528–46 (2016).

74. Ding, L., Worrell, G. A., Lagerlund, T. D., and He, B. Ictal source analysis: Localization and imaging of causal interactions in humans. *Neuroimage*, 34(2), 575–86 (2007).

75. Lu, Y., Yang, L., Worrell, G. A., and He, B. Seizure source imaging by means of FINE spatio-temporal dipole localization and directed transfer function in partial epilepsy patients. *Clin. Neurophysiol.*, 123(7), 1275–83 (2012).

76. Elshoff, L., Muthuraman, M., Anwar, A. R., et al. Dynamic imaging of coherent sources reveals different network connectivity underlying the generation and perpetuation of epileptic seizures. *PLoS One*, 8 (10), e78422 (2013).

77. Clemens, B., Puskás, S., Bessenyei, M., et al. EEG functional connectivity of the intrahemispheric cortico-cortical network of idiopathic generalized epilepsy. *Epilepsy Res.*, 96(1), 11–23 (2011).

78. Staljanssens, W., Strobbe, G., Van Holen, R., et al. Seizure onset zone localization from ictal high-density EEG in refractory focal epilepsy. *Brain Topogr.*, 30(2), 257–71 (2017).

79. Mormann, F., Andrzejak, R. G., Elger, C. E., and Lehnertz, K. Seizure prediction: The long and winding road. *Brain*, 130, 314–33 (2007).

80. Hughes, J., Devinsky, O., Feldmann, E., and Bromfield, E. Premonitory symptoms in epilepsy. *Seizure*, 2(3), 201–3 (1993).

81. Schulze-Bonhage, A., Kurth, C., Carius, A., Steinhoff, B. J., and Mayer, T. Seizure anticipation by patients with focal and generalized epilepsy: A multicentre assessment of premonitory symptoms.

Epilepsy Res., 70(1), 83–8 (2006).

82. Khambhati, A. N., Bassett, D. S., Oommen, B. S., et al. Recurring functional interactions predict network architecture of interictal and ictal states in neocortical epilepsy. *eNeuro*, 4(1), ENEURO.0091-16.2017 (2017).

83. Tauste Campo, A., Principe, A., Ley, M., Rocamora, R., and Deco, G. Degenerate time-dependent network dynamics anticipate seizures in human epileptic brain. *PLoS Biol.*, 16 (4), e2002580 (2018).

84. Iasemidis, L. D., Shiau, Deng-Shan., Chaovalitwongse, W., et al. Adaptive epileptic seizure prediction system. *IEEE Trans, Biomed. Eng.*, 50(5), 616–27 (2003).

85. Viglione, S S., and Walsh, G. O. Proceedings: Epileptic seizure prediction. *Electroencephalogr. Clin. Neurophysiol.*, 39(4), 435–6 (1975).

86. Lange, H. H., Lieb, J. P., Engel, J., and Crandall, P. H. Temporo-spatial patterns of pre-ictal spike activity in human temporal lobe epilepsy. *Electroencephalogr. Clin. Neurophysiol.*, 56(6), 543–55 (1983).

87. Iasemidis, L. D., Sackellares, J. C., Zaveri, H. P., and Williams, W. J. Phase space topography and the Lyapunov exponent of electrocorticograms in partial seizures. *Brain Topogr.*, 2(3), 187–201 (1990).

88. Lehnertz, K., and Elger, C. E. Can Epileptic Seizures be Predicted? Evidence from Nonlinear Time Series Analysis of Brain Electrical Activity. *Phys. Rev. Lett.*, 80(22), 5019–22 (1998).

89. Le Van Quyen, M., Soss, J., Navarro, V., et al. Preictal state identification by synchronization changes in

125

long-term intracranial EEG recordings. *Clin. Neurophysiol.*, 116(3), 559–68 (2005).

90. Mormann, F., Kreuz, T., Andrzejak, R. G., et al. Epileptic seizures are preceded by a decrease in synchronization. *Epilepsy Res.*, 53(3), 173–85 (2003).

91. da Silva, F. L., Blanes, W., Kalitzin, SN., et al. Epilepsies as dynamical diseases of brain systems: Basic models of the transition between normal and epileptic activity. *Epilepsia*, 44 (s12), 72–83 (2003).

92. Jirsa, V. K., Stacey, W. C., Quilichini, P. P., Ivanov, A. I., and Bernard, C. On the nature of seizure dynamics. *Brain*, 137 (8), 2210–30 (2014).

93. Stam, C. J. Modern network science of neurological disorders. *Nat. Rev. Neurosci.*, 15(10), 683–95 (2014).

94. Ponten, S. C., Bartolomei, F., and Stam, C. J. Small-world networks and epilepsy: Graph theoretical analysis of intracerebrally recorded mesial temporal lobe seizures. *Clin. Neurophysiol.*, 118(4), 918–27 (2007).

95. Kramer, M. A., Kolaczyk, E. D., and Kirsch, H. E. Emergent network topology at seizure onset in humans. *Epilepsy Res.*, 79(2–3), 173–86 (2008).

96. Geier, C., Lehnertz, K., and Bialonski, S. Time-dependent degree-degree correlations in epileptic brain networks: From assortative to dissortative mixing. *Front. Hum. Neurosci.*, 20(9), 462 (2015).

97. Takahashi, H., Takahashi, S., Kanzaki, R., and Kawai, K. State-dependent precursors of seizures in correlation-based functional networks of electrocorticograms of patients with temporal lobe epilepsy. *Neurol. Sci.*, 33(6), 1355–64 (2012).

98. Khambhati, A. N., Bassett, D. S., Oommen, B. S., et al. Recurring functional interactions predict network architecture of interictal and ictal states in neocortical epilepsy. *eNeuro*, 4(1), ENEURO.0091–16.2017 (2017).

99. Karoly, P. J., Ung, H., Grayden, D. B., et al. The circadian profile of epilepsy improves seizure forecasting. *Brain*, 140 (8), 2169–82 (2017).

100. Cook, M. J., O'Brien T. J., Berkovic, S. F., et al. Prediction of seizure likelihood with a long-term, implanted seizure advisory system in patients with drug-resistant epilepsy: a first-in-man study. *Lancet Neurol.*, 12(6), 563–71 (2013).

101. Park, Y., Luo, L., Parhi, K. K., and Netoff, T. Seizure prediction with spectral power of EEG using cost-sensitive support vector machines. *Epilepsia*, 52(10), 1761–70 (2011).

102. Gadhoumi, K., Lina, J.-M., Mormann, F., and Gotman, J. Seizure prediction for therapeutic devices: A review. *J. Neurosci. Methods*, 260, 270–82 (2016).

103. Freestone, D. R., Karoly, P. J., and Cook, M. J. A forward-looking review of seizure prediction. *Curr. Opin. Neurol.*, 30(2), 167–73 (2017).

104. Kiral-Kornek, I., Roy, S., Nurse, E., et al. Epileptic seizure prediction using big data and deep learning: Toward a mobile system. *EBioMedicine*, 1(27), 103–11 (2018).

105. Brinkmann, B. H., Wagenaar, J., Abbot, D., et al. Crowdsourcing reproducible seizure forecasting in human and canine epilepsy. *Brain*, 139 (6), 1713–22 (2016).

106. Beniczky, S., Karoly, P., Nurse, E., Ryvlin, P., and Cook, M. Machine learning and wearable devices of the future. *Epilepsia*, 62(Suppl. 2), S116–24 (2021).

107. Acharya, U. R., Hagiwara, Y., and Adeli, H. Automated seizure prediction. *Epilepsy Behav.*, 88, 251–61 (2018).

108. Smith, G. C., and Stacey, W. C. Graph theory for EEG: Can we learn to trust another black box? *Brain*, 142(12), 3663–6 (2019).

109. Kini, L. G., Bernabei, J. M., Mikhail, F., et al. Virtual resection predicts surgical outcome for drug-resistant epilepsy. *Brain*, 142(12), 3892–905 (2019).

110. Mtui, E., Gruener, G., and Dockery, P. Chapter 30. Electroencephalography. In *Fitzgerald's Clinical Neuroanatomy and Neuroscience.* 7th ed. Philadelphia: Elsevier. 2016. p. 289–97.

111. Javidan, M. Electroencephalography in mesial temporal lobe epilepsy: A review. *Epilepsy Res. Treat.*, 2012, 1–17 (2012).

112. Lindsay, K. W., Bone, I., and Fuller, G. Section, IV. Localised neurological disease and its management: A. Intracranial. In *Neurology and Neurosurgery Illustrated.* 5th ed. Churchill Livingstone; 2011. p. 217–388.

113. Granger, C. W. J. Investigating causal relations by econometric models and cross-spectral methods. *Econometrica*, 37(3), 424 (1969).

Chapter 9

A Neuroimaging Network-Level Approach to Drug-Resistant Epilepsy

Niels Alexander Foit, Fatemeh Fadaie, Andrea Bernasconi, and Neda Bernasconi

9.1 Introduction

Epilepsy affects approximately 1% of the population [1]. Although generally treatable, up to 30% of patients do not achieve seizure freedom from anticonvulsive medication alone. Due to its relationship with cognitive abilities [2], quality of life [3], and the associated risk of premature death [4], drug-refractory epilepsy should be treated promptly. Temporal lobe epilepsy (TLE) associated with mesiotemporal sclerosis [5] and extra-temporal lobe epilepsy related to focal cortical dysplasia (FCD) [6] constitute the most common refractory epilepsy syndromes. Surgical resection of these lesions remains the treatment of choice [7], with success rates approaching 80% [8]. By allowing the detection of epileptogenic lesions and offering system-level mechanisms of the disease process, MRI has shifted the field from electro-clinical correlations toward a multidisciplinary approach.

Lesional epilepsy is a prototypical example of a large-scale network disorder, with a structural brain lesion at its core [9]. A network perspective is of particular significance since structures within the epileptogenic network are thought to be involved in seizures as well as the maintenance of the disorder [10].

9.2 Methodologies to Study Brain Networks

9.2.1 Imaging Modalities

The brain is a hierarchically organized network [11], partitioned into interconnected areas involved in information processing [12]. Ongoing methodological advancements allow for noninvasive mapping of both structural and functional circuits in vivo. A network may be conceptualized as a collection of nodes and edges [13]. Nodes reflect anatomical or functional units, while edges represent connections based on the trophic relationship, white matter tracts, or functional associations.

Structural networks are usually inferred from diffusion MRI tractography [11]. Diffusion imaging provides information on the magnitude and directionality of water diffusion and is utilized to assess fiber architecture and white matter microstructural integrity [14]. Moreover, the use of tractography algorithms further allows for a reconstruction of fiber pathways along plausible diffusion trajectories, which demonstrate high reproducibility and have been cross-validated against anatomical tract-tracing studies in animal models [15]. Alternatively, covariance of morphological markers, such as gray matter volume or cortical thickness representing physical hardwiring may be used to sensitively assess structural connectivity between cortical areas [16]. Covariance patterns may reflect trophic and/or signaling interactions between brain areas and exhibit close overlap with networks derived from diffusion imaging and resting-state functional MRI (rs-fMRI), such as those subserving visual, language, memory, or other cognitive functions.

Functional connectivity is estimated from statistical associations of neurophysiological signals between brain regions, with time-series extracted from task-based or rs-fMRI [17]. These sequences are often included in presurgical evaluation

* The authors have nothing to disclose. This contribution was funded by CIHR MOP-57840 to AB and CIHR MOP-123520 to NB, Natural Sciences and Engineering Research Council (NSERC; Discovery-243141 to AB and 24779 to NB), Epilepsy Canada Jay and Aiden Barker grant (247394 to AB), Canada First Research Excellence Fund (HBHL-1a-5a-06 to NB) and the German Research Foundation (DFG, FO996/1-1 to NAF).

protocols, mainly to localize eloquent areas, e.g., hemispherical language dominance [18]. Resting state fMRI offers several advantages over task-based paradigms, e.g., reduced cognitive demand (patients are instructed to lie still, with their eyes closed) and high reproducibility among subjects [19]. However, its clinical yield compared to task-based measures still needs to be established.

9.2.2 Graph-Theoretical Metrics of Topology

Graph theory, a paradigm for the mathematical representation of complex systems, has received much attention in the neuroscience community in recent years as it represents a powerful formalism to quantitatively represent organizational patterns of brain networks [13]. Its application to neuroimaging data has revealed novel insights into both normal brain topology and its alterations in epilepsy [20]. In graph theory terms, a network comprises *nodes* (brain regions), which are interconnected through *edges* (structural or functional connections) [13]. Nodes may be defined as single voxels or, more often, as anatomical parcellations, and their pairwise associations are compiled into a connectivity matrix (or connectome) [21].

Based on similarity, groups of nodes can be arranged in clusters (or *modules*), demonstrating dense internal connectivity, but relative segregation from the rest of the network [22]. *Hubs* constitute pivotal nodes with a high degree of connectivity. The most common measures of connectivity are the *clustering coefficient*, which reflects hub connectional density within the local environment, *path length*, which describes the average number of connections between nodal pairs, and *degree*, which states the number of edges connecting a hub to other nodes [21]. The relative importance of a node within a specific network, namely the extent to which its immediate neighbors rely on that node for information, is referred to as *centrality*, and is measured by its *degree*. In the healthy brain, a small world configuration, combining high clustering with short path length, is well suited for efficient information transmission requiring minimal wiring and energy [23]. Another important organizational property, influencing dynamic interactions and contributing to higher level function, is the *rich-club* phenomenon, i.e., the tendency of central

nodes in the network to densely connect to each other [24]. *Controllability* may be an additional metric of particular interest in epilepsy, as it represents the ability to exert control, i.e., inducing shift from an initial state to a desired, final state [25,26]. Sparse inhomogeneous networks, which are commonly found in real-world complex systems, are generally considered most difficult to control, whereas dense and homogeneous networks can be controlled through just a few important driver nodes [27].

9.3 Epilepsy Is a Network Disorder

A network perspective seems particularly compelling to assess the complexity of epilepsy in vivo, since structures within the epileptogenic network are most likely involved in the generation and expression of seizures as well as the maintenance of the disorder [10]. Given their ability to noninvasively study networks in vivo, neuroimaging techniques offer a unique opportunity to capture the neurobiological complexity of these disorders at multiple levels [28]. Regarding disease subtypes, TLE is the most commonly studied syndrome from a network-level perspective. Widespread connectional reconfiguration has also been shown in epilepsies secondary to cortical malformations, particularly FCD. In addition to descriptive studies, initial evidence suggests that combining connectivity metrics with machine learning may identify salient features from high-dimensional imaging data sets that can be clinically useful [29].

9.3.1 Network Mechanisms of Temporal Lobe Epilepsy

TLE is the most prevalent drug-resistant seizure disorder. While traditionally viewed as a focal syndrome with hippocampal sclerosis as its histopathological hallmark, converging evidence from neuroimaging literature has shown distributed structural and functional anomalies in the neocortex and white matter, offering novel views on the neurobiology of this condition [28–31]. Indeed, a system-level approach to TLE is now a rapidly growing research area fueled by ongoing advances in network science [32]. Neuroimaging studies have revealed extensive structural and functional alterations affecting temporo-limbic and other large-scale networks. Network-level studies of pathology are also relevant for the understanding of cognitive dysfunction affecting memory, language, and executive domains, with growing evidence supporting the predictive value of structural and resting-estate functional connectome measures [32,33].

Graph-theoretical analyses of networks inferred from morphological covariance of cortical thickness and mesiotemporal volumes have revealed altered network topologies both locally and on a whole-brain level (Fig. 9.1) [34]. Compared to healthy individuals, patients deviate from a small world configuration toward a more regularized topology with increased path length, clustering, and altered distribution of hubs; they are also less resilient to targeted attacks. Overall, these alterations can be interpreted as reduced network efficiency impairing flow of information both globally and locally. Regularization of whole-brain network topology as well as pronounced shifts in the distribution of hubs and modularity were collectively reported across modalities, including structural MRI, diffusion MRI, and EEG-derived networks. Graph-theoretical studies also indicated reduced coupling between structural and functional networks, which may be partially modulated by disease duration [35]. Extensive anomalies have also been inferred from functional connectivity measures. Resting state functional MRI studies demonstrated reduced connectivity for mesiotemporal structures ipsilateral to the seizure focus, mostly involving associations between anterior and posterior hippocampus, and between anterior hippocampus and entorhinal cortex [36,37]. In addition to abnormal limbic circuitry, connectional derangements in TLE have also been documented within and between sensory-motor, attentional, episodic memory, working memory, and language networks, supporting the pervasive nature of the disease, affecting multiple systems [29]. Moreover, severity of functional connectivity alterations are clearly associated with disease duration, mirroring observations obtained from structural network investigations [38].

From a behavioral perspective, use of network-level MRI-derived mechanisms has advanced our understanding of disease-related cognitive impairment. Since normal cognitive functioning is highly dependent on the integrity of large-scale brain networks, it is very intuitive that neurocognitive disturbances commonly encountered in TLE result from disrupted network properties [39]. MRI-derived network mechanisms are therefore increasingly utilized to probe neurocognitive performance. To date, however, the vast majority of imaging studies have relied on the relationship between structural connectome measures and cognition [40]. In this regard, structural connectome metrics outperform hippocampal volumetry and tractography of large association fibers to predict memory and language impairment in TLE [41]. Network-level phenotyping is additionally utilized to identify disease-specific cognitive phenotypes in TLE [39]. Preliminary evidence suggests that functional connectivity parameters harbor particular potential to investigate dynamic cognitive processes, e.g., consolidation of declarative memory after surgery [42]. Moreover, material-specific neurocognitive abilities such as emotional perception in TLE were recently linked to functional network architecture disruptions in the mesiotemporal lobe [43]. Furthermore, network-parameters inferred from both resting-state and task-based fMRI combined with diffusion MRI derived are also increasingly harnessed to predict postoperative cognitive performance levels in epilepsy surgery candidates across several cognitive domains [44].

In parallel to evidence suggesting that combining connectivity metrics with machine learning may identify cognitive profiles, salient features from high-dimensional data sets can also serve as predictors of other clinical outcomes. For example, MRI-derived functional connectivity mechanisms have been used to predict treatment response in TLE based on patterns of thalamo-hippocampal functional connectivity [45]. While the resection of the lesion at the core of the epileptogenic network is generally sufficient to achieve seizure freedom after surgery, alterations of the structural connectome at distance may also modulate outcome [46]. Indeed, TLE patients with excellent seizure outcomes consistently display structural alterations close to the resected mesial temporal lobe. By analyzing connectivity patterns derived from rs-fMRI of temporo-limbic and default mode networks, a recent study was able to predict early seizure recurrence with high accuracy [47], while related work highlights the value of inter-hemispheric asymmetries to differentiate patients with favorable from those with suboptimal outcome [48]. Uncovering the complex interplay between the epileptogenic zone, the lesion, and whole-brain networks is likely to improve clinical decision-making [49].

A) Parcels

B) Structural covariance network construction

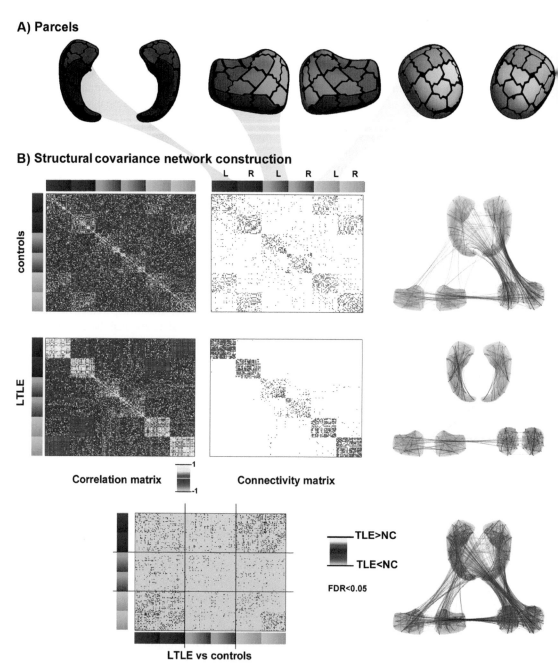

Figure 9.1 Mesiotemporal circuit representation based on volume covariance. A) High-resolution parcellation of the hippocampus (red), entorhinal cortex (green), and amygdala (yellow). B) Covariance network in controls and patients with left temporal lobe epilepsy (LTLE). (Left) High-resolution structural covariance matrices. (Middle) Binary network matrices thresholded at a density of 8% (threshold ensuring fully connected networks in all three groups). (Right) The corresponding network graphs. Color bars adjacent to the matrices signify the respective parcels as indicated in A, with red representing the left/right hippocampus (LH/RH), green the left/right entorhinal cortex (LE/RE), and yellow the left and right amygdala (LA/RA). Differences in inter-regional covariance between patients and controls are shown in the lower panel. Increases/decreases in patients relative to controls are shown in red/blue, corrected for multiple comparisons at FDR<0.05. Specifically, patients show decreased correlations between hippocampal and amygdalar subregions bilaterally, as well as between the left and right hippocampus. On the other hand, intra-hippocampal and intra-amygdalar covariance is increased within the same hemisphere. Excess in connectivity may be a consequence of axonal sprouting, a phenomenon commonly observed in both humans and models of limbic epilepsy. Conversely, decreases in inter-structure covariance may stem from the deafferentation of hippocampal connections.

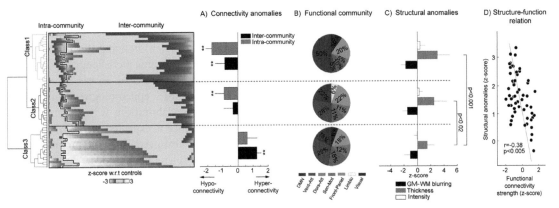

Figure 9.2 Connectome-based clustering and profiling of focal cortical dysplasia. After subdividing focal cortical dysplasia (FCD) Type II lesions into similarly-sized parcels, their connectivity to functional communities (i.e., canonical networks) were calculated. Applying hierarchical clustering to community-reconfigured connectome profiles identified three classes; in the re-ordered connectivity matrix, the flame scale indicates connectivity strength normalized with respect to healthy controls. A) Average z-scores of intra- and inter-community connectivity (**indicate difference at FDR<0.05 compared to controls); Classes show distinctive connectivity profiles: Class 1 is characterized by decreased intra- and inter-community connectivity, Class 2 by a selective decrease in intra-community connectivity, and Class 3 by increased intra- and inter-community connectivity. B) Proportion of functional communities across classes is maintained aside from default mode network that is more frequently associated to Class 1. C) Evaluation of structural anomalies (cortical thickness, gray and white matter interface blurring, and intensity) reveals distinct phenotypes across classes. D) The degree of structural changes negatively correlates to functional connectivity, with hyperconnectivity in parcels showing mild structural anomalies and marked hypoconnectivity in those with more severe structural compromise.

9.3.2 Network Mechanisms of Malformations of Cortical Development

Given the pivotal role of the lesion in the management of neocortical drug-resistant epilepsy, the vast majority of imaging studies of cortical malformations have focused on detection. A system-level approach has recently been triggered by studies showing the presence of widespread morphological abnormalities extending well beyond the primary lesion [50,51]. Similarly to TLE, graph-theoretical analysis of structural covariance networks has uncovered a more regularized network topology, as well as disrupted a rich-club configuration suggestive of inefficient global and excessive local connectivity [51]. Specifically, late-stage malformations, such as polymicrogyria and Type-I FCD, have been shown to selectively disrupt the formation of large-scale cortico-cortical networks, with a more profound impact on whole-brain organization than early stage disturbances of predominantly radial migration such as FCD Type-II, which likely affects a relatively confined cortical territory [51]. Applying hierarchical clustering to community-reconfigured connectome profiles identified lesional classes with distinct patterns of functional connectivity; hypoconnectivity

classes were mainly composed of FCD Type IIB, while Type IIA lesions were hyperconnected (Fig. 9.2) [50]. With respect to whole-brain networks, patients with hypoconnected FCD and marked structural damage showed only mild imbalances, while those with hyperconnected subtle lesions had more pronounced topological alterations. Multivariate structural equation analysis provided a mechanistic model of such complex, diverging interactions, whereby the FCD structural makeup shapes its functional connectivity, which in turn modulates whole-brain network topology [50]. Lesion-based functional connectivity models (i.e., connectivity from dysplastic tissue to the rest of the cortex) also demonstrated that network dysfunction can dissociate patients with favorable from those with suboptimal postsurgical seizure outcomes [50].

Network topology alterations were also found in studies probing cognition in FCD-related epilepsy. Utilizing functional MRI, studies investigating both adult and pediatric populations with frontal lobe seizures revealed extensive connectional derangements, involving language and auditory networks, working memory and the default mode network [52]. Other recent work has shown the ability of preoperative resting-state fMRI and white matter connectome markers to

131

predict postoperative cognition, particularly in relation to language [42].

9.4 Conclusion and Future Perspectives

Imaging methods that quantify noninvasively complex systems offer unprecedented opportunities to appraise system-level features of epilepsy. In parallel to a large body of descriptive studies, initial evidence suggests that combining connectivity metrics with machine learning may identify salient features from high-dimensional data sets to derive individual predictions. Network analysis is likely to reveal functional or structural biomarkers of cognitive functions that could be harnessed to predict neurocognitive functioning for

counseling of epilepsy surgery candidates during the preoperative phase. The integration of increasingly complex imaging techniques into routine practice remains a challenge. Success will be contingent to continued efforts in education and training of epileptologists, ultimately fostering close collaborations with research scientists. Open science is expected to catalyze clinical translation of advanced analytic methods [53]. A leading example is the ENIGMA-Epilepsy consortium [54], which has used meta- and mega-analysis techniques to assess group-level microstructure and network models of structural compromise across thousands of patients [55]. Knowledge derived from these large-scale studies is expected to set the basis of novel, clinically-applicable individualized disease biomarkers.

References

1. Fiest, K. M. et al. Prevalence and incidence of epilepsy. *Neurology*, 88, 296–303 (2017).

2. Bernhardt, B. C., Hong, S., Bernasconi, A., and Bernasconi, N. Imaging structural and functional brain networks in temporal lobe epilepsy. *Front. Hum. Neurosci.*, 7, 624 (2013).

3. Seiam, A.-H. R., Dhaliwal, H., and Wiebe, S. Determinants of quality of life after epilepsy surgery: Systematic review and evidence summary. *Epilepsy Behav.*, 21, 441–5 (2011).

4. Engel, J. What can we do for people with drug-resistant epilepsy? *Neurology*, 87, 2483–9 (2016).

5. Blümcke, I., Thom, M., Aronica, E., et al. International consensus classification of hippocampal sclerosis in temporal lobe epilepsy: A Task Force report from the ILAE Commission on Diagnostic Methods. *Epilepsia*, 54(7), 1315–29 (2013).

6. Blümcke, I., Thom, M., Aronica, E. et al. The clinicopathologic spectrum of focal cortical dysplasias:

A consensus classification proposed by an ad hoc Task Force of the ILAE Diagnostic Methods Commission1. *Epilepsia*, 52 (1), 158–74 (2011).

7. West, S., Nevitt, S. J., Cotton, J., et al. Surgery for epilepsy. *Cochrane Database Syst. Rev.*, 6 (6), CD010541 (2019).

8. Wiebe, S., Blume, W. T., Girvin, J. P., and Eliasziw, M. A randomized, controlled trial of surgery for temporal-lobe epilepsy. *N. Engl. J. Med.*, 345, 311–8 (2001).

9. Richardson, M. P. Large scale brain models of epilepsy: Dynamics meets connectomics. *J. Neurol. Neurosurg. Psychiatry*, 83, 1238–48 (2012).

10. Spencer, S. S. Neural networks in human epilepsy: evidence of and implications for treatment. *Epilepsia*, 43, 219–27 (2002).

11. Sporns, O., Tononi, G., and Kötter, R. The human connectome: A structural description of the human brain. *PLoS Comput. Biol.*, 1, e42 (2005).

12. Power, J. D., Fair, D. A., Schlaggar, B. L., and Petersen, S. E. The development of human functional brain

networks. *Neuron*, 67, 735–48 (2010).

13. Bassett, D. S., and Sporns, O. Network neuroscience. *Nat. Neurosci.*, 20, 353–64 (2017).

14. Jones, D. K., Knösche, T. R., and Turner, R. White matter integrity, fiber count, and other fallacies: The do's and don'ts of diffusion MRI. *Neuroimage*, 73, 239–54 (2012).

15. Conturo, T. E., Lori, N. F., Cull, T. S., et al. Tracking neuronal fiber pathways in the living human brain. *Proc. Natl. Acad. Sci. USA*, 96(18), 10422–7 (1999).

16. Alexander-Bloch, A., Giedd, J. N., and Bullmore, E. Imaging structural co-variance between human brain regions. *Nat. Rev. Neurosci.*, 14, 322–36 (2013).

17. Power, J. D., Cohen, A. L., Nelson, S. M.,et al. Functional network organization of the human brain. *Neuron*, 72, 665–78 (2011).

18. Abbott, D. F., Waites, A. B., Lillywhite, L. M., and Jackson, G. D. fMRI assessment of language lateralization: An objective approach. *NeuroImage*, 50, 1446–55 (2010).

19. Biswal, B. B., Mennes, M., Zuo, X. N., et al. Toward discovery science of human brain function. *Proc. Natl. Acad. Sci. USA*, 107, 4734–9 (2010).

20. van Diessen, E., Zweiphenning, W. J., Jansen, F. E., et al. Brain network organization in focal epilepsy: A systematic review and meta-analysis. *PLoS ONE*, 9(12), e114606 (2014).

21. Bullmore, E., and Sporns, O. Complex brain networks: Graph theoretical analysis of structural and functional systems. *Nat. Rev. Neurosci.*, 10, 186–98 (2009).

22. Rubinov, M., and Sporns, O. Complex network measures of brain connectivity: Uses and interpretations. *Neuroimage*, 52, 1059–69 (2010).

23. van den Heuvel, M. P., and Sporns, O. A cross-disorder connectome landscape of brain dysconnectivity. *Nat. Rev. Neurosci.*, 20, 435–46 (2019).

24. Colizza, V., Flammini, A., Serrano, M. A., and Vespignani, A. Detecting rich-club ordering in complex networks. *Nat. Phys.*, 2, 110–5 (2006).

25. Gu, S., Pasqualetti, F., Cieslak, M., et al. Controllability of structural brain networks. *Nat. Comm.*, 6, 8414 (2015).

26. Chari, A., Seunarine, K. K., He, X., et al. Drug-resistant focal epilepsy in children is associated with increased modal controllability of the whole brain and epileptogenic regions. *Commun. Biol.*, 5, 394 (2022).

27. Liu, Y.-Y., Slotine, J.-J., and Barabási, A.-L. Controllability of complex networks. *Nature*, 473, 167–73 (2011).

28. Tavakol, S. Royer, J., Lowe, A. J., et al. Neuroimaging and connectomics of drug-resistant epilepsy at multiple scales: From focal lesions to macroscale networks. *Epilepsia*, 60, 593–604 (2019).

29. Larivière, S., Bernasconi, A., Bernasconi, N., and Bernhardt, B. C. Connectome biomarkers of drug-resistant epilepsy. *Epilepsia* n/a,.

30. Gleichgerrcht, E., Kocher, M., and Bonilha, L. Connectomics and graph theory analyses: Novel insights into network abnormalities in epilepsy. *Epilepsia*, 56, 1660–8 (2015).

31. Caciagli, L., Bernhardt, B. C., Hong, S.-J., Bernasconi, A., and Bernasconi, N. Functional network alterations and their structural substrate in drug-resistant epilepsy. *Front. Neurosci.*, 8, (2014).

32. Balachandra, A. R., Kaestner, E., Bahrami, N., et al. Clinical utility of structural connectomics in predicting memory in temporal lobe epilepsy. *Neurology*, 94, e2424–35 (2020).

33. Reyes, A., Kaestner, E., Bahrami, N., et al. Cognitive phenotypes in temporal lobe epilepsy are associated with distinct patterns of white matter network abnormalities. *Neurology*, 92, e1957–68 (2019).

34. Besson, P., Dinkelacker, V., Valabregue, R., et al. Structural connectivity differences in left and right temporal lobe epilepsy. *Neuroimage*, 100, 135–144 (2014).

35. Chiang, S., Stern, J. M., Engel, J., and Haneef, Z. Structural-functional coupling changes in temporal lobe epilepsy. *Brain Res.*, 1616, 45–57 (2015).

36. Caciagli, L., Bernhardt, B. C., Bernasconi, A., and Bernasconi, N. Network Modeling of Epilepsy Using Structural and Functional MRI. In *Imaging Biomarkers in Epilepsy*, Bernasconi, A., Koepp, M., and Bernasconi, N. (eds.) Cambridge: Cambridge University Press. 2019. p. 77–94.

37. Bettus, G., Bartolomei, F., Confort-Gouny, S., et al. Role of resting state functional connectivity MRI in presurgical investigation of mesial temporal lobe epilepsy. *J. Neurol. Neurosurg. Psychiatry*, 81(10), 1147–54 (2010).

38. Haneef, Z., Chiang, S., Yeh, H. J., Engel, J., and Stern, J. M. Functional connectivity homogeneity correlates with duration of temporal lobe epilepsy. *Epilepsy Behav.*, 46, 227–33 (2015).

39. Hermann, B., Conant, L. L., Cook, C. J., et al. Network, clinical and sociodemographic features of cognitive phenotypes in temporal lobe epilepsy. *NeuroImage Clin.*, 27, 102341 (2020).

40. Rodríguez-Cruces, R., Bernhardt, B. C., and Concha, L. Multidimensional associations between cognition and connectome organization in temporal lobe epilepsy. *NeuroImage*, 213, 116706 (2020).

41. Kaestner, E., Balachandra, A. R., Bahrami, N., et al. The white matter connectome as an individualized biomarker of language impairment in temporal lobe epilepsy. *NeuroImage Clin.*, 25, 102125 (2019).

42. Audrain, S., Barnett, A. J., and McAndrews, M. P. Language network measures at rest indicate individual differences in naming decline after anterior temporal lobe resection. *Hum. Brain Mapp.*, 39, 4404–19 (2018).

43. Steiger, B. K., Muller, A. M., Spirig, E., Toller, G., and Jokeit, H. Mesial temporal lobe epilepsy diminishes functional connectivity during emotion perception. *Epilepsy Res.*, 134, 33–40 (2017).

44. Doucet, G. E., Rider, R., Taylor, N., et al. Presurgery resting-

state local graph-theory measures predict neurocognitive outcomes after brain surgery in temporal lobe epilepsy. *Epilepsia*, 56(4), 517–26 (2015).

45. Pressl, C., Brandner, P., Schaffelhofer, S., et al. Resting state functional connectivity patterns associated with pharmacological treatment resistance in temporal lobe epilepsy. *Epilepsy Res.*, 149, 37–43 (2019).

46. Bonilha, L., Jensen, J. H., Baker, N., et al. The brain connectome as a personalized biomarker of seizure outcomes after temporal lobectomy. *Neurology*, 84, 1846–53 (2015).

47. Morgan, V. L., Rogers, B. P., Anderson, A. W., Landman, B. A., and Englot, D. J. Divergent network properties that predict early surgical failure versus late recurrence in temporal lobe epilepsy. *J. Neurosurg.*, 1, 1–10 (2019).

48. Xu, Q., Zhang, Z., Liao, W., et al. Time-shift homotopic connectivity in mesial temporal lobe epilepsy. *Am. J. Neuroradiol.*, 35, 1746–52 (2014).

49. Foit, N. A., Bernasconi, A., and Bernasconi, N. Functional networks in epilepsy presurgical evaluation. *Neurosurg Clin N Am.*, 31(3), 395–405 (2020).

50. Hong, S.-J., Lee, H.-M., Gill, R., et al. A connectome-based mechanistic model of focal cortical dysplasia. *Brain*, 142, 688–99 (2019).

51. Hong, S.-J., Bernhardt, B. C., Gill, R. S., Bernasconi, N., and Bernasconi, A. The spectrum of structural and functional network alterations in malformations of cortical development. *Brain*, 140, 2133–43 (2017).

52. Vlooswijk, M. C. G., Jansen, J. F., Jeukens, C. R., et al. Memory processes and prefrontal network dysfunction in cryptogenic epilepsy. *Epilepsia*, 52(8), 1467–75 (2011).

53. Lhatoo, S. D., Bernasconi, N., Blumcke, I., et al. Big data in epilepsy: Clinical and research considerations. Report from the Epilepsy Big Data Task Force of the International League against Epilepsy. *Epilepsia*, 61(9), 1869–83 (2020).

54. Sisodiya, S. M., Whelan, C. D., Hatton, S. N., et al. The ENIGMA-Epilepsy working group: Mapping disease from large data sets. *Hum. Brain Mapp.*, 43(1), 113–128 (2020).

55. Larivière, S., Rodríguez-Cruces, R., Royer, J., et al. Network-based atrophy modeling in the common epilepsies: A worldwide ENIGMA study. *Sci. Adv.*, 6(47), eabc6457 (2020).

Chapter 10

Epilepsy as a Complex Network Disorder
Insights from Functional MRI

David Carmichael, Rory J. Piper, and Fraser Aitken

10.1 Background

10.1.1 A Brief Introduction to fMRI, Simultaneous EEG-fMRI and Their History in Epilepsy

Functional magnetic resonance imaging (fMRI) was conceived in the early 1990s due to the coincidence of two advances: (1) MRI scanner technology able to support fast echo-planar imaging imaging techniques with the required temporal stability and (2) the scientific knowledge that differences in the magnetic susceptibility of blood may be associated with MRI signal changes based on alterations in blood oxygenation levels. These elements, together with the assumption that changes in blood oxygenation and volume would accompany changes in neural activity in the brain, motivated research groups around the world to develop fMRI.

Soon after fMRI was used to make the first measurements of these signal changes in the visual cortex of humans [1,2], applications of fMRI in epilepsy were conceived. In 1993, Ives and colleagues first attempted to localize epileptic activity seen in electroencephalography (EEG) using fMRI, triggering the acquisition of scans when EEG events were visually detected to capture subsequent fMRI responses [3]. Supported by this initial work, EEG systems compatible with fMRI were developed, along with the signal processing needed to correct the artifacts associated with recording EEG and fMRI continuously. Unlike other early forms of resting state-MRI (rs-fMRI) (that used regional or voxel time series from the fMRI to correlate with other brain regions [4]), spontaneous brain activity recorded in the EEG was used to form a model of expected fMRI responses to the epileptiform activity. Those voxels that fitted the model of expected signal changes were then associated with the epileptiform activity. The primary purpose of these studies was to localize focal epileptic activity to aid presurgical evaluation. What became increasingly clear was that instead of a single focal region being active during a focal EEG event, instead a network of brain regions was often found. Although this was a somewhat disappointing outcome for the straightforward application of EEG-fMRI to provide surgical targets, it was entirely consistent with the now increasingly accepted idea that epilepsy, even epilepsy with focal-onset seizures, is a large-scale network disorder. What followed was a much more concerted attempt to understand the network interactions involved in epileptiform discharges that we will come back to later in the chapter. However, this early work suggested that the understanding of a complex interacting system was going to be vitally important to understand brain activity in epilepsy.

10.1.2 Resting State fMRI and Brain Networks

We do not provide a detailed or comprehensive description of rs-fMRI methods or their relative merits in this chapter. We rely instead on several key concepts being understood that can be found in numerous review articles, book chapters, or tutorials about rs-fMRI.

As detailed further in the review by Centeno and Carmichael [5], rs-fMRI may be used to interrogate networks in the following ways:

1. Seed-based correlation

    Functional connectivity may be implied by the correlation of fMRI signal from regions of interest (ROI) or voxels. This could be a "simple" correlation of average signal between selected areas (Fig. 10.1A), or correlation between the ROI (often termed the seed) signal to every voxel. An alternate approach is

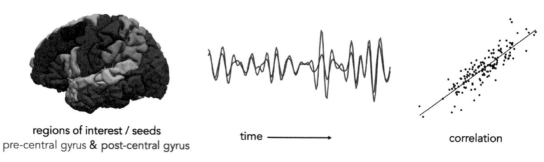

Figure 10.1A An example of seed-based correlation. The average fMRI signal in a time series of two (or more) regions can be measured and statistically compared to investigate functional connectivity.

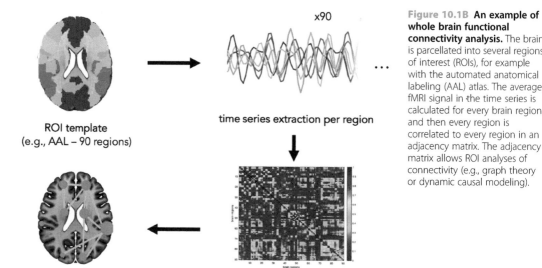

ROI template
(e.g., AAL – 90 regions)

time series extraction per region

analyses of connectivity
(e.g., graph theory or dynamic
causal modelling)

region-region correlation
adjaceny matrix

Figure 10.1B An example of whole brain functional connectivity analysis. The brain is parcellated into several regions of interest (ROIs), for example with the automated anatomical labeling (AAL) atlas. The average fMRI signal in the time series is calculated for every brain region, and then every region is correlated to every region in an adjacency matrix. The adjacency matrix allows ROI analyses of connectivity (e.g., graph theory or dynamic causal modeling).

to use an anatomical brain template to obtain the signal in every brain region, before correlating all of the brain regions signals to each other to form an adjacency matrix. This whole brain connectivity approach allows the "connectome" to be interrogated by using methods such as graph theory analysis (Fig. 10.1B) ((i) for examples of graph theory metrics) or dynamic causal modeling.

2. Spatial independent component analysis

A second frequently used rs-fMRI analysis method is a spatial independent component analysis (ICA) [6]. This method separates the fMRI image time series into a set of spatial maps (components) of covarying voxels with a single associated signal time course. This method does not require any spatial hypothesis or anatomical parcellation. The spatial components obtained can be derived and compared across groups of subjects.

An example of the use of the ICA approach is in identifying intrinsic connectivity networks (ICNs) [7], which are increasingly accepted as fundamental organizational aspects of brain architecture. The concept of ICNs is based on the discovery of functionally correlated fMRI time series data present during rest [4,8]. These early findings have been added to by data indicating the presence of ICNs in decompositions of fMRI data using independent components analysis. Many task-based studies have reported coactivation that appears markedly similar to that informed by the expected or canonical circuitry of resting state networks such as the default mode network (DMN) or the executive control network (see [9] for a review). The term "intrinsic connectivity network" therefore, expands upon the concept of resting state networks to include the set of large-scale functionally connected brain networks that can be captured in either resting state or task-based neuroimaging.

Regardless of whether a seed-based or spatial ICA approach is used, the researcher is required to make several choices, including:

1. One must choose between using an individual voxel or single brain region as a seed, a parcellation of the brain based on an atlas or driven by the data (e.g., using ICA).
2. The frequency range selected and a choice between fMRI signal magnitude (most studies) and phase.
3. How "connectivity" is established, via measurement of correlation, ICA, factorization, etc. Having made these choices, the result is a matrix representing connectivity at the spatial scale defined by choice 1 most often at the scale of tens of networks to hundreds of regions. This set of regions with a defined connectivity pattern can then be used to derive a wide range of metrics to describe the nature of the network, for example based on graph theory (see Fig. 10.1B) [10].

One further important detail is that the measures of functional connectivity can be either averaged over the whole scanning period or can be considered dynamic. In the latter case, dynamic information can be obtained by using a sliding window defining shorter epochs with connectivity measured in each. Other methods also allow for temporal changes in functional connectivity to be derived such as through utilizing phase information that will be described later in the chapter. Although the predominant approach is to derive a measure of functional connectivity from the data, the use of an underlying generative model is also possible.

It is important to carefully interpret connectivity results derived from indirect measures of brain activity such as fMRI and to, where possible, consider these results alongside elctrophysiological measures. [11]. The body of work looking at connectivity in EEG both scalp and invasive is

important context for fMRI-based connectivity studies. The availability of invasive EEG is a unique and useful feature of studies in patients with epilepsy owing to the availability of recordings from invasive monitoring for clinical purposes.

10.2 Network Alterations in Epilepsy from fMRI

Here we summarize the main findings from studies that aimed to determine network abnormalities in different epilepsy syndromes. We present a number of recent studies that are of relevance to the understanding of these syndromes in the context of complex systems.

10.2.1 Temporal Lobe Epilepsy

The epileptogenic network in temporal lobe epilepsy (TLE) is relatively well characterized, comprising several structures in the mesial temporal lobe (amygdala, hippocampus, adjacent cortex including entorhinal cortex), lateral temporal cortex, and extra temporal structures including thalamus and orbito-frontal cortex [12]. Connectivity maps seeding in these areas of the epileptogenic network have shown decreased connectivity within subregions in the epileptic temporal lobe, decreased connectivity between hippocampi, and decreased connectivity between the hippocampus and the orbito-frontal region, and decreased connectivity between the hippocampus and default mode network (DMN) [5].

Overall, decreased functional connectivity is the most common finding among those studies targeting the epileptogenic network. Hence, it is interesting to compare these findings with other measures of neuronal connectivity such as EEG where at least from intracranial data this is not always consistent. In one small study of five patients with TLE, intracranial EEG showed increased interictal connectivity in contrast to the decreased fMRI connectivity [13]. However, some studies have found local increases in connectivity using fMRI, and shown that connectivity can alter with disease duration in TLE [14].

One of the important findings from EEG-fMRI studies in TLE was the consistent perturbation of the DMN associated with interictal activity, where the DMN is deactivated during interictal discharges [15], just as it is during task activity. When recording EEG together with fMRI, a subtlety in interpretation may be required because the general finding of decreased static functional connectivity may in fact relate to changes in dynamics. A greater *variability* in functional connectivity (for example, between the DMN and hippocampus) has been shown using dynamic functional connectivity [16], commensurate with EEG-fMRI findings of consistent DMN deactivation with hippocampal spikes. Relating the two findings, local pathological activity within the epileptogenic network, some of which is likely to be interictal activity seen on EEG, may be causing downstream perturbations. The known interaction between the hippocampus and DMN during memory tasks also fits into this picture; patients' level of DMN deactivation was associated with a poorer performance [17], again consistent with the EEG-fMRI data showing greater variability in the dynamic connectivity of this network. This greater "within state metastability" [18] could also potentially perturb memory processes. Work showing reduced structural connectivity related to the severity of hippocampal sclerosis [19] also gives an underpinning for the reduction in coordination and connectivity between these key brain hubs. This begins to illustrate the complex interplay between structural alterations and functional dynamics between and within epileptic networks and ICNs.

10.2.2 TLE with Secondary Generalization

In this section, we will focus on a single, recent study while linking back to the previously mentioned fMRI and EEG-fMRI results. Studies using fMRI have investigated the circumscribed and bilateral brain networks that gives rise to generalized EEG patterns. TLE patients that suffer from generalization of their focal seizures, typically being bilateral tonic-clonic in nature, have a worsened prognosis including higher mortality rates. Therefore, a better mechanistic understanding is valuable for prognostication and, ultimately, improving treatment options.

The study by He et al. [20] has several elements that are both illustrative and interesting from the point of view of applying network science to epilepsy to derive some further understanding of the networks altered in patients with secondary

generalized seizures (Fig. 10.2). The hypothesis is that the basal ganglia acts as a control structure that acts to break thalamocortical generators of synchronous activity. There are few ways to access this circuitry in humans; even where invasive recordings are available, they will not widely nor consistently sample this network. Of the noninvasive methods that could be used, only fMRI has sufficient resolution and sensitivity to sample these deep-lying brain areas. One of the thorny methodological choices mentioned above is how to parcellate these regions and two approaches are used in tandem here. First, atlas-based regions were used; typically, these will have been generated using structural imaging and manual segmentation. However, the regions generated might not have a strong correspondence to functional subunits or lack the exact anatomical detail that is required for a given study. Therefore, larger regions can be used and subdivided into components that share similar spatio-temporal properties. Here, just as spatial ICA can be used at the whole brain level, it can also be applied within a particular brain region or area. This results in a data-driven parcellation that should reflect functional subdivisions. Validation is required for the parcellation to determine whether it is stable with respect to the number of subdivisions or components chosen. He et al. [20] derived a 21 region parcellation of the thalamic and basal ganglia circuitry (using data from the Human Connectome Project) and then applied this parcellation to the patient data. In addition to this custom parcellation of the basal ganglia and thalamus, a standard atlas-based cortical parcellation was performed, and the cortical regions were grouped to form a set of canonical resting state networks or ICNs. Then the connectivity between each subcortical region and each cortical parcel was summarized in terms of the distribution of connectivity across these canonical networks termed the participation coefficient. Put simply, this should show if the subcortical region is interacting across ICNs or with a select few. Here, there has effectively been an assignment of expected structure between the cortical parcels based on previous work. Additionally, network structure can also be defined using a variety of algorithms that factorize or cluster the nodes into groups that share connectivity or tend to interact with each other. This approach was used for the subcortical network, where a community

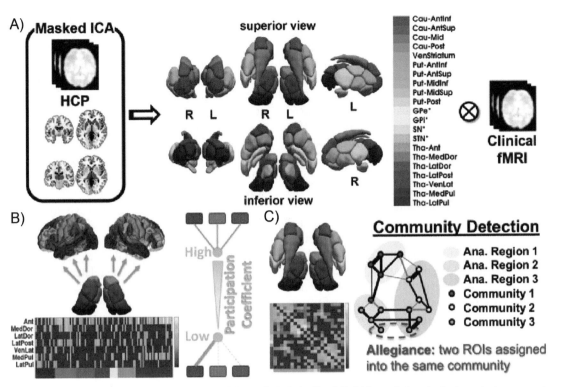

Figure 10.2 From He et al. Schematic overview of the analytical pipeline [20]. A) We applied masked independent component analysis (ICA) on an independent rs-fMRI data set from the Human Connectome Project (HCP, n = 100) to generate functional parcellations of the striatum (10 parcels) and thalamus (7 parcels). In addition, anatomical masks for GPe and GPi, STN, and SN were directly adopted from the ATAG atlas, yielding a final parcellation scheme of the basal ganglia-thalamus network with 21 regions of interest (ROIs) per hemisphere. These ROIs were then used to extract time series from the clinical rs-fMRI data collected in this study. B) Based on the Schaefer Atlas, we estimated thalamocortical functional connectivity between each thalamic parcel and cortical regions of interest, and then sorted them by seven predefined resting state networks. We used the participation coefficient to represent the distribution pattern of thalamocortical functional connections across different resting state networks. The more uniform the distribution, the higher the participation coefficient, and vice versa. C) We also estimated the functional connectivity matrix of the basal ganglia-thalamus network, on which we applied a community detection algorithm, to identify groups of regions of interest with higher preference for interacting with each other (i.e., communities). We used interregional integration to represent the probability of all the regions of interest from two different anatomical origins being assigned to the same community (i.e., allegiance) over iterative applications of this algorithm (specifically, 1,000 optimizations of a modularity quality index).

detection algorithm was applied to determine modules of nodes with the network. Here, again there are various methodological choices to navigate to determine the appropriate algorithm and the number of modules, factors, or communities that they are separated into. These functional network measures were assessed in a group of patients with TLE separated into those with and without focal to bilateral tonic-clonic seizures (FBTCS) with the latter further divided into those patients with and without a recent history of these seizures. Patients with a recent history of FBTCS were found to have a higher participation coefficient than those without in the ipsilateral medial-dorsal thalamic nuclei. This means that these brain regions were more widely connected

across the different ICNs rather than being functionally segregated. This could mean that there is more of an "open circuit" where cortical–cortical communication is facilitated. However, it must be noted that this is in the inter-ictal state and does not necessarily mean greater connectivity overall because the measure of participation coefficient is sensitive to changes in the distribution of connectivity rather than in its strength.

As highlighted above, EEG-fMRI and fMRI studies have shown that there is, in general, a reduction in functional connectivity in TLE, for example, with the DMN, with a failure to reduce its connectivity during a task. Earlier studies in TLE using ICA-based approaches did find disruptions to ICNs and patients with secondary generalized seizures did not show normal activity in the DMN [21]. The increased participation coefficient found by He et al. is potentially consistent with this – a failure to segregate networks appropriately would lead to both findings. One possible interpretation could be that the *spatial* organization of the ICNs is perturbed in FCTSG patients so that the community structure defined from healthy subject data no longer matches that found in patients so that distributed connectivity across these networks is found consistently. In the case of FCTSG, the thalamus was implicated in the reduction of this ability leading to the elevated participation coefficient. The value of the participation coefficient overall is remarkably high across subcortical regions, patient, and controls – close to full connectivity – it is not obvious that this is a realistic scenario and would benefit from validation. Interestingly, one other functional connectivity study in nonlesional children with TLE where EEG was recorded noted that increased connectivity and abnormally anticorrelated thalamic activity was detected only in the patients with abnormal electroencephalograms [22]. It is interesting to speculate whether greater temporal variance in connectivity (as found by Laufs et al. [16] for a TLE cohorts between the DMN and hippocampus) could also explain the findings in FBTCS, where the participation coefficient could represent either less distinction between ICNs (a kind on intra-state metastability increase) and/or a different switching regime between states (a more global alteration in metastability).

Differences were shown in the basal ganglia and thalamic networks, where patients with recent FCTSG had increased interaction between putamen and globus pallidus internus, and decreased interaction between the latter and the thalamus, compared to the other two patient groups. This was found to be a change in network structure that was not readily seen by just looking at functional connectivity strength. In a previous study in a more mixed group of temporal and extra temporal children, the thalamus, hippocampus, and caudate were found to be weaker hubs if the subjects had secondarily generalized seizures [23].

In summary, this interesting study accessed functional connectivity in a large group of patients in brain regions using fMRI that would be difficult to study with any other methodology.

Plausible alterations in the interaction between the basal ganglia and thalamus were found in TLE patients who have secondary generalized seizures. Alterations in thalamocortical structure were also seen. Both of these findings would not be apparent by simply looking at connectivity strength between regions but are related to topographic changes in connectivity. The complexity of network analysis can make it difficult to relate a difference back to physiological arguments; the typically more abnormal EEG features seen clinically in patients with FBTCS may relate to some of the differences in fMRI connectivity found. This speaks to the future use of measures that help to define the dynamics generating these findings, and understanding if, and how, altered dynamics in the interictal state relate to secondary generalized seizure generation.

10.3 Temporal Lobe Resection: Predicting Outcomes Using fMRI-Derived Networks

Temporal lobe resection (TLR) for the treatment of drug-resistant TLE is an attractive application of network neuroimaging research since, compared to other focal epilepsy surgery paradigms, there are a limited number of variables to control for. TLE, as described in Section 10.2.1, disrupts a relatively well-understood brain network and the variations of TLR surgical approaches are somewhat limited. This section describes the recent studies that demonstrate that seizure freedom following TLR may be predicted or, at least, explained by networks, and TLR may alter or allow compensation of abnormal brain networks through "plasticity." Although fMRI studies are the focus of this chapter, it is worth mentioning that there have been several complementary studies that have used diffusion MRI to demonstrate the utility of a networks approach in questions around TLR and seizure freedom [24].

Another study by He et al. [25] showed with presurgical rs-fMRI that the degree centrality and eigenvector centrality of both the ipsilateral and contralateral thalami was significantly higher in patients who were not seizure free following TLR when compared to those who were seizure free. This builds on the idea that wider pathological functional networks that involve these subcortical structures may not be disconnected by TLR alone and may not deliver an optimal therapeutic effect. With further development, functional networks could be used as a biomarker of surgical success and surgical candidacy.

A study by González and colleagues [26] investigated 26 adults with TLE using fMRI and graph theory network analysis and showed that, compared to controls, there was an abnormal loss of negative correlation between the thalamus and occipital lobes. Furthermore, 19 patients who underwent TLR for TLE with favorable seizure outcomes showed partial recovery of thalamic-occipital and thalamic-brainstem connectivity. The authors concluded that the disrupted thalamic arousal networks may recover following "successful" epilepsy surgery. These studies also direct more interest toward deep brain stimulation of the thalamus as a complementary therapy for drug-resistant epilepsy [27]. Although not specific to TLE, fMRI-derived network studies have also found utility in interrogating the networks altered by deep brain stimulation (DBS) of the thalamus [28,29].

fMRI and network analysis has been applied to several applications in surgery for TLE, including the preoperative determination of the dominant hemisphere for language processing [30]. These include a number of examples of studies that have examined language reorganization following TLR for TLE. A 2012 study [31] showed that, in 44 patients with TLE undergoing neuropsychological assessments and fMRI before and 4-months after TLR, left TLE showed postoperative reorganization of language networks to the frontal lobe and posterior hippocampal remnant. Foesleitner et al. showed, based on 28 patients undergoing TLR, that pre- and postoperative fMRI revealed bihemispheric alterations in language networks [32]. There was a decrease in fronto-temporal connectivity in patients with either right or left TLE and TLR. The patients with left TLE and preoperative atypical language dominance had better postoperative verbal fluency and naming performance. For those with right TLE, there was an association with left frontal language dominance and better semantic and verbal fluency pre- and postoperatively.

Overall, a range of studies have suggested that network properties may have predictive utility. For these to be translated it is necessary to put these studies together and form a consistent approach in a large group, with data shared across centers, to determine their predictive value in a reproducible manner. Currently, the relative complexity and variety of network analyses makes comparison and determination of true efficacy difficult to assess.

10.3.1 Extra Temporal Lobe Epilepsy (xTLE)

Extra temporal epilepsy (xTLE) provides a significant network analysis challenge as compared to TLE, owing to the relative heterogeneity of patient characteristics, such as etiology and spatial location of abnormalities. In this respect, some more general whole brain measures of alterations to network structure are a potential route to generalizable findings where interrogation of local networks related to the epileptogenic zone will be highly individual. Some of the most interesting and important formative work in this area has also been performed in a pediatric setting. This is most likely due to the greater prevalence of xTLE cases with drug-resistant seizures, motivating studies to improve understanding and, ultimately, treatment options in this group. Within the epileptogenic areas and network there is evidence of increased connectivity [33] which, although enhanced by, is not simply related to transient EEG activity [34].

In frontal lobe epilepsy (FLE) patients and control children aged 8–13 years old, rs-fMRI was used to investigate alterations in network structure and how this related to cognitive performance. The brain was parcellated into 83 regions and thresholded connectivity matrices were summarized via a range of network measures. Furthermore, cognitive testing was used to relate the alterations in global network structure to performance. The main finding was that an increased modularity was seen in the patients, this means their network structure was more insular with increased intra- but reduced inter-module connectivity [35]. Although not directly investigated in the same study, this could be due to a lower connectivity between the modules via hubs such as the thalamus, as was measured by Ibrahim et al. [23]. Is this the opposite effect to the study above by He et al. [25] described in Section 10.3, where in TLE an increase in the participation coefficient was found? Perhaps these two results can be rationalized not only by the potential differences between TLE and FLE, adults and children, but also because the FLE patients showed a clear difference in the module structures themselves. Two separate frontal-temporal and frontal-parietal networks were seen in healthy controls and patients with equivalent cognitive performance, but in patients with lower cognitive performance these two modules coalesced into a single module demonstrating that abnormal modular organization of the brain is associated with impairment. This kind of spatial coalescence would be expected to result in a higher participation coefficient when measured across canonical brain networks. Therefore, it is potentially a similar process in FLE as compared to the TLE patients with FBTCS. This relationship between functional connectivity and cognitive performance was also demonstrated using an alternative analysis by Ibrahim et al., again in children in a heterogeneous group including both TLE and FLE where inter-network segregation was associated with higher full-scale intelligence quotient scores [36].

As highlighted above, much of the literature has focused on TLE patients because they are easier to study owing to the consistent spatial network that is typically affected, allowing for group studies where the machinery typically developed for cognitive neuroscience can be employed. Extra temporal epilepsy is more challenging in this regard owing to variable lesion location and etiology. So far, patient groups in the papers described in this section have not been defined based on pathology, although a sizable proportion of focal xTLE patients, particularly in pediatric surgical series, will have a malformation of cortical development such as focal cortical dysplasia (FCD).

In this section, a paper by Hong et al. will be described [37]. Here, connectivity was examined in patients with FCD type II. Again, much of the processing is familiar from the papers already described in this chapter. A brain parcellation was made of the neocortex into 78 regions based on the AAL atlas [56]. These were subdivided into 1,000 approximately equally sized areas in a group of control subjects and FCD type II patients. Epilepsy lesions were manually segmented and then in each patient where the cortical parcel volume was >50% lesion it was assigned to be a lesion parcel. Parcels within a lesion were then merged where they had high similarity in terms of their signal time course. This resulted in a total of 55 parcels across 27 patients, these were then compared in terms of their connectivity to the rest of the cortex. Again, the concept of communities was used where across subjects, the main networks or typical ICNs were defined. Then the connectivity of the lesion parcels was separated into intra- and inter-community components. These were then clustered (after a "trick" of deriving a distance measure between each connectivity vector using dynamic time warping that allows for differing vector lengths). Finally, standard whole brain measures of network topography were calculated. The key findings were that the FCD II lesions showed different patterns of both increased and decreased connectivity. The lesion parcels could be grouped into classes: decreased intra- and inter-community connectivity (Class I), a selective decrease in intra-community connectivity (Class II), and both increased intra- and inter-community connectivity (Class III). These different classes were related to structural abnormalities and global network features. Class I and II lesions were characterized by hypoconnectivity and greater visible structural anomalies on structural MRI. These were also associated with relatively little impact on global network abnormalities (e.g., modularity, path length, and clustering coefficient) in contrast to the group studies described earlier by Ibrahim et al. [36] and Vaessen et al. [35], respectively. In contrast, the structurally less affected regions (at least as apparent on MRI) had hyperconnectivity intra and inter-community (Class III) and a much greater impact on global network properties. The latter group were generally small FCDIIa lesions and therefore it is plausible that the nature of the lesions at the microscopic scale is important. It is perhaps surprising that the scale of the MRI abnormality has an inverse relationship to alterations in network topography. One of the key clinical questions relates to the epileptogenicity of these abnormalities and it is an intriguing possibility that the abnormalities at the level of cell types and cortical architecture lead to quite different manifestations in terms of functional connectivity.

10.3.2 Generalized Genetic Epilepsy (GGE)/Idiopathic Generalized Epilepsy (IGE)

A number of EEG-fMRI studies have now characterized the networks involved in the generation of generalized spike wave (GSW) epileptic activity that is the hallmark of GGE/IGE syndromes. Common findings across studies show activation of a cortico-subcortical network composed of the mid-frontal regions, thalami, caudate, and cerebellum during the occurrence of generalized spike-waves. Although now taken for granted, this was an important finding – that there was a widespread but not all-encompassing involvement of the neocortex in human GSW. Around this time there was also substantial progress made in understanding the pathophysiology of GSW in animal models that indicated a focal cortical generation of discharges. In parallel came the identification of key genetic abnormalities that were shared between the various clinical syndromes (JME, JAE, CAE, GTCS, etc.) suggesting a similar substrate. An excellent summary of findings from experimental models can be found in Lüttjohann and van Luijtelaar [38], with the most important concept being that "GSW are not primary generalized and are not sudden and unpredictable events." A network neuroscience perspective can identify alterations in network topography that might be relevant, but it does not obviously allow access to these key questions: are GSW predictable or have a predisposing state and is this a localized phenomenon? To attempt to address these requires knowledge of the timing of GSW occurrence as the marker of the state change, which requires an EEG recording. Second, it is necessary to understand the dynamic changes in network structure.

In the study of Tangwiriyasakul et al., EEG and fMRI data were obtained simultaneously in a group of patients with IGE [39]. In the studies described in more detail until this point, the correlation between signal time courses was made over periods of five or more minutes and then these connectivity matrices used for subsequent analysis. This process can be made dynamic, such as in the study of Laufs [16] in TLE mentioned earlier that used a sliding window approach. Nevertheless, there is a choice between temporal resolution and stability of the result that depends on the window size chosen. An alternative approach is to instead utilize the instantaneous phase of the signals, an approach more familiar in EEG and MEG data analysis. Here, the fMRI data is filtered, with a passband in the range of fMRI physiological signal changes before being Hilbert transformed. This provided a phase value

at each spatial location for each time point giving an instantaneous time resolved matrix for 90 brain regions. Here, rather than correlation, connectivity between regions was assumed when the phase lay within a certain range. The overall phase within regions, networks, or globally can be assessed to give a measure of synchrony. To derive measures of network topography, the phase value matrix can be binarized keeping only connections within a predefined phase range and making these connections equal to one. This binarized version can then be used for graph-based analysis as before, however, there will be a value for every time point. Using this approach 95 GSW from 20 patients were measured and investigated in terms of network changes time-locked to GSW events (Fig. 10.3). Eigenvector centrality (EC), a measure of nodal importance or influence within the network, was assessed for each region over time. Significant EC was found during discharges, and for 20s after EEG offset in a widespread network involving frontal, parietal, and occipital cortex similar to that found in prior EEG-fMRI studies. In the 6s before the GSW the sensorimotor network showed significant connections to the prefrontal and precuneus brain regions. Interestingly, significantly elevated EC was also found in a sensorimotor network in the minute before discharge onset. Furthermore, with or without GSW these two networks showed elevated synchrony in patients compared to controls. This could be interpreted as an altered baseline state of high sensorimotor synchrony that facilities GSWs, with events being initiated following an interaction between the sensorimotor and key nodes in the network involved in GSW generation. There is significant literature regarding sensorimotor involvement in GSW generation from animal models [38]. In addition, imaging studies have confirmed structural abnormalities in connectivity between sensorimotor and frontal regions [40], and it is consistent with the clinical syndrome of JME one of the GGE family of syndromes with myoclonic jerks as a defining feature. This study is therefore important in that it used dynamic analysis both to reveal the changes associated with GSW and indicated that a predisposing peri-ictal state existed in humans as suggested by the animal model literature. Additionally, network abnormalities that were not time-locked to GSW were found. This altered background may have only been uncovered because the networks were defined heuristically

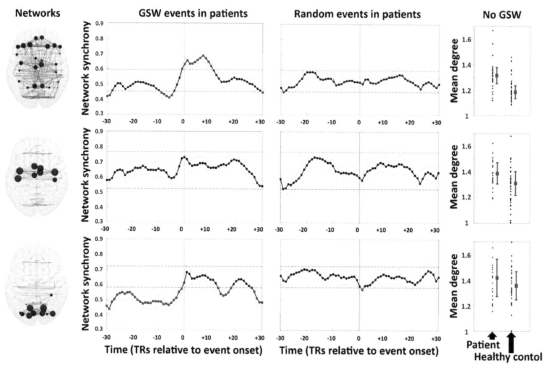

Figure 10.3 **From** Tangwiriyasakul et al., 2019 [41]. **Time course of normalized synchrony in three canonical brain networks before, during, and after GSW events or random events.** We present three rows of data, one for each network. (Top) GSW network. (Middle) Central sensorimotor network. (Bottom) Occipital network. Networks: cartoons of the distribution of network edges and hubs of each of these networks. Table 10.1 shows the anatomical locations of nodes in each network. GSW events in patients: the group mean normalized network synchrony at each TR (its standard error). The x-axis shows time indicated in TRs from TR30 to TR + 30 (one TR lasts 2.16 s). The y-axis is group mean normalized network synchrony. The vertical red line marks the GSW onset (TR = 0). The light green lines represent the 99% CI of the group mean normalized network synchrony, estimated from the 96 random event epochs from the functional MRI runs without GSW. Significantly high/low synchrony is highlighted in red. Random events in patients: control synchrony time courses for epochs time-locked to random events without GSW in patients. The vertical red line marks the random event onset (TR = 0). No GSW: average network synchrony (in terms of normalized mean degree) averaged within each network over the entire 296 TR functional MRI runs for all functional MRI runs without GSW in patients, and for healthy controls. The red square is the median, whiskers show 25th and 75th centiles; black squares are each individual subject. Note that average synchrony is higher in patients than controls in the GSW network and in the central sensorimotor network, over the entire 296 TR epochs without GSW events. Average synchrony in the occipital network does not differ between patients and healthy control subjects.

based on the time-locked analysis although there is increasing evidence from EEG [41] and MEG [42] of similar findings.

This study may provide a potential therapeutic mechanism – if the sensorimotor network synchrony can be reduced, will the occurrence of GSW likewise be altered? There is just a single study looking an N-back spatial memory task using EEG and fMRI [43]. This showed that there was an interaction with the task and GSW occurrence, with a greater rate of GSW associated with task difficulty. Whether this corresponded to greater synchrony in a corresponding sensorimotor or GSW network is purely speculative. This task involved sensory-motor areas as it required the use of a joystick and demonstrated an interaction between the GSWs and the task activated network, although there was not a clear direct effect of GSW on task performance. It is also intriguing to consider if a similar analysis would reveal a pre-ictal or permissive state in focal syndromes and how this might relate to the alterations in network properties found to date.

In summary, many aspects of our understanding of genetic generalized epilepsy are changing, in part driven by network measurements demonstrating circumscribed regions, predisposing network abnormalities, and changes prior to electrographic activity. It is clear that we must consider how generalized discharges arise from altered dynamic processes, that are shaped by complex interactions not just within the brain

Table 10.1. Network terminology terms discussed in the current chapter

Term	Definition
Brain network	Brain regions connected with one another by anatomical or functional measures.
Canonical brain network	A set of brain regions that form a network and are associated with a particular function or state. An example is the default mode network (DMN).
Characteristic/distance path length	The reachability matrix describes whether pairs of nodes are connected by paths ("reachable"). The distance matrix contains lengths of shortest paths between all pairs of nodes. The characteristic path length is the average shortest path length for the network.
Community detection/ structure	A graph theory method that identifies sets of nodes (e.g., brain regions) that are densely connected to one another as a "community" / a network that has multiple groups of highly connected nodes.
Complex network	A network that has nontrivial structure and can produce complex behavior not apparent from the individual nodes. Community structure, "scale free" are types of complex networks.
Connectome	At term that typically refers to a comprehensive description of the connectivity of the brain.
Degree centrality	A graph theory measure that describes the number of other nodes that a node is connected to.
Dynamic causal modeling	A Bayesian method of network analysis of dynamic signals and aims to infer causal relationships in networks or compare potential network structures.
Eigenvector centrality	A graph theory measure that indicates the influence that a particular node has on a network. The eigenvector centrality of a node increases in proportion with (a) the number of nodes connected to it, and (b) how connected those nodes are.
Functional connectivity	Two (or more) regions of the brain are thought to be functionally connected if they share temporal signal characteristics, e.g., they are correlated or synchronous.
Global network integration	A graph theory measures that uses path length as an index of information transfer efficiency.
Graph theory	A branch of mathematics and computer science that represents how systems are connected and behave. In this case, nodes indicate anatomical elements (e.g., brain regions), and edges represent the relationships between nodes (e.g., connectivity).
Hub	A highly connected/important node that makes it important to the larger network in which it resides. Defined in a number of ways such as a node with high centrality or degree.
Metastability	A particular dynamic state where there is spatial and temporal integration and segregation of activity leading to the formation of transiently stable states.
Minimum spanning tree	Subset of the edges of a connected, edge-weighted undirected graph that connects all the vertices together, without any cycles and with the minimum possible total edge weight.
Modularity	A graph theory measure that is related to community structure. It describes the degree to which a network is "modular" or comprises of a set of highly connected sub-networks with relatively few connections between the sub-networks.
Network topology	Network topology is the structure (either physical or theoretical) of a network.

Table 10.1. (*cont.*)

Term	Definition
Normalized leaf number	A graph theory measure. The number of nodes with a degree centrality of 1 divided by the total number of nodes in the network.
Parcellation	Describes the partition of the brain into distinct regions or clusters of imaging voxels.
Path length	Describes the level of integration relating to the number of discrete steps between nodes (or edges) that are needed to move from one node to another.
Robustness	A graph theory measure. The capacity of a network to sustain its features and performance when it is perturbed, for example, when a node is removed.
Transitivity	A measure of connectivity of a given region to it neighbors.

but also with the environment and factors such as sleep, cognitive load, and medication.

10.3.3 Cognitive fMRI in Epilepsy and Network Interactions

Initially, fMRI was primarily used with cognitive tasks to localize brain functions. Naturally, this work was also quickly taken up in epilepsy applications with cognitive tasks to delineate brain structures relevant to surgery. One of the main applications is in the identification of language areas. For TLE, the main aim is to identify language lateralization and this approach has largely been adopted (and has largely replaced the WADA test) in centers specializing in epilepsy surgery because it is noninvasive, cheaper, and repeatable. Particularly for temporal lobe resections, both language and memory function before and after surgery have been extensively studied. This is not the focus of this chapter and interested readers are directed to review articles, e.g., [44]. These studies do have direct relevance in two areas. First, they highlight one cautionary element for fMRI studies in general where although language lateralization is reliably elicited, the network of brain regions that is active (and variable) during various tasks involving language only partially spatially overlaps with knowledge gained from invasive monitoring such as awake cortical stimulation procedures. This highlights that brain networks involved in language processing in fMRI are not necessarily essential for language in an individual. Similarly, fMRI may not always delineate this core network – an absence of fMRI changes in a region cannot be taken as

license to resect while sparing language function. This is in part due to some of the limitations of fMRI, where, for example, poor signal quality in basal temporal areas might obscure any fMRI signal changes that can be seen with careful noise correction [45].

10.3.4 Antiseizure Medications and fMRI-Derived Networks: A Known Unknown

One fascinating but problematic aspect is the influence of anti-seizure medications on the results of connectivity studies using fMRI, where they can be both a potential global and/or local modulator of particular networks or brain regions. The effects are likely to be heavily dependent on factors such as the medication's presumed mechanism of action and, for example, the regional distribution of receptor densities. In a recent study on brain connectivity, carbamazepine treatment had a region-specific effect on the limbic circuit and thalamus network [42]. In previous pharmaco-fMRI studies [46], medication reduced abnormal network activations in the temporal lobe. In contrast, both sodium valproate and levetiracetam appear to restore the fMRI activation patterns in genetic generalized [47] and focal epilepsies [48], respectively. The effects of medication therefore require careful consideration and still require considerable further investigation to understand the complex interaction between underlying pathology, medication, and the resulting modification of brain dynamics. In particular, for fMRI, medication can potentially alter both the neural activity directly and its expression in fMRI signals via physiological parameters such as vascular reactivity. In whole brain network connectivity parameterization such as graph theoretic measures, the exact nature of this influence might be harder to predict and account for. It certainly can be dramatic; a study by Joules et al. [49] investigated ketamine-induced changes in degree centrality along with pre-treatment with lamotrigine or risperidone. There was a strong effect of ketamine with a large shift in degree centrality from cortical to subcortical hubs. This shift was moderated by risperidone but not lamotrigine showing that it was the NMDA receptor blockade rather than downstream glutamatergic effects that were responsible. This also illustrates the complexity of anticipating changes in connectivity patterns with polytherapy that can be common in drug-resistant epilepsy. To understand and account for medication effects is an important endeavor and the relatively modest volume of work to date (for an example see [50]) has demonstrated disease-medication interactions.

10.3.5 Vagus Nerve Stimulation (VNS): Predicting Treatment Outcome from fMRI Network Measures

Vagus nerve stimulation (VNS) is an empirically based method for treating drug-resistant epilepsy, VNS therapy involves repeated stimulation of the vagus nerve via implanted electrodes and is beneficial for around 50% of patients. Although considered a relatively minor procedure compared to other epilepsy surgeries, VNS implantation still poses surgical risk, has significant costs, requires device maintenance and battery replacement, and may not be an effective therapy for all patients. There is a requirement, therefore, to develop methods to pre-operatively predict those patients who will be responders to VNS therapy. This section details recent findings related to fMRI-derived networks that have been used to predict patient's response to VNS.

The mechanism of action of VNS in seizure mediation is still not completely resolved (for a review of the neural circuit influenced in VNS see [51]). By various mechanisms, VNS causes widespread alteration to interacting cortical and subcortical networks that influence the probability of seizures or their severity. fMRI was first used for

this purpose in the early 2000s to perform functional studies to interrogate the brain networks manipulated by implanted VNS systems (see, for example, [52]). Early studies found brain regions more active in patients that responded to VNS, including the cingulate cortex, basal ganglia and insular, and especially thalamic regions. Owing to safety considerations in relation to patients with implanted VNS devices, post-implantation MRI studies are relatively few. To avoid such safety issues, there has been an increase in research attempting to find potential markers of response based on brain connectivity patterns obtained prior to implantation.

Under the idea that the therapeutic effects of VNS may be mediated by afferent projections from the thalamus, Ibrahim and colleagues [23] examined the hypothesis that intrinsic thalamo-cortical connectivity may be altered in patients more responsive to the treatment. The study obtained rs-fMRI data from 21 children diagnosed with drug-resistant epilepsy prior to implantation of VNS and compared connectivity measures to postoperative seizure frequency defined as "good" or "bad." The study identified two thalamic ROIs (left and right) in patients and assessed time series correlations with all voxels in the brain to generate first level connectivity maps. Mixed effects, higher levels analysis was then performed to contrast first level connectivity maps between patients more responsive to VNS to those less responsive with the general linear model included controlling for age and sedation (some patients required sedation in the scanner). Following this analysis, a machine learning technique termed support vector analysis [53] was applied to predict the likely success of VNS. Inputs for the support vector machine (SVM) model were clusters from time series data demonstrating significant connectivity to both thalamic ROIs plus anterior cingulate cortex and the left insula. These data were then used to train a model that produces predictions for the response to VNS in new patient data and a SVM classifier that provides data regarding the optimal hyperplane (maximum level of separation between all data points of one class from the other class) was built. As hypothesized, results of these different analysis techniques pointed toward a key role of intrinsic thalamocortical connectivity in the level of therapeutic effects conferred by VNS. When the left thalamus was used in a seed-voxel analysis, two significant clusters were identified in patients with

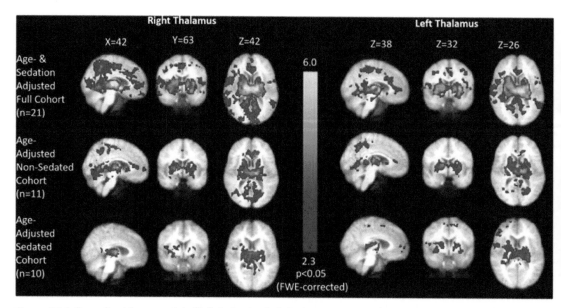

Figure 10.4 **Generalized linear model of left thalamic whole brain connectivity regressed against selected covariates.** In patients with good seizure response to VNS, the left thalamus is significantly more strongly connected to the anterior cingulate and bilateral operculo-insular cortices as well as the parietooccipital junction and peri-Rolandic cortex (top panel). This effect was dissociable from age-related differences in connectivity to the left thalamus (second panel). There was no significant sedation effect or interaction (lower panel). All clusters shown are significant at p < 0.05 following FWE-correction for multiple comparisons. Figure and caption taken with permission from [23].

a good response to VNS, indicating enhanced thalamocortical connectivity in patients associated with good VNS response as opposed to a bad response. Furthermore, when the right thalamus was correlated with all voxels, patients exhibiting a good response to VNS showed greater connectivity between the ROI and anterior cingulate cortex and the ventromedial prefrontal cortex (see Fig. 10.4). Finally, based on this data the SVM classifier analysis was able to predict with 86% accuracy the likelihood of a patient providing a good response to VNS, thus reinforcing results from imaging data indicating that patients with increased intrinsic thalamocortical connectivity patterns may respond more effectively to VNS. However, while providing convincing findings that this pattern may predict treatment response, it is not clear that this is related directly to how VNS might normalize connectivity and reduce seizure severity. It is plausible that this study identifies intact circuitry that allows the VNS to be effective as opposed to an abnormality that is a treatment target. Studies measuring connectivity before and after VNS implantation are important to differentiate between these possibilities but, at least using MRI, are currently limited by safety considerations.

Mithani et al. acquired structural and functional connectomic data using diffusion tensor MRI (DTI) and rs-MEG to test the theory that responsiveness to VNS may be related to intrinsic connectivity variability in patients [54]. The study tested 56 children diagnosed with drug intractable epilepsy who in contrast to those in [23] had received VNS insertion previous to data acquisition (within the past three years) and a minimum of a year of follow up symptom assessment sessions. Results from structural connectomic DTI analysis, showed differences between patients responsive to VNS. In VNS responders, they observed increased fractional anisotropy in left-lateralized limbic, association, and projection fibers, including the internal and external capsules, parts of the corona radiata, posterior thalamic radiation, and fornix. Interestingly, results from functional connectivity analyses were also consistent with these differences. Here, rs-MEG data indicated greater functional connectivity in exactly the same brain regions as found to have increased fractional anisotropy in the DTI analysis. Overall, while results do show some differences with those of [23], they are consistent in that they also report increased structural connectivity between thalamic and other brain regions and also build on these findings by relating structural connectivity to functional connectivity.

In summary, previous work has indicated that it may be possible to predict the likely success of VNS based on measures of fMRI network connectivity patterns. In particular, networks involving thalamic connectivity do appear to be predictive of a better outcome. However, although increased thalamic connectivity patterns may be a helpful marker in ascertaining the likely success of VNS, the fact that it was found both before and after implantation in the outlined studies means question still persist about how VNS actually mediates seizure activity. In the future, experimental paradigms that can safely accommodate in situ fMRI acquisition may be able to answer this question more effectively that may in future better inform the value of predictive data.

10.4 Summary and Conclusions

In this chapter, we have described a wide range of examples of large-scale network alterations in different forms of epilepsy, assessed using fMRI. There is evidence that in both focal and generalized epilepsy there are regional alterations within the systems involved in the generation of pathological activity and this has refined our understanding of pathological networks. A particular strength of fMRI is the ability to access deep-lying brain regions that are hard to characterize by other means and to understand their interaction with large-scale brain activity. This was exemplified by observations showing how the basal ganglia and thalamus were altered in their interactions with typical large-scale brain networks in patients with TLE that have secondary generalized seizures. In addition to this, there are a large volume of studies that have found differences in the large-scale networks or ICNs that are not directly associated with seizure generation.

A common theme is an alteration to the modularity or community structure of ICNs in different syndromes. In simple terms this amounts to a disruption to the coherent network organization of the brain where there is a difference in the ability of brain regions to coalesce into the coherent networks thought to subserve effective brain function. Some of these effects can be directly attributed to ongoing pathological activity; in TLE, interictal discharges were associated with DMN changes where transient activity is

recorded. On the one hand a difference in modularity maybe due to a structural reorganization, on the other hand, changes in the dynamics of the system when temporally averaged could result in similar measures. Hence, increasingly, studies have been instead looking at the dynamics of large-scale networks rather than considering the brain's network organization as a stationary system over a period of minutes. In patients with generalized epilepsy, mirroring some aspects of studies in animal models, changes associated with GSW indicated that a predisposing peri-ictal state existed in humans. Overall, these studies are moving toward an understanding that the pattern of brain dynamics is that of a carefully tuned system able to form transiently stable states as part of a rich dynamic repertoire and this is affected by the various disease processes.

Work to date to understand large-scale network alterations in epilepsy has too often been siloed with cognitive task-based fMRI, EEG-fMRI, and functional connectivity based largely on resting state data developing relatively independently with too little overlap or cross-referencing. Data from studies of pharmacological alterations and drug naive patients are needed to determine effects solely related to disease processes. However, this literature is far from complete. Further, the difficulty of evaluating results from multiple data sets of modest size within individual centers may lead to bias and is often compounded by variable analysis pipelines and a wide range and variable metrics used to measure network alterations. This makes it challenging to combine results into a coherent picture.

A practical clinical endpoint of this research is predicting clinical outcome of surgery or stimulation and some evidence that measurement of the brain's network structure is predictive has been presented. Again, a greater modularity, perhaps reflecting more normal dynamics was predictive of success. Accounting for the nonstationarity and state-dependence of functional connectivity are likely to be important factors in the search for potential connectivity-derived biomarkers Laufs et al., [16] particularly in the context of stimulation [55].

It is clear that these multi-factorial relationships cannot be understood by looking at the individual nodes of the system, receptor pharmacology, or any other individual aspect of the particular underlying pathology. It is likely also too

149

superficial to conceptualize epilepsy simply as a "network disease." Instead, it might be more helpful to think of the brain as a complex system with the possibility for emergent behavior at multiple scales that can lead to the familiar clinical features. Focal epilepsy, for example, perhaps is sometimes a circumscribed pathological region. However, it participates more strongly with anatomically connected regions and its activity is constrained by its surroundings and controlled by many factors. Characterizing these dynamic interactions and utilizing ongoing rapid developments in imaging and electrophysiological recordings to characterize them across spatial and temporal scales will be critical to understanding and ultimately better treating epilepsy in the individual.

References

1. Belliveau, J. W., Kennedy, D. N., McKinstry, R. C., et al. Functional mapping of the human visual cortex by magnetic resonance imaging. *Science*, 254(5032), 716–9 (1991).

2. Kwong, K. K., Belliveau, J. W., Chesler, D. A., et al. Dynamic magnetic resonance imaging of human brain activity during primary sensory stimulation. *Proc. Natl. Acad. Sci. USA*, 89 (12), 5675–9 (1992).

3. Ives, J. R., Warach, S., Schmitt, F., Edelman, R. R., and Schomer, D. L. Monitoring the patient's EEG during echo planar MRI. *Electroencephalogr. Clin. Neurophysiol.*, 87(6), 417–20 (1993).

4. Biswal, B., Yetkin F. Z., Haughton, V. M., and Hyde, J. S. Functional connectivity in the motor cortex of resting human brain using echo-planar mri. *Magn. Reson. Med.*, 34(4), 537–41 (1995).

5. Centeno, M., and Carmichael, D. W. Network connectivity in epilepsy: Resting state fMRI and EEG-fMRI contributions. *Front. Neurol.*, 5, 93 (2014).

6. McKeown, M. J., Jung, T. P., Makeig, S., et al. Spatially independent activity patterns in functional MRI data during the Stroop color-naming task. *Proc. Natl. Acad. Sci. USA*, 95 (3), 803–10 (1998).

7. Seeley, W. W., Menon, V., Schatzberg, A. F., et al. Dissociable intrinsic connectivity networks for salience processing and executive control. *J. Neurosci.*, 27(9), 2349–56 (2007).

8. Xiong, J., Parsons, L. M., Gao, J. H., and Fox, P. T. Interregional connectivity to primary motor cortex revealed using MRI resting state images. *Hum. Brain Mapp.*, 8(2–3), 151–6 (1999).

9. Smith, S. M., Fox, P. T., Miller, K. L., et al. Correspondence of the brain's functional architecture during activation and rest. *Proc. Natl. Acad. Sci. USA*, 106(31), 13040–5 (2009).

10. Sporns, O. Graph theory methods: Applications in brain networks. *Dialogues Clin. Neurosci.*, 20(2), 111–20 (2018).

11. Murta, T., Leite, M., Carmichael, D. W., Figueiredo, P., and Lemieux, L. Electrophysiological correlates of the BOLD signal for EEG-informed fMRI. *Hum. Brain Mapp.*, 36(1), 391–414 (2015).

12. Jiang, W., Li, J., Chen, X., Ye, W., and Zheng J.. Disrupted structural and functional networks and their correlation with alertness in right temporal lobe epilepsy: A graph theory study. *Front. Neurol.*, 8, 179 (2017).

13. Bettus, G., Guedj, E., Joyeux, F., et al. Decreased basal fMRI functional connectivity in epileptogenic networks and contralateral compensatory mechanisms. *Hum. Brain Mapp.*, 30(5), 1580–91 (2009).

14. Morgan, V. L., Abou-Khalil, B., and Rogers, B. P. Evolution of functional connectivity of brain networks and their dynamic interaction in temporal lobe epilepsy. *Brain Connect.*, 5(1), 35–44 (2015).

15. Laufs, H., Hamandi, K., Salek-Haddadi, A., et al. Temporal lobe interictal epileptic discharges affect cerebral activity in "default mode" brain regions. *Hum. Brain Mapp.*, 28 (10), 1023–32 (2007).

16. Laufs H., Rodionov R., Thornton R., et al. Altered fMRI connectivity dynamics in temporal lobe epilepsy might explain seizure semiology. *Front. Neurol.*, 5, 175 (2014).

17. Stretton, J., Winston, G. P., Sidhu, M., et al. Disrupted segregation of working memory networks in temporal lobe epilepsy. *Neuroimage Clin.*, 2, 273–81 (2013).

18. Deco, G., Kringelbach, M. L., Jirsa, V., and Ritter P. The dynamics of resting fluctuations in the brain: Metastability and its dynamical cortical core. *Sci. Rep.*, 7, 3095 (2017).

19. Voets, N. L., Beckmann, C. F., Cole, D. M., et al. Structural substrates for resting network disruption in temporal lobe epilepsy. *Brain*, 135(8), 2350–7 (2012).

20. He, X., Chaitanya, G., Asma, B., et al. Disrupted basal ganglia-thalamocortical loops in focal to bilateral tonic-clonic seizures. *Brain*, 143(1), 175–90 (2020).

21. Lui, S., Ouyang, L., Chen, Q., et al. Differential interictal activity of the precuneus/posterior cingulate cortex revealed by resting state functional MRI at 3T in generalized vs. Partial seizure. *J. Magn. Reson. Imaging*, 27(6), 1214–20 (2008).

22. Mäkinen, V. T., May, P. J., and Tiitinen, H., The use of stationarity and nonstationarity in the detection and analysis of neural oscillations. *Neuroimage*, 28(2), 389–400 (2005).

23. Ibrahim, G. M., Sharma, P., Hyslop, A., et al. Presurgical thalamocortical connectivity is associated with response to vagus nerve stimulation in children with intractable epilepsy. *Neuroimage Clin.*, 16, 634–42 (2017).

24. Sinha, N., Wang, Y., Moreira da Silva N., et al. Structural brain network abnormalities and the probability of seizure recurrence after epilepsy surgery. *Neurology*, 96(5), e758–71 (2021).

25. He, X., Doucet, G. E., Pustina, D., et al. Presurgical thalamic "hubness" predicts surgical outcome in temporal lobe epilepsy. *Neurology*, 88(24), 2285–93 (2017).

26. González, F. J., Chakravorti, S., Goodale, S. E., et al. Thalamic arousal network disturbances in temporal lobe epilepsy and improvement after surgery. *J. Neurol. Neurosurg. Psychiatry*, 90(10), 1109–16 (2019).

27. Fisher, R., Salanova, V., Witt, T., et al. Electrical stimulation of the anterior nucleus of thalamus for treatment of refractory epilepsy. *Epilepsia*, 51(5), 899–908 (2010).

28. Warren, A. E. L., Dalic, L. J., Thevathasan, W., et al. Targeting the centromedian thalamic nucleus for deep brain stimulation. *J. Neurol. Neurosurg. Psychiatry*, 91(4), 339–49 (2020).

29. Middlebrooks, E. H., Grewal, S. S., Stead, M., et al. Differences in functional connectivity profiles as a predictor of response to anterior thalamic nucleus deep brain stimulation for epilepsy: A hypothesis for the mechanism of action and a potential biomarker for outcomes. *Neurosurg. Focus*, 45 (2), E7 (2018).

30. Doucet, G. E., Pustina, D., Skidmore, C., et al. Resting-state functional connectivity predicts the strength of hemispheric lateralization for language processing in temporal lobe epilepsy and normals. *Hum. Brain Mapp.*, 36(1), 288–303 (2015).

31. Bonelli, S. B., Thompson, P. J., Yogarajah, M., et al. Imaging language networks before and after anterior temporal lobe resection: Results of a longitudinal fMRI study. *Epilepsia*, 53(4), 639–50 (2012).

32. Foesleitner, O., Sigl, B., Schmidbauer, V., et al. Language network reorganization before and after temporal lobe epilepsy surgery. *J. Neurosurg.*, 134(6), 1694–1702 (2020).

33. Stufflebeam, S. M., Liu, H., Sepulcre, J., et al. Localization of focal epileptic discharges using functional connectivity magnetic resonance imaging: Clinical article. *J. Neurosurg.*, 114(6), 1693–7 (2011).

34. Iannotti, G. R., Grouiller, F., Centeno, M., et al. Epileptic networks are strongly connected with and without the effects of interictal discharges. *Epilepsia*, 57(7), 1086–96 (2016).

35. Vaessen, M. J., Braakman, H. M. H., Heerink, J. S., et al. Abnormal modular organization of functional networks in cognitively impaired children with frontal lobe epilepsy. *Cereb. Cortex*, 23 (8), 1997–2006 (2012).

36. Ibrahim, G. M., Morgan, B. R., Lee, W., et al. Impaired development of intrinsic connectivity networks in children with medically intractable localization-related epilepsy. *Hum. Brain Mapp.*, 35 (11), 5686–700 (2014).

37. Hong, S.-J., Lee, H.-M., Gill, R., et al. A connectome-based mechanistic model of focal cortical dysplasia. *Brain*, 142 (3), 688–99 (2019).

38. Lüttjohann, A., and van Luijtelaar G. Dynamics of networks during absence seizure's on- and offset in rodents and man. *Front. Physiol.*, 6, 16 (2015).

39. Tangwiriyasakul, C., Perani, S., Centeno, M., et al. Dynamic brain network states in human generalized spike-wave discharges. *Brain*, 141(10), 2981–94 (2018).

40. Vulliemoz, S., Vollmar, C., Koepp, M. J., et al. Connectivity of the supplementary motor area in juvenile myoclonic epilepsy and frontal lobe epilepsy. *Epilepsia*, 52(3), 507–14 (2011).

41. Tangwiriyasakul, C., Perani, S., Abela, E., Carmichael, D. W., and Richardson, M. P. Sensorimotor network hypersynchrony as an endophenotype in families with genetic generalized epilepsy: A resting-state functional magnetic resonance imaging study. *Epilepsia*, 60(3), e14–9 (2019).

42. Routley, B., Shaw, A., Muthukumaraswamy, S. D., Singh, K. D., and Hamandi, K. Juvenile myoclonic epilepsy shows increased posterior theta, and reduced sensorimotor beta resting connectivity. *Epilepsy Res.*, 163, 106324 (2020).

43. Chaudhary, U. J., Centeno, M., Carmichael, D. W., et al. Imaging the interaction: Epileptic discharges, working memory, and behavior. *Hum Brain Mapp.*, 34(11), 2910–7 (2013).

44. Haag, A., and Bonelli, S.. Clinical application of language and memory fMRI in epilepsy. *Epileptologie*, 30, 101–8 (2013).

45. Tierney, T. M., Weiss-Croft, L. J., Centeno, M., et al. FIACH: A biophysical model for automatic retrospective noise control in fMRI. *Neuroimage.*, 124, 1009–20 (2016).

46. Wandschneider, B., and Koepp, M. J. Pharmaco fMRI: Determining the functional anatomy of the effects of medication. *Neuroimage Clin.*, 12, 691–7 (2016).

47. Vollmar, C., O'Muircheartaigh, J., Barker, G. J., et al. Motor system hyperconnectivity in juvenile myoclonic epilepsy: A cognitive functional magnetic resonance imaging study. *Brain*, 134(6), 1710–9 (2011).

48. Wandschneider, B., Stretton, J., Sidhu, M., et al. Levetiracetam reduces abnormal network activations in temporal lobe epilepsy. *Neurology.*, 83(17), 1508–12 (2014).

49. Joules, R., Doyle, O. M., Schwarz, A. J., et al. Ketamine induces a robust whole-brain connectivity pattern that can be differentially modulated by drugs of different mechanism and clinical profile. *Psychopharmacology (Berl.)*, 232(21–22), 4205–4218 (2015).

50. Haneef, Z., Levin, H. S., and Chiang, S. Brain graph topology changes associated with anti-epileptic drug use. *Brain Connect.*, 5(5), 284–91 (2015).

51. Eljamel, S.. Mechanism of action and overview of vagus nerve stimulation technology. In *Neurostimulation: Principles and Practice*. Oxford, UK: John Wiley & Sons, Ltd. 2013. p. 111–20.

52. Lomarev, M., Denslow, S., Nahas, Z., et al. Vagus nerve stimulation (VNS) synchronized BOLD fMRI suggests that VNS in depressed adults has frequency/dose dependent effects. *J. Psychiatr. Res.*, 36(4), 219–27 (2002).

53. Cortes, C., and Vapnik, V. Support-vector networks. *Mach. Learn.*, 20(3), 273–97 (1995).

54. Mithani, K., Mikhail, M., Morgan, B. R., et al. Connectomic profiling identifies responders to vagus nerve stimulation. *Ann. Neurol.*, 86(5), 743–53 (2019).

55. Li, L. M., Violante, I. R., Leech, R., et al. Brain state and polarity dependent modulation of brain networks by transcranial direct current stimulation. *Hum. Brain Mapp.*, 40(3), 904–15 (2019).

56. Tzourio-Mazoyer N, Landeau B, Papathanassiou D, Crivello F, Etard O, Delcroix, N, et al. Automated anatomical labeling of activations in SPM using a macroscopic anatomical parcellation of the MNI MRI single-subject brain. *Neuroimage.* 15: 273–89 (2002). doi: 10.1006/nimg.2001.0978

Index